Methods of Modifying
SPEECH BEHAVIORS

Second Edition

Second Edition

Methods of Modifying SPEECH BEHAVIORS

Learning Theory in Speech Pathology

DONALD E. MOWRER
Arizona State University

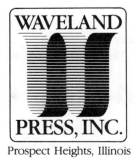

WAVELAND
PRESS, INC.
Prospect Heights, Illinois

I would like to dedicate this book to my dear wife Yvette; my sons Jacques, Alan, and Patrick; and to my daughters Sue, and Christine.

For information about this book, write or call:

Waveland Press, Inc.
P.O. Box 400
Prospect Heights, Illinois 60070
(708) 634-0081

Preface

In everyday practice, the speech and language pathologist constantly works toward remediating certain speech and language problems. Until recently, however, little was written about "how to do" therapy. *Methods of Modifying Speech Behaviors* was designed to systematically examine the underlying theories and recommended methods for clinical practice in a methods or clinical practicum course in the communication disorders curriculum.

As with the first edition, this book presents important learning theories and methods useful for daily clinical practice. By reading about learning theories, clinicians can better select effective procedures to insure success with their clients. Likewise, understanding these approaches can help clinicians grasp the aims of commercially prepared materials or programs; thus, guide the clinician in selecting appropriate commercial programs for a given purpose. The reader will find critiques of commercially available materials throughout chapters. Hopefully, this will be a starting point for therapists in choosing or developing their own materials.

This revision reflects a reorganization of materials into seven units to promote better understanding and retention. Lists of objectives appear at the beginning of each unit and a list of suggested assignments is included to clarify the activities. Likewise, 20–30 questions appear at the end of each unit (except Unit 7). My students responded enthusiastically to knowing what might be expected of them in future examinations.

To extend a student's experience beyond the textbook and into the speech clinic itself, one 60-minute tape is available free upon adoption to instructors. Free duplication rights are granted for educational use by your students. The student simply listens to selections of actual, unrehearsed therapy sessions with clients, then fills in the exercises for that session. Questions are asked in each session; and an answer key is provided for checking answers. Since speech requires listening; and speech/language clinicians must refine their listening skills, the tapes should assist them in mastering these skills. This allows the students to practice their clinical skills.

The following major changes have been made: an addition to chapter 2, "Basis of Scientific Methodology," on magic and superstition. Since magic prevails widely even today, it's important for clinicians to understand its lure. Secondly, the chapter on counseling and psychotherapy now examines the speech/language pathologist's job in assisting clients through the grieving process. Third, chapter 9, "Application of Programming Techniques" in speech pathology, covers three new programs: two in stuttering, one in voice.

Perhaps the most significant change in this edition has been the addition of chapter 12 on the application of behavior therapy, techniques, selected case studies. It shows clinicians how to use behavior therapy to change the speech behaviors of individuals with communication problems. In reading these documented case studies the reader learns how the methods can be used. As you will see, sticking to a strict behavioral model is not always easy. It may be necessary to stray from the strictly defined scientific method in order to be an effective clinician.

It is my hope that the revised edition will better serve instructors and students alike. By working through the exercises, I hope students may take away some problem solving skills to use in their public schools and clinics.

Acknowledgments

The two individuals who were most influential in changing my thinking about speech therapy methodology are Robert Baker and Richard Schutz, both professors in educational psychology at Arizona State University during the 1960s. Several other professors in the psychology department at ASU, I. Goldiamond, A. Staats, J. Michaels, and L. Meyerson, also provided excellent leadership as professors whose classes I attended.

During my professional growth a large number of colleagues have been very supportive in helping me develop and clarify educational strategies. Most influential was Dr. Bruce Ryan. Others include Jan Costello, Jim Bryden, Tom Johnson, Kathy Gordon, and Doris Bradley.

Finally, I wish to thank Jean Krikorian for typing the manuscript; Tom Hutchinson for his editorial assistance, and my wife Yvette for correcting my spelling errors, not to mention her valuable moral support during the eight months while this manuscript was in preparation. I have learned much in researching the material in this book, and I hope it is beneficial to the reader.

A special thanks to Bruce Ryan who provided many helpful comments concerning the revised edition of this text. I would also like to thank Kathy Kenney and James Case for their case study contributions to chapter 12.

Contents

Methods of Modifying
SPEECH BEHAVIORS

Second Edition

Unit 1

Philosophy of Education and the Scientific Method

Objectives

The first objective of this unit is to help you identify and define four educational philosophies; second is learning how these philosophies influence the behavior of speech/language pathologists. Third, you will be able to describe three theories of learning and trace their effects on how speech/language pathologists provide services.

The fourth objective is to help you identify four basic principles of the scientific method and describe their application in speech and hearing pathology. Fifth, you will be able to cite instances in which the principles of the scientific method have been violated. Finally, you will be able to identify limitations of the scientific method as applied to human learning.

Suggested Assignments

Read chapters 1 and 2 in preparation for class discussion. Lecture material will review the basic philosophies of education, theories of learning, and basic elements of the scientific method. Various theories and practices that violate the scientific method will be identified.

First, speed-read chapters 1 and 2 before you attend class to prepare for a discussion of each section, then carefully reread the text. Make notes in the margins where appropriate. This way you can review the important points of your lecture notes and text before being tested on the material. Be sure to answer all of the study guide questions at the end of the unit. Follow this study procedure in other chapter assignments and you should be able to master the material.

The second assignment will involve an outside reading selected from the references found at the end of Unit 1. In each of these readings, some principles of the scientific method are violated. You are to select one reading and write a four- to six-page critique showing how principles of the scientific method were violated.

1

Philosophical and Educational Foundation of Speech Therapy Methodology

Recently while visiting a public school I overheard a speech clinician reprimand a young child who apparently was inattentive during the therapy session. The monologue went something like this:

"All right, Bobby, stop fooling around. Let's get to work. We're not here to play, you know. I'm here to help you learn to speak better. Someday you'll appreciate what I'm doing for you. Now let's go through these words again. Say them after me slowly just like I do."

Two days later I visited a speech clinician in another school engaging three children in the following conversation:

"I've got a new game today for you all and I know you all are really going to like it."

"Oh boy, how do you play it?"

"Can I be firtht Mith Jay?"

"No me!"

"Now wait a minute, you'll all get a chance to play. First we'll have to learn the rules. Here, Becky, you put these papers on the start square."

Later that day another speech clinician working with one child was heard saying: "Great. Fine. Good job. Yes. Not quite. That's it. Put your tongue up higher."

The child was responding rapidly, and for the most part, correctly.

It is not difficult to find examples of the diverse methods employed by speech clinicians throughout the United States. All are aimed at modifying some aspect of an individual's speech behavior. But why such diversity, especially when many of the children appear to have similar speech problems? One wonders if there shouldn't be one right way of conducting speech therapy.

Diversity in the behavior of speech clinicians can be understood by viewing instructional methodology as an outgrowth of educational and social philosophies. These philosophies have their roots buried deeply in early Greek and Roman culture. They have been modified profoundly during periods of epic change in governments, science, and religious beliefs throughout the centuries. Aristotle, Plato, Galileo, Bacon, Rousseau, Locke, James, Marx, and Dewey are but a few of the philosophers and scientists who have molded and changed our thinking not only within our educational framework but also in the life-style each of us chooses to live.

When a speech clinician tells a child to get down to work because it's good for him, she's reflecting a philosophical viewpoint which can be traced to the early teachings of Aristotle, St. Thomas Aquinas, and Maritain and still later, to essayists Royce, Emerson, and Hutchins. A different philosophical track is reflected by the clinician who encourages diversity in children's language usage where standard English is viewed as an alternative option to the child's present dialect. Plato, St. Augustine, and Bacon, followed much later by Dewey, Pierce, and James, contributed greatly to the development of a philosophy which encouraged cultural change.

Philosophies of Education

Although no textbooks about the correction of speech problems were written before the eighteenth century, many historical references about the nature and treatment of these problems have been found. Stuttering was mentioned in hieroglyphics dating back to the twentieth century B.C. (Clark & Murray, 1965). Aristotle pointed out the disadvantage of misarticulating consonant sounds. Demosthenes, plagued with a speech impediment, placed pebbles in his mouth to help him overcome his problem. During the Middle Ages speech handicapped individuals were frequently ridiculed and put on exhibition, while the deaf were secluded from public places, destined for a solitary life in an institution. Clearly deviances of speech have been considered a definite handicapping condition—a condition requiring change.

Bringing about changes in articulation habits was accomplished mostly through individual tutoring before the twentieth century. A student met with his teacher and practiced lessons in elocution with emphasis on voice projection, correct breathing patterns, and body posture. Although most of the drill books used for these vocal exercises no longer exist, the few that do suggest a great deal of syllable and word repetition was used. Lessons were conducted in much the same way as music instruction of that period. The instructor demonstrated a model which was copied by the student and practiced until the student's performance matched that of the instructor.

Speech instructors had little tolerance of deviances of speech patterns. There was a right and a wrong way of speaking, and it was important for everyone to speak in a certain, prescribed way. But differences in articulation were not the only concern. Many educators were greatly disturbed over the fact that America was a nation of poor spellers—our presidents included; and the dialectical patterns arising in the Southern states caused further alarm. It was feared that if speech and writing skills were not standardized, Americans would one day be unable to understand each other. Since much of the communication between distant points was written, it was felt the most practical way to standardize was through educating children in uniform reading and writing skills. If children spelled the same way, chances were they would also pronounce words in a similar fashion. Thus, Noah Webster produced his famous "Blue-backed Speller" in an attempt to standardize the pronouncing and spelling of English words; and it was used in virtually all schools during the eighteenth and nineteenth centuries.

Perennialism: The prevailing educational philosophy of the eighteenth and early nineteenth centuries was Perennialism, a belief that there is a permanence throughout time. There are universal truths which never change, and it is up to the schools to see that these truths are taught. The development of the intellect, especially of the nation's teachers, was emphasized. Thomas Jefferson as well as other wealthy landowners of the aristocracy strongly favored this educational viewpoint.

The Perennialist was not particular about the means used to instill these universal truths. The end justified the means. If it was felt punishment would expediate conveying information, then it was used without compunction. Wrapping the knuckles with stout rulers, standing dunce-capped children in the corner, and providing generous swats to the behind were frequently used procedures designed to drill in the facts of reality. A Perennialist educator, for example, would sanction the Spanish Inquisition on the basis that the end result, purging evil, justified use of any means. The Christian Crusades of the Middle Ages were justified on the same basis.

A speech teacher holding this philosophy could easily endure hours of painful vocal drills during elocution lessons. Whether or not the child enjoyed these lessons was of little or no concern to the Perennialist. The end result, "correct" speech, was the single, important objective. Perennialists are strong proponents of pragmatism. If it works, it's good. Speech teachers who worked with stutterers would employ any method that appeared to work. Breathing and rhythm exercises were widely used in schools for the treatment of this disorder. When Van Riper (1973) reflected the treatment he received for his stuttering as a youth, he recalled attending a school where the daily routine was so rigorous he became physically ill and was forced to terminate the treatment program.

Essentialism: Closely associated with Perennialism is the more traditional view, Essentialism. Proponents of Essentialism maintain that children should be taught the basic skills needed for daily life. These skills consist of a firm mastery of the academic basics, especially reading, writing, and mathematics. Academic standards are established based upon the tried and tested heritage of skills, facts, and laws of knowledge that come to us from modern civilization. Policies are determined by society, interpreted by boards of education, and handed down to the teacher to instill in the child.

Essentialism prevailed in America during the late nineteenth and early twentieth centuries and may account in part for the tremendous industrial growth during that period. The individual was subservient to the will of the society, which at that time meant industry. Schools were "mass education factories."

According to this educational philosophy, prescribed standards had to be met whether or not the child was interested; it was felt interest followed hard work. William Bagley, an outspoken proponent of Essentialism during the 1920s, believed it was good for children to begin with effort since effort had some moral good connected with it. Simply set the standards and make children come up to them. Those who could not meet the school's standards should attend nonacademic special schools. This philosophical position was greatly responsible for the establishment of residential schools for the deaf and mentally retarded set in rural environments, away from centers of academia.

Surprising as it may seem most schools today are dominated by a philosophy which embraces Essentialism. For example, if a child finishes second grade, he is expected to pass standardized tests at the second-grade level. Those of authority in education who represent our present-day society determine what the standards should be, and the goal of every teacher is to see that the children in their class attain these standards. This idea that all children conform to certain standards is designed to strengthen the society through common understanding.

It is interesting to note that two strong proponents of Essentialism, William Bagley and John Keith, wrote a brief introduction to Helen Peppard's (1925) early text, *The Correction of Speech Defects*. In the introduction Bagley and Keith suggest that one cause of the increasing number of children who have speech problems may be the neglected use of phonetics in the schools, which emphasize "content" instead of "form." They point out the necessity of correcting minor speech defects, which on the surface appear to be insignificant, but in actuality may interfere with the effectiveness and happiness of the individual. The implication here is that if one does not conform to accepted speech standards, he will be unable to live a happy, fulfilling life.

Peppard begins her book with a section on preparing the child for life by teaching him proper speech habits and suggests that if teachers fall short of this aim, they will be sending these children forth into the world as handicapped individuals. Teachers, as leaders and models in the community, must possess distinct, correct enunciation and have full, resonant speaking voices, both qualities resulting from the strong influence of Essentialism. The child is educated and fitted for life by those who know what is important in our modern society. Clear, articulate speech will enable him to better adjust to and be accepted by society.

The work ethic advocated by the Essentialists is prevalent throughout Peppard's book. The laborous vocal drills call for hard work and great mental effort on the part of the child. The child is motivated by a desire for accomplishment, but if this interest cannot be aroused, Peppard states, "We may have to resort to other means of control." Thus, we see a tinge of Perennialism in that the end justifies the means. The "other means of control" Peppard referred to more than likely is a hefty dose of punishment in the form of verbal reprimand or threat. Still, Peppard is quick to point out that praise is necessary to stimulate a child's effort. The remaining sections of Peppard's book analyze various speech problems and offer suggestions for their correction, i.e., tongue placement cues, breathing exercises, word and sentence drills.

Evidence of the Essentialist's philosophy can be found among the writings of most so-called traditional textbooks in the field of speech pathology. Much attention is given to the description and treatment of various speech disorders, but the ever-present implication is to help children conform to speech patterns set by society.

Progressivism: About the time of the French and American Revolutions, there was a sweeping surge of interest in the freedom of the individual, especially the underdog. Rousseau lectured that the individual was born good but could be corrupted by society, an idea foreign to both Perennialists and Essentialists. Pestalozzi was experimenting with a new educational format at that time, a philosophy that maintained children, if left alone, would develop into happy, well-adjusted adults. Its chief translator to the American school system was John Dewey, who was responsible for the Progressive movement in our school system.

Dewey was strongly influenced by psychologists of the early twentieth century who were investigating individual differences among children. Dewey felt these individual differences should be included in developing the school curriculum. He believed the purpose of education was not to standardize thinking based upon principles of the past but to help the child cope with the culture he would have to enter as an adult. There were, according to Dewey, no such things as common needs of all children or universal goods. The needs of children were relative, i.e., relative to the child and his community. Schools were seen as instruments of cultural change, always in a state of fluctuation.

The school's job was to keep pace with an ever-changing society. Progressivists are rather vague about identifying ultimate educational goals since it is impossible to predict what the society will be in the future; consequently, one of the basic differences between Essentialism, Perennialism, and Progressivism lies in the goal of education. The former two philosophies clearly identify the goal as fixed in a set body of facts while the latter philosophy embraces an open-ended, ever-changing view of educational goals.

A second major difference between these philosophies concerns how children are educated. Recall the Essentialist's viewpoint that interest follows effort. Dewey felt it should be just the opposite. If you first secure the child's interest, effort will follow. He stressed the importance of motivating the child through things which interest children. It was during the late 1930s and 1940s that aquariums, live animals, plants, and microscopes appeared in elementary school classrooms. Teachers discovered that as children became interested in the classroom goldfish and pet rabbits, then science, mathematics, and reading could be introduced with ease. Rather than forcing the child to learn, the child was enticed to learn with activities and stimuli designed to arouse his interest.

One of the most immediate influences the Progressive school of thought had upon speech therapy was in the area of motivating children. Speech clinicians were encouraged to use games as means of securing a child's interest in an activity. Once the child was involved in playing a game, the clinician could introduce speech activities which would allow the child ample opportunity to practice saying sounds in a variety of contexts. Drill became taboo. Learning new speech habits was supposed to be fun, not work.

Social Reconstructionism: Following on the heels of the Progressive movement, as an inevitable growth from it, evolved the Social Reconstructionist philosophy. The aim of this philosophy was to envisage and assist in the birth of a new cultural design. It advocated a radical approach to education, one which would result in the building of a new civilization dedicated to the fulfillment of values established by the people. A major aim was to work toward consensus of group ideas. Once these ideas are established, then schools translate the ideas to students. Social Reconstructionists wish to teach children not what society is or how to live in it, but what it should be. They propose to draw up a "blueprint" of the emerging, ideal society and use these blueprints as the curriculum. Utopian societies, such as the one B. F. Skinner (1948) described in *Walden II*, reflect the philosophy of the Social Reconstructionist, where the individual is viewed as the creator of culture.

While this educational philosophy is too new to have attained widespread popularity, it has influenced the thinking of many linguists, who in turn influence speech pathologists. For example, current controversy exists concerning dialectical patterns among minority groups. Black dialect, for instance, is viewed by the linguist as a correct and legitimate language system because it follows certain phonological and syntactical rules just as standard English does. Yet, listeners outside the boundaries of this dialectical region experience difficulty understanding the speech of its inhabitants. The question is how should black dialect be treated in schools? The Essentialist and Perennialist would insist that standard English be used both in speech and in reading materials. They would discourage the use of any special dialects. The Progressivist would accept black dialect as a second language, while the Social Reconstructionist would encourage the use of the new dialect as an emerging speech pattern. Reading books at all grade levels, written in black dialect, would be adopted in preference to standard English. Even different spelling would be incorporated. Noah Webster would turn over in his grave at this!

Unfortunately, most speech clinicians have been concerned chiefly with the technology of *how* to change speech patterns, rather than giving thought to whether or not they should be changed. It will be increasingly difficult to maintain the Essentialist viewpoint of education as minority groups strive to maintain their individuality and identity through language usage. One organization, The American Speech and Hearing Association, could provide speech clinicians with leadership regarding an educational philosophy, but this organization seems intent chiefly with seeing that clinicial services in speech and hearing are of high quality. This is certainly an important goal, but unless we, as a profession, begin to grapple with philosophical issues involved in education, we will remain simply highly trained technicians whose job it is to carry out the dictates of the educator-philosophers.

One example may clarify this point. A large percentage of children seen by public school speech clinicians lisp. These children are usually enrolled in speech therapy classes, if not while they are in first grade, certainly by the time they reach second' or third grade. They are given anywhere from 10 to 30 hours of instruction designed to teach "correct" articulation of /s/. Yet, we know lisping does not impair intelligibility of the intended message. If one holds that all children should meet certain perscribed standards of performance and it is the job of the schools to see that these standards are upheld (Essentialism), then the clinician is quite justified in her efforts to remediate the lisping speech. If, on the other hand, lisping is considered acceptable speech behavior, perhaps reflecting change in speech patterns (Progressivism and Social Reconstructionism), then attempts to change lisping are unnecessary. We should tolerate, indeed, foster individuality rather than suppress it. Our basic philosophical position dictates which behaviors we choose to modify.

Learning Theory
in Education

While our philosophy dictates what our general objectives will be, it has been the responsibility of learning theory to provide us with tools and strategies for modifying specific behaviors. For example, suppose we agree that it is important to "correct" lisping. Some method of accomplishing this task must be selected. How do we proceed? Do you simply tell the child to speak correctly or provide some special training and, if so, what type of training? The method we select to change the behavior will depend upon what we know about modifying human behaviors as well as our "gut-level" feelings. There are fairly clear-cut educational strategies used in speech therapy, most of which can be traced to contemporary learning theorists. Once the basic learning theory upon which a speech clinician operates is identified, we can understand the teaching strategy of that clinician. We can also predict how the clinician will teach and, perhaps, how she will react to a different educational strategy.

But before we analyze educational strategies employed by speech clinicians, it is important to identify the major learning theories developed during, and prior to, the twentieth century.

Prescientific Theories

Although few, if any, speech clinicians today would support a mental discipline concept, traces of this belief in the early treatment of both stuttering and articulation problems can be found. This theory held that learning is a process of disciplining the mind. Animals differed from humans in this respect. Animals had bodies but not minds, while only humans had both. The mind of a human, considered as separate from the body, was akin to a muscle. The more practice you gave the mind, the better it became. Educators of the nineteenth century followed this principle.

The adage "Spare the rod and spoil the child" developed from the mental discipline approach. Humans were believed to be basically evil or conceived in sin, and the task of education was to "civilize" them through strict discipline and hard work.

Fortunately, this approach was discredited, chiefly through the work of Edward Thorndike and Robert Woodworth, two Columbia University psychologists. The results of their experiments with animals and humans indicated that drilling or training in certain tasks did not improve the faculties for performing those tasks. The theory of mental discipline was considered untenable.

A second prescientific theory which developed more out of philosophical attitude than psychological theory concerned learning through unfoldment. The romantic naturalism of Rousseau viewed humans as naturally good; humans became corrupt because of the evil influences of society. The Swiss educational reformer, Pestalozzi, and the German educator, Froebel, developed Rousseau's ideas within an educational setting and adopted a "hands off" approach. It was felt children were basically good and should be encouraged to indulge freely in their impulses, interests, and feelings. Much emphasis was placed on the needs of the child, which were unique at each stage of development. Some speech clinicians today endorse this basic belief as reflected in free-play speech therapy sessions. These clinicians feel that if the child is free to express himself, his communication skills will improve as he matures. They believe the cause of his problem rests in frustrating communication situations, which inhibit his speech development.

Scientific Schools of Psychology

Four men were primarily responsible for the introduction of the scientific method in psychology. They were Ernst Weber, Gustav Fechner, Herman von Helmholtz, and Wilhelm Wundt, all German scientists with a common core interest in physiology. Weber's contribution was the use of systematic experimentation in psychology. Fechner developed psychophysical methods of measurement. Helmholtz's aptitude was in the area of exact experimentation in sensory physiology. Finally, Wundt had a unique ability to organize various trends of psychology into a scientific body of knowledge.

One of Wundt's students, E. B. Tichener, brought many of these new ideas to the United States and began the school of *structuralism*. Tichener felt that human experience was the subject of psychology, and introspection, or self-analysis, was the means of studying these experiences. An individual could step outside of his skin, so to speak, and objectively analyze sensations, images, and affective states. But American psychologists were not content to confine their study to introspection of consciousness; consequently, structuralism as a school of psychology weakened and finally collapsed. Nevertheless, Tichener's work firmly established psychology as a science.

The study of the mind as it functions in adapting the organism to its environment was the emphasis of the school of *functionalism*. Charles Darwin and William James laid the groundwork for this movement, followed by John Dewey, leader of the progressive movement in education, James Angell, and Harvey Carr. Functionalism spans from 1850 to the present time. In fact, present-day American psychology is mainly functionalistic because of the heavy emphasis on learning, testing, perception, and other functional processes. Today, functionalism is no longer considered a school of thought, but has been absorbed into contemporary psychology.

Behaviorism had its beginnings while structuralism was at its peak and during the time functionalism was developing into a mature system. The young, American psychologist, John Watson, well-grounded in the functionalistic movement, became highly interested in animal behavior research. Watson rebelled against the mentalistic concepts of the structuralist. Concepts such as "mind," "consciousness," and "image" had no place in his scientific methodology. He also refused to accept the elusive terminology of the functionalist movement. "Emotion," "volition," and "process" were concepts that could not be included in a science of behavior. He preferred to deal with behavior strictly on a stimulus-response level. From a stimulus, a scientist should be able to predict the response and vice versa. Watson, with his deterministic, mechanistic, and superscientific attitude toward human nature, barred the concept of the mind. Behaviorism was to have one of the strongest influences in the development of speech therapy, as I shall show later in this text.

An anti-analytic school of psychology sprang up, again born in Germany, under the leadership of Max Wertheimer, Wolfgang Köhler, and Kurt Koffka, about the time Watson was dealing some deathblows to structuralism and functionalism. This new school, *Gestalt psychology,* first took issue with Wundt's structuralism and then revolted against behaviorism. Basically, Gestaltists held that the whole is greater than the sum of its parts. For example, in education it was demonstrated that once classroom experiences were arranged into meaningful wholes, insight would occur. When the student understood the concept, he could apply it correctly to many problems. Learning of this type was considered far superior to rote drill and memorization tasks usually provided in school. The Gestalt school had its greatest influence in the fields of education and perception, especially the latter. An articulation therapy program, as we shall see, was constructed from principles of Gestalt psychology.

Finally, a movement which is not clearly a school of psychology because it developed outside of the academic circles was called *psychoanalysis.* Psychoanalysts have shown little interest in sensation, attention, perception, or learning, which have been targets of other schools. Their aim was to develop constructs which would enable them to provide therapy to neurotic and psychotic patients. Nevertheless, psychoanalysis as a nonexperimental, clinical technique has had a powerful influence upon modern psychology. Sigmund Freud, the German physician, pioneered its development as he became aware that patients with bizarre behavior problems appeared to be suffering from mental conflicts and frustrations existing in their mind. Treatment of the behavioral symptoms failed to produce beneficial results. These patients were encouraged to "talk out" their problems through free association or by dream analysis. The analyst helped the patient understand and cope with his feelings and experiences in a new light. Subsequently, Alfred Adler and Carl Jung extended and modified Freud's ideas, and their work strongly influenced interest in educational child psychology and child development theory. Two areas where this movement has contributed substantially in speech therapy has been in the treatment of stuttering and psychogenic voice problems.

The various schools of psychology collapsed by 1940 simply because it no longer became feasible to regard the entire science of psychology as belonging to one school. The result was specialization, so that contemporary psychology now includes certain "miniature systems" which encompass research findings in the separate areas of learning, perception, intelligence, personality, and model construction. The remaining section of this chapter will deal with only one of these systems as it relates to speech therapy methodology, that of learning theory.

Theories
of Learning

Contemporary learning theory in psychology has been strongly influenced by the various schools of psychology presented in the previous section. Proponents of each school adopted definite views regarding the nature of learning, some agreeing across schools, others representing conflicting points of view. But rather than describe each school's position with regard to learning theory, it is more practical to group these viewpoints into two major theories: (1) association theories, and (2) cognitive theories. Association theories include both the functionalists and the behaviorists, while cognitive theories embrace chiefly the Gestalt psychologists. Methodology in speech therapy has been influenced by both of these positions.

Association Theories

Association theory of learning holds that certain relationships are formed between stimuli and responses when they occur in close proximity of time. Aristotle formed his laws of memory based upon principles of association. His laws were the foundation of the eighteenth and nineteenth century British empiricists. The writings of Berkeley, Hume, Hartley, Mill, and other scientist-philosophers of that time set the stage for empirical investigation in psychology. Ebbinghaus, a German psychologist, attempted to scientifically investigate the nature of learning. His carefully controlled experiments concerning the nature of memory were the beginning of scientific investigations into human behavior.

Pavlov's classical conditioning: *Classical conditioning* is the term applied to the work conducted by Ivan P. Pavlov in which he studied learning through association, using animals as subjects. This was the first instance where conditioning was studied with scientific rigor. Pavlov presented meat to his dogs and measured the salivation response following this presentation. Then he sounded a bell simultaneously with the presentation of the meat. Salivation continued from the dog's mouth. Finally, only the bell was sounded, and this stimulus alone produced salivation; an association had been made between the bell and the meat. Pavlov maintained learning had occurred.

Brutten and Shoemaker (1967) drew directly from classical conditioning techniques as one of their important techniques for the treatment of stuttering. They argued that neutral stimuli, such as certain speaking situations, words, or sounds, become paired with "negative emotion," or fluency failure, and soon these neutral stimuli themselves are sufficient to produce the disfluency reaction. The neutral stimuli become the conditioned stimuli, and the resultant disfluency the conditioned response.

Brutten and Shoemaker present a therapy model to reverse this classical conditioning of disfluent speech through deconditioning and counterconditioning—deconditioned stimulus (the feared situation) followed by absence of unconditioned stimulus (the negative emotional reaction). Thus, the associations built up between the previously neutral stimuli and the negative consequences are weakened in an effort to return the conditioned stimuli back to their neutral state.

Counterconditioning adds one more element to the model. Instead of following the conditioned stimulus with just absence of negative emotion or a neutral condition, a new response is substituted. This new response is one of positive emotion or pleasant feelings. It is felt the speech clinician should arrange conditions so that stimuli which offer fewest negative emotional reactions are presented first, followed by positive responses, such as fluent utterances. The conditioned stimulus, therefore, evokes a new and different response which is positive instead of negative.

Van Riper (1973) also suggests the use of both deconditioning and classical conditioning as important therapeutic techniques in the treatment of stuttering. Many clinicians employ these methods in stuttering therapy but often do not identify their methods as classical conditioning. Few, if any, speech clinicians have applied classical conditioning procedures in articulation therapy.

Thorndike's instrumental conditioning: E. L. Thorndike's (1898) early monograph concerning animal intelligence clearly established a new trend in learning theory which continues to be a major influence in educational methodology today. His subsequent experimentation and published works resulted in the formulation of certain "laws of learning" within the framework of *instrumental conditioning*.

Perhaps his best known laws are the Law of Effect and the Law of Exercise (Thorndike, 1911). The first law stated that if the events following a connection between a stimulus and a response are satisfying, the strength of the connection is increased. When it is followed by unsatisfying results, the connection is weakened. This strongly resembles what many refer to today as *reinforcement*. The Law of Exercise simply states that repeated responding strengthens association bonds. Thorndike later modified this law to the effect that knowledge of results must accompany the repeated practice. His third law, Law of Readiness, refers to a preparatory set on the part of the organism. If the organism is prepared for a specified behavior, that behavior pattern will be rewarding; but when the organism is forced to do what it does not wish to do, the experience is annoying. In addition to his three primary laws, Thorndike identified several subsidiary laws and principles, such as multiple responses, set, selective responses, response by analogy, and associative shifting. These five subsidiary laws plus the three broader laws constitute Thorndike's fundamental, systematic views on learning.

Thorndike was a prolific writer. Two of his best known books, *Human Learning* (1931) and *The Fundamentals of Learning* (1932), were significant and promising contributions to the field of education. They came at a time when the Progressive movement in education was beginning. Throndike's theories fit nicely as a methodological network within this philosophical movement. In retrospect, Thorndike was heralded as the leader of educational psychology in the 1930s, as was Skinner thirty years later during the 1960s.

Turning to developments in speech therapy during this period of the early '30s, an influential program in speech pathology was rapidly developing at the University of Iowa. Carl Seashore, a well-known psychologist and dean of the graduate school, encouraged his doctoral student, Lee Edward Travis, to head the University of Iowa Speech Clinic. This Travis did, bringing a background of training from several disciplines including psychology, speech, physics, psychiatry, neurology, and otolaryngology.

Three doctoral candidates, Johnson, Bryngelson, and Van Riper, were among the first graduates of this program and were to become leaders in designing methodology in speech therapy. Both Johnson and Van Riper were talented writers as well as researchers and both published widely. They were strongly influenced by Travis, whose position with respect to mental hygiene and personality adjustment is reflected in Johnson and Van Riper's subsequent publications about the nature and treatment of stuttering. Johnson devoted the majority of his efforts to the area of stuttering, while Van Riper addressed a broader area of speech pathology. Van Riper was one of the few authors who spelled out in detail a specific methodology for the correction of articulatory problems. His early textbook, *Speech Correction: Principles and Methods* (1937), is probably, in its revised form, the most popular and widely used college text on that subject today.

One reason Van Riper's text has remained so popular is that he states in clear and concise terms a practical methodology for the remediation of speech problems. The methods he proposed were easy to understand and could be replicated in a step-by-step fashion. As a student, Van Riper was exposed to Thorndike's educational methodology and theory, which he later incorporated into his first book. Many of Thorndike's principles of learning were based upon research findings from experiments with animals as well as with human subjects. Van Riper had only to apply these principles with slight modification to the correction of speech problems.

Thorndike identified six tasks he felt were important for the teacher to follow:

1. identify the specific elements of the learning tasks.
2. determine the particular response desired for each stimulus.
3. present the tasks from simple to complex.
4. present the tasks in a way most likely to evoke the correct response.
5. reward the correct response.
6. provide ample practice for the correct response to occur followed with reward.

Thorndike pointed out additional principles affecting the learner. He felt they should be prepared to learn, or be in the correct "set." This is equivalent to the concept that an organism should be motivated before learning can take place. The learner should be rewarded either intrinsically through satisfaction or extrinsically by praise. The ability for the organism to distinguish between relevant, stimulus conditions was also important. Finally, Thorndike maintained that although punishing the learner failed to weaken connections, it might serve to direct the organism toward the correct response.

Analysis of Van Riper's early book and revised editions of the same text reveal many striking similarities to Thorndike's tenets, especially in Van Riper's section on articulation disorders. Van Riper feels that the clinician must first convince the individual that he has a problem. This would be analogous to Thorndike's preparatory set. Van Riper proceeds to break down speaking into its smallest, component parts, beginning with ear training, discrimination, production of sound in isolation, nonsense syllables, words, sentences, and conversational speech, following Thorndike's task presentation from simple to complex. The importance of reward is stressed by Van Riper and usually consists of verbal praise. Mild forms of punishment were suggested when an individual responded incorrectly. Punishments suggested were requiring the child to remove a pencil from behind the left ear to behind the right ear contingent on an incorrect response, or putting one's foot in a trash can. Punishment in these forms was more a reminder than a reprimand as Thorndike had suggested.

Van Riper was very critical of textbooks that suggested drill in the form of monotonous word or sentence repetition. He felt this was an old educational concept, no longer supported by modern, educational practice and theory. "Motivation, maturation, discrimination and application to life situations are indispensable to any therapy" (Van Riper, 1937). It is clear to see Thorndike's influence here.

Following on the heels of Van Riper's first text about speech therapy, a sizable number of similar books were written, also designed for use as college texts. Each presented a methodology for the correction of articulation disorders similar to the analytic method suggested by Van Riper. It is not possible to determine whether the authors followed Van Riper's lead with regard to methodology or whether they operated from the same Thorndikian theory. Whatever the case may be, the methodology is practically identical. These authors include Fairbanks (1940), Johnson et al. (1942), Berry and Eisenson (1942), and later Anderson (1953), Van Riper and Irwin (1958), and Carrell (1968).

All of these books have been revised, some as many as five times. Most of them, especially Van Riper's text, are still used today as college textbooks, and the methodology contained therein is taught to the majority of students majoring in speech pathology.

While Thorndike's emphasis on bonds or connections, his elementary account of transfer of training, the mechanical operation of the Law of Effect, and his rote-drill conception of human learning are considered greatly oversimplified by learning theorists today, there can be little doubt of his extensive influence on the teaching profession, especially speech clinicians. If we were to pick two individuals who have had the greatest impact upon methodology in speech pathology, other than the area of stuttering, they would be Thorndike, for his identification of principles of learning, and Van Riper, for his application of these principles to speech therapy.

Another example of the use of instrumental conditioning in speech therapy is found in the work of Brutton and Shoemaker (1967). In addition to using classical conditioning to alter basic emotional responses of the stutterer, instrumental conditioning was employed to alter the stutterer's coping behaviors. The authors point out that both types of conditioning are practically inseparable. During instrumental conditioning the subject is told precisely what behaviors will be rewarded and which will not be rewarded. During therapy, disfluent utterances go unrewarded, while fluent speech is rewarded with social praise. The authors also draw upon current learning theory to substantiate their methodological system.

Rejecting Thorndike's Law of Effect as well as several of his other learning principles, the behaviorist, Guthrie (1952), presented his *substitution theory,* sometimes referred to as a contiguity theory. To Guthrie, the only prerequisite to learning, indeed his only law of learning, involved the principle of contiguity. The pairing of a stimulus with a response results in one-trial learning, which is established at full strength at the time of pairing. There is no need to practice a response since practice or repetition will not improve the response. It is the particular combination of cues and responses that is learned. Good performance results from the association of correct responses with appropriate cues or stimuli.

Since to Guthrie contiguity in time is the only important element in learning, reward and punishment play little or no part in determining whether or not learning occurs. Motivation is given little importance, only that it serves to initiate some activity. Forgetting occurs not from disuse, but from interpolated activities which interfere with original learning.

It is difficult to find speech clinicians who subscribe to Guthrie's model of learning. Although some authors give no attention to providing rewards to a subject, this does not mean they would be opposed to providing appropriate rewards for good performance. One who appears to use a method similar to what Guthrie would recommend is Eugene McDonald (1965), author of a text about correcting articulation. The fact that McDonald barely mentions reinforcement, his stress on contiguity, his insistence that the child be provided the widest association of correct motor responses to syllable or word stimuli, plus his disconcern for motivating subjects could clearly place him in Guthrie's camp. But McDonald points out that many effective techniques have been developed for improving articulation and suggests that the reader should study these techniques. Perhaps McDonald did not wish to restate these techniques or he may not have been familiar with learning theory to the point of outlining a methodology. On the other hand, it is possible he was following Guthrie's model. It would seem likely McDonald did not feel it was necessary to tie his articulation strategy to any one system of learning theory. He makes no references to learning theorists in his text.

Clark Hull's book, *Principles of Learning,* appeared in 1943, followed by a revision, *Essentials of Behavior,* and a final 1952 publication, *A Behavior System.* In these books, Hull presents a highly integrated set of postulates, theorems, and corollaries explaining how learning occurs. Hull presented his theory in complex mathematical terms, and unless the reader has a wide background in both learning theory and mathematics, he would be in no position to understand Hull's theory. Only a gross simplification of his position will be presented here.

A firm behaviorist, Hull was in basic agreement with Thorndike concerning the importance of contiguity of stimuli, responses, and reinforcement. He felt learning could occur only when the organism was first in a state of tension, or a "drive state." When a contiguous response results in drive reduction (reinforcement), the resultant is a change in the structure of the nervous system of the organism. So in the future when a similar stimulus occurs, there is a strong probability the previously paired responses will also occur. If the organism's drive state is zero, no response can be evoked. There is a direct relationship between the number of reinforced, contiguous repetitions of the stimulus-response relationship and strength of the habit or degree of learning. He also identified unobservable, intervening variables which affect both certain antecedent and consequent responses. These unobservable events helped Hull account for observable behaviors. In Hull's later work he introduced incentive motivation as an important variable in learning. The greater the person's incentive to learn, the greater the learning.

The central concept in Hull's system remained that of reinforcement. He identified both primary and secondary reinforcers in much the same light as they are conceived today. Hull's attempt to formulate exacting quantitative laws governing human behavior had a powerful influence on emerging learning theory in psychology.

The application of Hull's reinforcement theory in the classroom would include

1. high degree of order and systematic presentation of material
2. skills developed from simple to complex
3. clear understanding of the stimuli and responses to be associated
4. stimulating environment
5. providing artificial incentives in the form of secondary reinforcers after learning new skills was established
6. practice to build up desired habits

It is not surprising that Hull's learning theory is seldom mentioned in speech therapy literature. His texts are extremely complex and difficult to understand because of his pedantic language and mathematical models. His name is referred to only once by Irwin and Griffith (1973), who authored a chapter in a book dealing with the treatment of articulation disorders. Hull is mentioned briefly as one who supports the contention that the behavior that is reinforced is the behavior that is learned. Although speech pathologists seem not to have drawn directly from Hullian theory, his influence upon developments in psychology have had far-reaching effects. Other contemporary learning theorists have modified, and perhaps communicated more effectively some of his basic tenets.

Skinner's operant conditioning: It has been pointed out that Thorndike concentrated on stimulus-response connections, Guthrie relied heavily on analyzing the response, and Hull interjected an intervening variable between the stimulus and response to account for learning. B. F. Skinner's system focused entirely on responses. His was a system of descriptive behaviorism in which theory played little part. Skinner felt most of our learning results from a special kind of conditioning which is called *operant conditioning*. He differentiated between classical conditioning of the Pavlovian type, in which eliciting stimuli could be clearly identified, and operant conditioning, in which the stimulus might be identifiable but certainly irrelevant to the understanding of operant behavior. He felt psychologists gave too much attention to classical conditioning and the stimulus conditions involved.

Skinner adopted a kind of instrumental conditioning experiment by placing a rat in his "Skinner Box" and observing the frequency of its bar-pressing response when food pellets were released, contingent on the response. From these data and other carefully controlled laboratory experiments, Skinner postulated his law of acquisition, which said if reinforcement follows an operant behavior, the strength of the behavior is increased. This finding is strikingly similar to Thorndike's Law of Effect or Hull's Postulate 4, the difference being Skinner makes no assumption about pain-pleasure consequences of reinforcement nor does he interpret reinforcement as a kind of drive reduction. While Thorndike and Hull attempted to explain what was happening, Skinner merely offered a description.

In any descriptive system measurement of the behaviors being studied is of critical importance. In effect the data *are* the system, provided these data are predictable and lawful. Skinner used rate of response as his basic measure of conditioning by computing the number of responses emitted per unit of time. Laws of learning are derived directly from response rates. He carefully observed events which increased or decreased rate of response.

Skinner is probably best known for his work with various schedules of reinforcement (Skinner & Ferster, 1957). He points out that given certain schedules of reinforcement, one can predict not only what effect they will have upon rate of response during training, but also what effects will occur after reinforcement is discontinued.

Motivation, or drive, is discussed in terms of deprivation, which Skinner feels activates the organism. There would be little opportunity for conditioning a rat's operant responses if the animal was well fed. Thus, Skinner defines drive in terms of the number of hours of deprivation.

Skinner (1957) also outlined procedures for shaping new response classes in both animals and humans. He called this procedure *successive approximation*. Extinction, generalization, and secondary reinforcement were other concepts he elaborated.

In addition to his research in animal and human behavior modification, Skinner also grappled with philosophical and ethical issues involved in controlling human behavior (Skinner, 1953). His own research demonstrated that much human behavior is subtly controlled by others. The fundamental problems is *who* should control behavior, and *what* behaviors do they have a right to control? Many who feel threatened by Skinner's concept of the controlled individual reject Skinner's entire system. They consider humans as having a "free will," unencumbered by past experiences. At present, Skinner's views on the destiny of humans are quite controversial.

Although Skinner's first book was published in 1938, it was not until the 1950s with the addition of more publications that his work became well known. By 1960, Skinner's views had tremendous impact upon departments of psychology across the country. Application of principles he had carefully formulated filtered into the educational system, and by the 1970s, almost every teacher had some contact with "behavior modification," derived either directly or indirectly from Skinner's work.

And yet, this filtering process has been slow. It seems that educational application lags 30 to 50 years behind psychological research and theory. Speech clinicians also seem to lag behind psychological theory. Only in recent years has Skinner's descriptive behaviorism been applied in speech therapy as a system for the effective modification of speech behaviors.

One of the problems has been there are so few materials written in speech pathology outlining Skinner's principles of learning as applied to correction of speech problems. As a consequence, university speech therapy training programs must rely upon revised editions of textbooks in speech therapy that were written in the 1930s and 1940s. The revisions usually include a few pages incorporating some principles adapted from current learning theory. For example, Johnson et al. (1967) inserted five pages in their 1967 revised edition to discuss Skinner's theory of operant conditioning as it applied to speech as a learned behavior. Van Riper and Irwin (1958) devoted two pages to shaping speech responses, a process recommended by Skinner. Perkins (1971) in a more recent text on speech therapy presented wider coverage of methodology based upon current learning theory.

Skinner's influence is seen more clearly in the works of authors who published journal articles or book chapters during the late 1960s and early 1970s. Journal articles by Brookshire (1967), Holland (1967), Mowrer (1969), and McReynolds (1970) clearly outline Skinner's principles and their application to speech therapy. One of the few textbooks outlining operant procedures used in speech therapy was published in 1968, edited by Sloane and MacAulay (1968). Irwin and Griffith (1973) drew heavily upon operant conditioning procedures, as did Mowrer, Baker, and Schutz (1968) and Mowrer (1973), in their development of programs for the remediation of articulation errors.

A sizable number of researchers have employed operant conditioning as a treatment of stuttering. Goldiamond (1965), Mowrer (1971), Ryan (1970), and Shames and Egolf (1976) are a few who have designed instructional programs based upon operant procedures to reduce stuttering behaviors. The modification of certain language skills also has been reported by several authors using operant conditioning (Gray & Ryan, 1973; Risley et al., 1972).

Next to Thorndike, it can be said without reservation that the work of Skinner and his associates has made a substantial impact upon methods used by speech clinicians to remediate communication problems. Aside from the emphasis placed on operant conditioning, many clinicians are using a much more rigorous, scientific model in conducting therapy. Characteristic of this procedure is a careful specification of behavioral objectives, precise measurement of behaviors before, during, and following therapy, systematic management of reinforcement schedules, and use of programmed instructional techniques.

Cognitive Theories

Rejecting the concept that learning consisted of associations between stimuli and responses, Gestalt psychologists emphasized understanding and intellectual interpretation of sensory experiences in the learning process. They felt learning occurred in organized patterns, and it is the patterns we learn, not the specific details of the task. A great deal of learning comes through insight when there is a sudden restructuring of the "field relationship," or environmental conditions. Grasping situations as a whole was stressed as more meaningful than understanding of its parts. Thus, this was a synthetic approach to learning as opposed to the associationistic, analytic method of learning through building up a series of stimulus-response connections.

Two psychologists were chiefly responsible for introducing Gestaltism to education: Kirt Lewin (1938) and Edward Tolman (1932, 1942). Lewin, often viewed as a neo-Gestaltist, felt within each person there exists a field of forces, his life space. It consists of the people he knows, objects around him, his thoughts, internal tensions of a physiological nature, as well as psychological tensions. Behavior results from an interplay of all these forces. Any changes in behavior result from forces in the structure of his cognitive field or from his inner needs or motivation. These behavioral changes may occur suddenly, as in the case of insightful learning or, in some cases, a great deal of repetition may be required. Motivation is held as being very important as a tension system of an individual. Motivation is satisfied when the goal is achieved. Reward comes from the internal satisfaction the individual receives from attaining the goal, thus reducing inner tension.

Lewin focused on the individual rather than on groups of subjects. He had little regard for statistics, which buried the individual among the masses. He was considered a social psychologist in that most of his work involved human subjects, especially children. Several of his experiments involved topics of concern to educators. For example, he found that democratic groups were far more productive than were authoritarian groups. His writings and concepts have had considerable influence in the fields of social, child, and experimental psychology.

As a direct outgrowth of Lewin's field-theory plus the writings of those who initiated the orthodox Gestalt movement (Wertheimer 1945; Köhler, 1929; Koffka, 1935), Backus and Beasley (1951) devised a therapeutic approach for the correction of articulation errors in children. The authors also drew upon the works of practitioners Karen Horney and Carl Rogers. A chief complaint of Backus and Beasley is that carry over, or generalization of the new speech response, is often a problem with traditional, analytic speech correction procedures. These problems, according to the authors, can be overcome if children are placed in ideal conditions for learning so that they will continue to learn after formal instruction ends. A child does not learn speech in a sequence of isolated sounds, nonsense syllables, words, and connected speech, but learns sounds as conversational speech units, as wholes, not isolated parts.

The job of the speech clinician is to create a special environment in which the child can restructure articulation patterns. The special environment includes a group of children who are motivated to converse with one another and with the teacher. Little stress is placed on repetition. Through speaking with others in carefully structured situations, the child perceives an overall organization of the total speaking process. Building feelings of belonging, personal worth, and social skills go hand in hand with modifying the speech behavior. Children are not labeled as stutterers, cerebral-palsied individuals, or as poor speakers, so no attempt is made to group children homogeneously.

Motivation is an important key to success, but that motivation must come from *within* an individual, not from another person. As Lewin put it, there must be an "inner tension" within the individual before learning can take place. Reward in the form of praise for speech attempts should be given in abundance, according to Backus and Beasley. The child's feeling of success should first come from the clinician, then from the entire group, which usually consists of from eight to ten children.

This procedure is a unique one since it is such a radical departure from more traditional therapy approaches. Along with the Gestalt approach to teaching articulation skills, Backus and Beasley rely heavily upon principles of good mental hygiene. Although this type of therapy has never become very popular among practicing speech clinicians, many adapt parts of Backus and Beasley's strategy into their own style of teaching.

Aside from Lewin, Edward Tolman also adapted principles of Gestalt psychology to the field of learning, but he also attempted to combine them with behaviorism, a seemingly impossible task. Tolman's "Sign-Gestalt" concept resulted from his many studies with animals. He found animals running a maze learned certain "signs" along route which they organized into a molar behavior pattern. Introduce a shorter route to the goal and the rat proceeded directly to the goal without having to be reinforced many times for this new behavior. To Tolman, the rat had a "cognitive map" of getting to the goal along the shortest possible route. Therefore, he felt repetition and reinforcement had little to do with learning. Practice alone does not result in learning. It is, however, necessary to provide confirmation that a goal has been reached, but this does not mean reinforcement is to be provided. Tolman's concept of place learning and latent learning have been of greatest interest to psychologists. Many of his other terms like *sign Gestalts, cognitions,* and *expectations,* and his terms for a set of intervening variables have been criticized frequently.

No direct evidence or reference to Tolman's learning theory can be found in the literature about articulation therapy. Inspection of methodology reveals little, if any, direct influence. Perhaps his terminology was too vague or his procedures too impractical to be applied to articulation behaviors. Van Riper (1971) devotes only two sentences to Tolman's concepts of cognitive mapping—one-trial learning and exploratory learning—in his discussion of cognitive learning theories of stuttering. Apparently Festinger's (1957) cognitive dissonance theory seems to have had more influence on the few investigators who view stuttering as a cognitive learning problem.

Theories of Psychotherapy and Counseling

Although not a learning theory in its own right, the field of psychotherapy and its milder form, counseling strategies, have had an influence on methods used in speech therapy. One could argue that the methodology has developed from, or relies heavily upon, cognitive learning theory, but it is possible to employ techniques devised by operant conditioning psychologists for changing behavior in the counseling situation.

Van Riper (1937) devoted a chapter of his book to psychotherapy and its use in speech correction. His definition of psychotherapy ranged from simple suggestions to profound psychoanalysis. The amount of psychotherapy needed varies from individual to individual, according to Van Riper. Emphasis is placed on helping the individual understand his problem and vent negative feelings and frustrations in an attempt to help him gain insight into the nature of his problem and take the necessary steps toward correcting it. Often it is felt the individual can accomplish this himself from within. The clinician only serves as a catalyst in these situations. Van Riper also pointed out the benefits of group therapy as an effective means of helping children develop proper attitudes about their speech.

Van Riper was no doubt strongly influenced by Travis (1931), himself a psychologist who wrote extensively about the application of psychotherapy to stutterers as well as a general counseling approach. The work of Barbara (1954) and Glauber (1958) represents two authors who applied psychotherapy treatment methods to stutterers in a systematic way. The psychoanalytic literature dealing with stuttering is too extensive to cover here. Most speech clinicians are reluctant to use a treatment method based on psychoanalytic theory because they lack the training necessary to conduct it. What filters down to them is an awareness of the complexity of stuttering and the need for counseling. Hence, many stutterers are simply referred to psychologists, either solely for therapy or at least as a supplemental part of therapy. Certainly a large number of speech clinicians use counseling strategies in some form or other during the course of therapy with stutterers, probably with the idea of helping the stutterer better understand and cope with his problem. The basic idea here, coming from the Gestalt school, is that once a person gains insight into his problem, he will be in a better position to solve it.

Drawing from counseling procedures developed by Carl Rogers (1942, 1951), several speech clinicians devised nondirective methods for treating articulation problems. One of the first clinicians to formalize a nondirective approach was Hejna (1960). It was designed for use with children who do not respond to usual therapy methods and who may have emotional problems associated with their speech problem. Hejna's basic premise is that every individual has the ability to solve his own conflicts with indirect assistance from the clinician. The task of the clinician is to create an atmosphere in which the individual feels completely accepted and free to express himself. As the child works through his hostilities and frustrations by engaging in play therapy, the removal of restraint allows him, through self-discovery, to make better adjustments to his environment. Speech patterns can improve automatically as the child progresses toward self-realization.

This type of therapy is radically different from those which have developed from associationistic learning theories. There is no formal attention to reinforcement, rate of learning, generalization of response classes, forgetting, stimulus presentation, or any of the other factors about which associationists are vitally concerned. Nondirective clinicians are concerned with feelings, attitudes, needs, and those attributes which contribute to good mental health.

Analysis of
Procedures Used by
Practicing Speech Clinicians

Some data are available regarding the different remedial procedures used by speech clinicians. Although these data were collected from questionnaires, they provide an indication of the effects learning theory has had upon remedial procedures used in speech therapy. One comprehensive study conducted by Chapman et al. (1961) was part of a nationwide study of speech and hearing practices in public schools. The limitations of this study are one, it was conducted before speech clinicians were exposed to Skinner's operant conditioning model, and two, the procedures identified in the study were selected by a study committee and do not necessarily represent those actually used by clinicians.

Analysis of the data the authors collected did not appear to indicate the existence of any strong school of therapeutic thought. Speech clinicians tended to be rather eclectic in their choice of procedure. Results of a factor analysis of all procedures used in articulation therapy indicated that a highly structured drill approach emphasizing speech sound production was favored. This was followed by a factor made up of psychological counseling in the form of directive counseling, nondirective counseling, play therapy, and psychotherapy. Factors relating to stuttering therapy were not clearly marked because of extreme distortion of the distributions and because of the high incidence of clinicians working with few stutterers.

From an analysis of remedial procedures used, it was apparent that games were the vehicles for teaching speech sounds as opposed to use of speech drills. Counseling was preferred as a descriptive term for the speech clinician's activity rather than psychotherapy. The percentage of clinicians who neither provide counseling nor psychotherapy was surprisingly high.

Interviews were conducted with many of the clinicians in an attempt to uncover some basic, overall philosophy concerning use of remedial procedures. The conclusion was that speech clinicians select the method they feel is appropriate for the individual child. This could be viewed as an eclectic approach, or an attempt to select the best procedure from a large pool of procedures. The clinicians reported that research studies and tradition were key factors leading to the choice of remedial procedures. Chapman et al. speculated about the influence clinical training might have on the remedial procedures used. It was suggested clinicians might use a limited number of procedures because of inadequate exposure to a wide variety of approaches.

Finally, clinicians were asked to list the publications they felt were most helpful to them in determining remedial procedures. Books heading the list were written by Van Riper, Fairbanks, Travis, West et al., Johnson et al., and Berry and Eisenson. All of these books stressed Thorndike's learning theory. Near the end of the list were books by Backus and Beasley and Rogers, showing some influence of Gestaltism and counseling.

This finding is not surprising. It is extremely doubtful that speech clinicians have time to dig deeply into the writings of the learning theorists to extract strategies to assist them in teaching speech skills. This seems especially true of practicing speech clinicians in view of the fact Chapman et al. (1961) found that lack of time for therapy was a chief complaint of the clinicians surveyed in their study. Speech clinicians must be satisfied, for the most part, with: (1) what they learn during their training, (2) reading books and journals, (3) attending workshops, (4) continuing education programs, and (5) conversing with other clinicians. Little wonder speech clinicians describe their approach to remedial procedures as "eclectic."

Current Trends of
Learning Theory in
Speech Pathology

During the years following the 1961 survey, speech clinicians were gradually introduced to a learning theory based upon Skinner's operant conditioning model. It is difficult to ascertain the impact this learning theory has had upon speech therapy, but it is safe to say most speech clinicians have some working knowledge of this theory commonly referred to as *behavior modification*. Considering the increasing number of studies published in professional journals in speech and hearing pathology, as well as a growing number of books outlining techniques of operant conditioning, it is safe to say that this learning theory presently plays a major role in determining instructional strategies used by speech clinicians.

An additional indication of the growth of the behavior modification movement is illustrated by the organization of small groups of professionals whose sole purpose is to foster the knowledge and use of behavior modification procedures in speech therapy. One group of about forty professionals met annually during the early 1970s publishing a now defunct publication called *Feedback*. A similar organization, active in the state of Ohio, the Association for Precision Speech Therapy and Communications Technology, presently boasts about seventy-five members. Their publication is entitled *Apstractions*. It is anticipated that similar organizations may be established in other states. Workshop lecturers who present information about behavior modification in speech therapy are in high demand across the country. Whether this movement will have a lasting effect upon methodology used by speech clinicians or will be a passing, educational fad remains to be seen. But judging from proponents of this current learning theory, it seems likely the former will be true.

Future Development
in Learning Theory

The search continues for more precise definitions and critical tests of fundamental conditions of learning. The issue of reinforcement divides many learning theorists. Reinforcement is no longer an explanation of learning as Thorndike conceived of it. Guthrie and Tolman discredited its importance, and Skinner saw it only as a descriptive principle, not in terms of drive reduction. Hull's theory was the last surviving fortress of reinforcement as a principle factor responsible for habit strength. But even Hull abandoned his original position in favor of a drive-stimulus-reduction explanation.

Current research and theories concerning the role of reinforcement and drive seem to be widely separated. Of those who favor a stimulus-response analysis of learning, some feel reinforcement is not necessary, but contiguity explains why learning occurs. They cite instances of latent learning, incidental learning, and learning under conditions of no reward to support their belief. Those who feel reinforcement is necessary have difficulty explaining why it increases learning. Some feel it supports drive-reduction theory. Others see reduction as playing little part and hold that different types of reinforcement operate differently depending on the situation. The role of reinforcement is a complex issue, one not likely to be solved easily within the next decade.

It is safe to say that the behavioristic movement started by Watson over 70 years ago will predominate learning theory for years to come. But contrary to Thorndike's views, we will no longer find theorists who attempt to combine all learning into one theory as if there was some magic formula to explain learning in general. "Miniature" theory systems have grown increasingly important, so we can look forward to refinement in certain aspects of learning. We can also look forward to increasing precision and quantification of learning theories which grow out of experimental data rather than speculation.

On the other hand, we can also look forward to a growing interest on the hidden, nonbehavioral aspects of the learning process that have been identified as *intervening variables*. Topics relating to self-controlled behavior and motivation also appear to be promising areas of study.

One conclusion seems certain. The scientific method will prevail as a process for investigating *how* learning occurs. Speech clinicians, especially those who write textbooks, must continue their efforts to remain current in the area of learning theory for it is primarily through books such as these and the professors who use them that theory is passed on to practicing speech clinicians.

BIBLIOGRAPHY

Anderson, V., & Newby, H. *Improving the child's speech*. New York: Oxford University Press, 1953.

Backus, O., & Beasley, J. *Speech therapy with children*. Boston: Houghton Mifflin, 1951.

Barbara, D. A. *Stuttering: A psychodynamic approach to its understanding and treatment*. New York: Julian, 1954.

Berry, M., & Eisenson, J. *The defective in speech*. New York: F. S. Crofts, 1942.

Brookshire, R. H. Speech pathology and the experimental analysis of behavior. *Journal of Speech and Hearing Disorders*, 1967, *32*, 215–227.

Brutten, E. J., & Shoemaker, D. J. *The modification of stuttering*. Englewood Cliffs, N.J.: Prentice-Hall, 1967.

Carrell, J. *Disorders of articulation*. Englewood Cliffs, N.J.: Prentice-Hall, 1968.

Chapman, M. E., Herbert, E. L., Avery, C. B., & Selmar, J. W. Clinical practice: Remedial procedures. *Journal of Speech and Hearing Disorders*. Monograph, 1961, *8*, 58–77.

Clark, R. M., & Murray, F. M. Alterations of self concept: A barometer of progress in individuals undergoing therapy for stuttering. In D. E. Barbara (Ed.), *New directions in stuttering*. Springfield, Ill.: Charles C Thomas, 1965.

Fairbanks, G. *Voice and articulation drillbook*. New York: Harper, 1940.

Festinger, L. *A theory of cognitive dissonance*. Evanston, Ill.: Row, Peterson, 1957.

Goldiamond, I. Stuttering and fluency as manipulatable operant response classes. In L. Krasner & L. Ullman (Eds.), *Research in behavior modification*. New York: Holt, Rinehart & Winston, 1965.

Glauber, I. P. The psychoanalysis of stuttering. In J. Eisenson (Ed.), *Stuttering: A symposium*. New York: Harper & Row, 1958.

Gray, B., & Ryan, B. *A language program for the nonlanguage child*. Champaign, Ill.: Research Press, 1973.

Guthrie, E. R. *The psychology of learning*. New York: Harper, 1952.

Hejna, R. *Speech disorders and non-directive therapy*. New York: Ronald Press, 1960.

Holland, A. Some applications of behavioral principles to clinical speech problems. *Journal of Speech and Hearing Disorders*, 1967, *32*, 11–18.

Hull, C. *Principles of behavior*. New York: Appleton-Century-Crofts, 1943.

Hull, C. *Essentials of behavior*. New Haven, Conn.: Yale University Press, 1951.

Hull, C. *A behavior system*. New Haven, Conn.: Yale University Press, 1952.

Irwin, J., & Griffith, F. A theoretical and operational analysis of the paired stimuli technique. In W. Wolfe & D. Goulding (Eds.), *Articulation and learning*. Springfield, Ill.: Charles C Thomas, 1973.

Johnson, W., Brown, S., Curtis, J., Edney, C., & Keaster, J. *Speech handicapped school children*. New York: Harper & Row, 1942.

Johnson, W., Brown, S., Curtis, J., Edney, C., & Keaster, J. *Speech handicapped school children* (3rd ed.). New York: Harper & Row, 1967.

Koffka, K. *Principles of Gestalt psychology*. New York: Harcourt, Brace, 1935.

Köhler, W. *Gestalt psychology*. New York: Liveright, 1929.

Lewin, K. *Contributions and psychological theory*. Durham, N.C.: Duke University Press, 1938.

McDonald, E. *Articulation testing and treatment: A sensory-motor approach*. Pittsburgh, Penn.: Stanwix House, 1965.

McReynolds, L. Contingencies and consequences in speech therapy. *Journal of Speech and Hearing Disorders*, 1970, *35*, 12–24.

Mowrer, D. E. Evaluating speech therapy through precision recording. *Journal of Speech and Hearing Disorders*, 1969, *34*, 239–244.

Mowrer, D. E. *Technical research report S-1: Reduction of stuttering behavior*. Tempe, Ariz.: Arizona State University, 1971.

Mowrer, D. E. Behavioral application to modification of articulation. In W. Wolfe & D. Goulding, (Eds.), *Articulation and learning: New dimensions in research, diagnosis and therapy*. Springfield, Ill.: Charles C Thomas, 1973.

Mowrer, D. E., Baker, R., & Schutz, R. Operant procedures in the control of speech articulation. In H. Sloane & B. MacAulay (Eds.), *Operant procedures in remedial speech and language training*. Boston: Houghton Mifflin, 1968.

Peppard, H. *The correction of speech defects*. New York: Macmillan, 1925.

Perkins, W. H. *Speech pathology: An applied behavioral science*. St. Louis, Mo.: C. V. Mosby, 1971.

Risley, T., Hart, B., & Doke, L. Operant language development: The outline of a therapeutic technology. In R. L. Schiefelbusch (Ed.), *Language of the mentally retarded*. Baltimore: University Park Press, 1972.

Rogers, C. R. *Counseling and psychotherapy*. Boston: Houghton Mifflin, 1942.

Rogers, C. R. *Client-centered therapy*. Boston: Houghton Mifflin, 1951.

Ryan, B. An illustration of operant conditioning therapy for stutterers. In M. Fraser (Ed.), *Conditioning in stuttering therapy: Applications and limitations*. Memphis, Tenn.: Speech Foundation of America, 1970.

Shames, G., & Egolf, D. B. *Operant conditioning and the management of stuttering: A book for clinicians*. Englewood Cliffs, N.J.: Prentice-Hall, 1976.

Skinner, B. F. *Walden II*. New York: Macmillan, 1948.

Skinner, B. F. *Science and human behavior*. New York: Macmillan, 1953.

Skinner, B. F., *Verbal behavior*. New York, New York: Appleton-Century-Crofts, 1957.

Skinner, B. F., & Ferster, C. *Schedules of reinforcement*. New York: Appleton-Century-Crofts, 1957.

Sloane, H. N., Jr., & MacAulay, B. D. (Eds.), *Operant procedures in remedial speech and language training*. Boston: Houghton Mifflin, 1968.

Thorndike, E. L. Animal intelligence: An experimental study of associative processes in animals. *Psychological Monograph*, 1898, *2*, no. 8.

Thorndike, E. L. *Animal intelligence*. New York: Macmillan, 1911.

Tolman, E. C. *Purposeful behavior in animals and men.* New York: Appleton-Century-Crofts, 1932.

Tolman, E. C. *Drive's toward war.* New York: Appleton-Century-Crofts, 1942.

Travis, L. E. *Speech pathology.* New York: Appleton-Century, 1931.

Van Riper, C. *Speech correction: principles and methods.* Englewood Cliffs, N.J.: Prentice-Hall, 1937.

Van Riper, C. *The nature of stuttering.* Englewood Cliffs, N.J.: Prentice-Hall, 1971.

Van Riper, C. *The treatment of stuttering.* Englewood Cliffs, N.J.: Prentice-Hall, 1973.

Van Riper, C., & Irwin J., *Voice and articulation.* Englewood Cliffs, N.J.: Prentice-Hall, 1958.

Wertheimer, M. *Productive thinking.* New York: Harper, 1945.

2

Basis of Scientific Methodology

Early Attempts to Control
Natural Phenomena

The Need for Control

Early primitive people had many needs, fears, hungers, and weaknesses. Their lives could be snuffed out without reason. They recognized a life force and attributed human characteristics to objects, living or not. The lion was brave, the hyena cowardly, the river was calm or could be angry, the sun provided heat and light, and was most powerful of all. Everything in their environment had a spirit like people, good and evil; and each spirit can be influenced, like people could be influenced. If the river was angry, it would overflow its banks. If it did not rain, the sky spirits were angry, just like one person could become angry with another.

A powerful force or magic was needed to subdue the spirits and persuade them to yield to the will of the people; to provide rain and sunshine for crops, mild winters, good hunting. Magic rituals to the spirits were used to reduce pain or eliminate disease or other catastrophes that plagued them.

Magic became too time consuming for everyone to practice, so one person in the tribe was appointed to spend all of his time making magic. The tribal magician held secret knowledge about cures and spells; as his rituals became more complex and stylized, he became the most powerful member of the tribe. These individuals performed white magic to do good to the people of the tribe. Later, black magic was used to wake evil spirits and gradually a set of taboos were adopted for each tribe so as not to offend evil spirits. Violate the taboos and punishment followed.

An elaborate system of taboos existed and continue to persist today in many primitive societies. These taboos are used in order to avoid bad consequences. For example, the Ewe-speaking peoples of the Slave Coast believe that the inner spirit of a person leaves the body and returns through the mouth. Thus, opening the mouth, becomes a dangerous event for another spirit may enter the mouth if one is not careful. In order to protect one's spirit, great care must be taken when eating or drinking. The Zafimanelo of Madagascar lock their doors when eating and allow no one to see them eat. This gives them control over other spirits entering their mouth. One king ordered his 12-year-old son quartered after the son had inadvertently seen his father drink. Taboos exist for showing one's face, menstruating, spitting, cutting nails and hair, using certain words, viewing sacred grounds, and meeting strangers—just to mention a few. An essential part of all taboos is the fear of offending some spirit. Only the best magicians had the power to protect someone who violated a taboo.

Those in charge of the tribal magic ceremonies were expected to perform magic acts, using spells to constrain spirits or gods and sway them to obey the will of the magician. The use of symbolic prayers and objects during religious ceremonies elevated the magician to an important position in the religious community. As time went on, the magician took the title of priest and continued in his former capacity. In societies where the magicians were not successful or powerful, the members felt it better just to beg for favors of the gods. In these tribes a high priest was appointed to placate the gods and the magician was lowered to a lesser position. All rulers called upon their high priests and magicians for counsel and they held important positions in the society. In Egypt, both held posts of equal importance. Effigies and painted images, the bystanders of magicians, were part of every religious ritual.

While civilization spread, bringing the religions of Mesopotamia and Egypt with it, a new religion gained prominence among Canaanites led by Abraham. The tribes came from the Mesopotamian city of Ur around 2000 B.C. and believed in a single deity, Yahweh or Jehovah, an abstract god who could not be influenced by even the best magician. This new religion shunned all forms of formalized magic rites and was constantly being threatened by surrounding cultures that practiced magic. Many of the Israelites, as these Canaanites were later called, continued to practice magic and consult with magicians. The Old Testament relates the story of Aaron, brother of Moses, who threw his rod down before Ramses II. The rod instantly turned into a live snake. The Pharoah's own magicians Jannes and Jambres duplicated Aaron's feat with their own rods. These two snakes were consumed by Aaron's snake. We know that the Egyptian cobra can be made motionless by applying a pressure point just below its neck. It is surprising that Aaron, a believer in Yahweh, would resort to magic tricks.

The ancient Greeks devised their own art of divination such as *chiromancy* in which the shape and lines of the hand foretell the future, length of life, and character of a person. They also practiced *numerology* to foretell the future by determining numbers associated with heavenly bodies and letters of the alphabet, so knowing the date of your birth and letters in your name one could foretell future events.

It was in ancient Greece that the power of magic came under question with the conflict between astrology and astronomy and the realization that the Chaldean astrological maps were incorrect. Euclid challenged the art of numerology. Knowledge of scientific laws of nature conflicted with magic formulas. Medical knowledge was substituted for magical healing rituals. This struggle between science and magic has continued until today and is still present.

The ancient Romans were firmly convinced of the efficacy of magic. Black magic flourished along with the official religions of Rome. Common was the use of vexes, casting malicious spells, and worship of evil spirits.

The Roman emperors were worried about the growing power of the magicians and made efforts to ban the practice of magic or consultations with magicians. Yet they were highly superstitious, wearing magic *amulets* to ward off evil spirits, and they consulted with astrologers before making decisions. But they were not successful, not even the introduction of Christianity could erase these ancient beliefs. Christians were forced to an uneasy coexistence with pagan religions and mystic cults. They searched for ways to compete with the old gods and idols and found what they wanted by reaching back to ancient Greek beliefs in a Satan, or devil, as the Prince of Darkness and creator of evil in the battle for the hearts and souls of mankind. The devil was not a Christian invention. He was Pazuzu, king of evil spirits in Mesopotamia; Baal-zebub, lord of the flies, among the Philistines; Satan, ruled the underworld to the Israelites. But none of these evil doers played as important a role as that assigned by the Christian church followers. They said the Devil and his horde of evil followers lay in wait to ensnare the innocent into sinning. They reiterated the evils of the Devil to create a dread and loathing of him. But despite efforts of the early Christians to instigate a fear of the Devil, people began to personify him, identify with him, create a mystique that gave the Devil a godlike status in another religion, the antichristian cult of Satanism.

According to the temptation story in the Gospel of Matthew, Satan was powerful enough to dominate the world. This power appealed to many and gave rise to the Black Mass celebrated by Satan's followers. Hundreds of religious sects, cults, beliefs, and rituals were a source of constant trouble to the Christian during medieval times. One of the better known sects was Cabalism. Followers of this sect used formulas, figures, and arithmetic combinations of letters and numbers to cast spells and perform all manner of sorcery. Magical symbols played an important role, the circle, triangle, cross, which Christianity adopted, the swastika, and the five-sided pentagram.

The lure of sorcery was extremely popular during the eleventh and twelfth centuries to the thousands of suffering people. It offered them a way to achieve power and the promise of control over their plight in life. Many flocked to established sorcerers requesting magic spells. Others sought to be a sorcerer's apprentice so they could learn the power of the occult.

Attempts to Discourage Use of Magic

During the first ten centuries of its existence, Christianity suffered from continuing belief in magic. By the eleventh century, the church was more powerful and launched an attack to get rid of magicians and wipe out the practice of magic. In 1233, Pope

Gregory IX established the Inquisition to stamp out magic practices. Tortures were used to extract confessions out of suspected sorcerers.

In England white witches or Wiccas brewed herbs for the sick and had no connection with Satan. They used their power for good works. Black witches or Satanists were supposed to be able to fly and used their power to bring harm to others. They were believed to curdle milk, stop hens from laying, cause a ripening field to wither and die, make a person sicken and die, or make people fall in or out of love.

In 1484, Pope Innocent XIII issued an edict condemning witchcraft, and an attempt was made to destroy every trace of witchcraft. In the years between 1400 and 1700 an estimated one million persons were punished for witchcraft, sorcery, magic, and other heresies. The Puritan witch hunts spread to Massachusetts reaching its peak in 1692 with the death of twenty witches. In Europe, conjurers who performed slight of hand tricks with human confederates were suspect even though they said they had nothing to do with Satan.

Also suspect were alchemists, who searched for a way to turn metal into gold and bring youth to the aged. Although alchemy had its roots among the ancient Egyptian metallurgists, it was not practiced much in Europe until the fourteenth century. Magic, science and religion were at odds with one another and the alchemist remained in the secrecy of his laboratory. Some achieved fame, like the sixteenth century German-Swiss alchemist and physician, Paracelsus, often described as the father of medicine and Jon Lowenstern, who isolated phosporous. Eventually, chemistry, metallurgy and other sciences replaced alchemy but people could not give up the art of *divination*. During the thirteenth and fourteenth centuries, astrology, numerology and chiromancy had been practiced for centuries. Several other types had fallen into disuse, namely:

1. haruspicy—predicting the future by examining the entrails of sacrificed animals.
2. cleromancy—prediction by casting lots.
3. aeromancy—observing atmospheric conditions.
4. crystallomancy—crystal ball gazing.
5. rhabdomancy—using small sticks or divining rods especially in finding water.
6. geomancy—throwing handfuls of dirt into the air to note the pattern or figures made when it fell to earth.

Late in the fourteenth century another art of divination appeared, cartomancy or predicting future events by reading tarot cards.

By the end of the sixteenth century a renaissance of thought spurred by the discovery and conquest of unknown lands caused a rebirth of intellectual curiosity and mechanical speculation not evidenced since ancient Greek and Roman times. Science was at the threshold of a new age.

Nevertheless, interest in the occult and many forms of divination continued in new forms. Examples are

1. metoposcopy—using markings on the forehead to predict future events.
2. physiognomy—predicting from characteristics and expressions of the human

face or body type. As late as the 1940s, the psychologist Sheldon claimed he could predict human behavior and temperament from analyzing and measuring body types such as the mesomorphy, endomorphy, and ectomorphy. This theory has been criticized extensively.

3. mesmerising—grew from the work of Franz Mesmer, an eighteenth century physician who claimed he could heal the sick with his hands. From his work sprung faith healing and hypnosis and research into telepathy and spiritualism.

During the eighteenth and nineteenth centuries, clairvoyance and clairaudience, seeing and hearing beyond normal vision and hearing limits, traced back to Greek oracles, gained renewed interest. In this century continued research is conducted chiefly at Duke University into extrasensory perception, an area scoffed by most present day scientists.

As scientific thought prevailed, interest in the occult as well as black and white magic subsided but many remnants of these arts prevail today. The magician adopted his full stature as an entertainer whose purpose was to amuse and amaze his audience. Yet even today, within a mile or so of any university, you can have your future told by a diviner in the parlor of a tumbledown house for a fee of from $5 to $10. Or you can pick up any newspaper and study the predictions about today's events in the astrology section or you may even say some prayers in the hopes of increasing your test scores. We have not been able to completely eliminate the influence of the past 4000 years of sorcery.

The methods of scientific investigation were introduced a scant 400 years ago. In comparison to human appearance in the Western Hemisphere some 300,000 to 400,000 years ago, it can be safely said that science is still in its infancy. Yet with respect to human knowledge about the world and the ability to control naturalistic events, the last 400 years has represented a gigantic step forward, unparalleled in history. Progress in scientific technology within the past 80 years has been truly phenomenal. What early settler in Western United States would have dreamed of crossing the entire country in a few hours? Within the past ten years, advances in the area of electronic technology alone have completely revolutionized many aspects of our daily life. Practically every phase of human life is in some way influenced by scientific methodology, whether it be in the fields of medicine, agriculture, education, industry or, as we shall soon see, athletics.

Current Use of the Scientific Method in Education

The application of scientific methodology in education has also had a profound effect upon methods of teaching, especially since 1960. O. R. Lindsley (1964) coined the term *precision teaching* to describe a functional model for the management of classroom behavior, utilizing a science-based rationale. In this model a teacher is described as a scientist whose area of study is the behavior of students in a school setting. Frank Hewett (1968) speaks of his use of scientific methodology in education as the *engineered classroom* and views teachers as "engineers" who plan a successful program of remediation for students. *Prescriptive teaching,* a procedure developed by Lawrence Peter (1965), directly applies scientific methodology to diagnosis and treatment of problems children experience in learning.

This movement to incorporate scientific methodology in education had its beginning in the field of special education and has now spread to many other sectors of education as a basic modus operandi of regular classroom instruction. Techniques and procedures used in the treatment of communication disorders have also been influenced as a direct result of recent application of scientific methodology in education. For example, a number of articles and books describing the application in speech therapy of procedures based upon scientific methodology have appeared recently (McReynolds, 1970; Holland, 1967; Brookshire, 1967; Mowrer, 1969; Sloane & MacAulay 1968).

The rigors of this methodology have permeated research endeavors for many decades. The application of these same rigors to therapeutic procedures in speech pathology is long overdue. The following discussion should provide the reader with a basic rationale necessary for the application of the scientific method to therapeutic procedures.

Scientific Attitudes

Basically, the scientist seeks to discover why things happen the way they do. He carefully observes and records events in his environment and attempts to identify simple, functional relationships which may exist between these events. Finally, he subjects his findings to examination by replicating the relationships to establish verification.

Four fundamental attitudes of science inherent in this general description are (1) empiricism, (2) determinism, (3) parsimony, and (4) scientific manipulation (Whaley & Surratt, 1968). While these are certainly not the only characteristics of a scientific approach for solving problems, they are most basic to an understanding of the methods of the scientist.

Empiricism

The most useful tools we have for investigating the world about us are our senses of touch, taste, hearing, smell, and sight. We use these senses often aided by precision instruments, such as the microscope, telescope, recorder, computer, and the like, to make accurate observations about events in our environment. Empiricism is synonymous with observation. A good auto mechanic uses an empirical method when he troubleshoots an engine failure; a doctor who examines a patient uses empiricism.

Observation: One of the main reasons astronauts were sent to the moon was to bring back rock samples so that scientists could observe them firsthand. As you might suspect, highly sophisticated instruments were used to allow far more detailed observation than the human senses alone could perform. From these observations we have learned more about the origin of the universe.

Galileo made countless observations from the Tower of Piza while formulating his laws of motion. Darwin's chief source of scientific information evolved from his observations. Observation is the foundation of the scientific method. It is the major prerequisite to the establishment of an empirical law.

But conclusions drawn from faulty observations may lead the observer farther away from the truth. Before the time of Columbus, humans observed that the earth was flat and concluded if a ship were to sail far enough away from the continent, it would surely plunge off the edge into space. Also, people believed to be possessed by the devil were either put to death or jailed. Other widely held beliefs were people with high foreheads were more intelligent than people with low foreheads, and that the study of Latin increased one's ability to learn other subjects.

The problem with these observations is that no one actually observed the event or phenomena firsthand. No one ever observed the world to see if it was flat. They looked at only one part of it. No one ever observed the intelligence of people with high and low foreheads or bothered to test the learning ability of those who had and those who had not had Latin. I am reminded of the story of the blind men who were asked to describe an elephant. The one who felt the elephant's leg said, "An elephant is like a tree trunk;" another felt its tail and replied, "An elephant is like a rope;" and so on. Each observed the elephant from different locations, so naturally, their conclusions regarding what an elephant was like were correct individually but wrong collectively.

But conclusions from observation can be faulty. For example, consider John Taylor's 1859 book, *The Great Pyramid: Why Was It Built?* He felt an Israelite acting on divine orders built it, not an Egyptian. He found mathematical truth in its measurements. Divide the height into twice the length of a side of its base and you get a close approximation of *pi* (the ratio of circumference to diameter of a circle). He felt the measuring device for the pyramid was the Biblical "cubit" used by Noah in building the ark. He found a score of bibliographic references to support his views. Isaiah 19:19–20, "In that day shall there be an altar to the Lord in the land of Egypt . . . and it shall be a sign and for a witness unto the Lord of Hosts." He felt the Pyramid symbolized the true Church with Christ as the topmost stone. The pyramid symbol has been popular in Christian mystical lore and was adopted by the founding fathers on the reverse side of the U.S. Seal.

In 1864, University of Edinburgh astronomer Charles Smyth, enthusiastic about Taylor's theories, wrote a 664-page book, *Our Inheritance in the Great Pyramid*. He found the length of the base divided by the width of a casing stone equals 365″ (days in a year). The casing stone measured 25″ and Smyth concluded this was the sacred cubit. He defined the "Pyramid inch" as $\frac{1}{25}$ of the width of the casing stone, the smallest unit of measurement used in its construction. It is exactly $\frac{1}{10,000,000}$ of the earth's polar radius (other casing stones were later found, all of different widths). He applied the Pyramid inch to every measurable portion of the Pyramid to find historic and scientific proofs.

Multiply the pyramid's height by 10^9 to equal the distance from earth to the sun. Similar multiples of its length equals the earth's mean density, period of precision of its axis, mean temperature of earth's surface, etc. He formulated an outline of history symbolized by Pyramid's internal passages. When measured in Pyramid inches, one inch equals one year, the world was created about 4,004 B.C. Dates of the Flood, Exodus, and when Pyramid was built, etc. could be determined. The beginning of a slope of Grand Gallery marks birth of Christ, also his atonement at age 33, descent to Hell, and Resurrection.

Competent archeologists at that time came up with different measurements including the most basic base length. Later, more accurate measurements disagreed, so Smyth took an average, or picked the one that fit best.

Smyth felt that the number five was a very important number. There were five corners to the Pyramid and five sides. The Pyramid inch was $\frac{1}{5} \times \frac{1}{5}$ of a cubit. He also made the point that five was a symbol of God's work. Humans have five extremities, there are five books of Moses and twice five Commandments.

But suppose we look at this magic number as applied to the Washington Monument according to facts stated in the World Almanac. The monument is 555 feet and 5 inches high, its base is 55 feet square, the windows are 500 feet from the base, multiply the base times 60 (five times 12 months of the year) and it equals 3,300 (divisible by five), the exact weight of the capstone in pounds. Washington has two times five letters. The weight of the capstone times the length of the base equals the speed of light (181,500). The decision to print a pyramid on the U.S. Seal was made by the Secretary of the Treasury (25 letters) on June 15, 1935. As you can see, you can find all sorts of facts and "truths" if you only look hard enough and juggle the right figures.

Smyth spent 20 years of his life making exact measurements of the Pyramid in an effort to discover scientific truths. His work was carried on by many others. Dozens of volumes about Pyramid measurements and their significance appeared in many languages. An International Institute for Preserving and Perfecting weights and measures was established in 1879 to make our measurement system conform to the sacred Pyramid. Their goal was to combat the atheistic metrical system being taught in France at that time.

A periodical, *The International Standard*, was published during the 1880s. Its president, a civil engineer, prided himself in having an arm exactly one cubit in length. Articles published in this periodical denounced the French metric system.

A colonel J. Garnier wrote a book in 1905 which proved by the Pyramid measurements that Christ would return in 1920. Charles Taze Russell, founder of Jehovah's Witnesses, published a book in 1891, *Studies in the Scripture,* about biblical prophecy using evidence from Pyramid. He said the Pyramid clearly revealed invisible second coming of Christ in 1874 followed by 40 years of Harvest when true members of the Church rallied round Russell's leadership. After 1914, the dead will arise to be given a second chance to accept Christ; those who accept will live forever in a world cleansed of evil. The true meaning of "witnesses" is "millions now living will never die." They were called Russellites. When 1914 brought nothing but a World War, they lost thousands of members. Certain portions of Russell's book were changed. The 1910 version, "The deliverance of the saints must take place some time before 1914," changed to " . . . must take place very soon after 1914."

Judge J. F. Rutherford succeeded Russell after he died in 1916. Eventually he discarded Pyramidology and in the November 15 and December 1, 1928 issues of the *Watchtower* said the so-called altar in Egypt was inspired by Satan to mislead the faithful. Today, the Witnesses still believe the millennium is about to dawn but they have set no date.

A work published in 1924, *Pyramid: Its Divine Message* is the size of the *Encyclopedia Britannica!* This demonstrates how easy it is to work over massive amounts of data and emerge with a pattern that is nothing more than product of the human brain. Consciously or unconsciously, preconceived dogmas twist and mold the objective facts into forms that support those dogmas. We can all make exact observations, but it's what we do with them that is important!

The point is that for an observation to be valid, it must be *public*. We must all agree on what is being observed and make sure that it is being observed accurately. It is also important that *repeated* observations be made. This allows us to establish credulity of our observations. The chance for error in a single observation is far greater than it is for a hundred observations. Since validity of observation is so crucial to the scientific method, observations have moved away from the naturalistic setting to the well-controlled laboratory. Precision recording instruments have taken the place of our senses. As psychology developed into a science, it was expected that observations of behavior would be conducted first under carefully controlled laboratory conditions. Also, animal behavior would be studied first because their past experiential histories could be controlled as well. Pavlov studied dogs; Tolman and Guthrie cats and rats; and pigeons were Skinner's choice. From countless thousands of observations, psychologists were able to arrive at certain irrefutable conclusions about animal behavior.

Operational Definition: As a logical follow up of the observations of animals, social and behavioral psychologists began setting up systematic observation procedures for the study of human behavior. One of the first problems encountered was the inadequacy of the language used to describe human behavior. For example, we commonly use the term *aggressive behavior* when referring to a child who continually fights with, or bothers, other children. If a psychologist asked three untrained observers to count the number of aggressive behaviors exhibited by a particular child during a 5-minute period, each observer might report a different number of aggressive behaviors. Since their individual interpretations of the word aggression differ, they would not be counting the same behaviors. It is not until the psychologist clearly defines specific behaviors exhibited by the child that results of the three observers coincide. When aggressive behaviors include instances of specific, observable events, such as shoving, punching, hitting, kicking, biting, and the like, we can expect a much higher percentage of agreement.

When we observe someone doing something, we say she's operating on her environment. Sometimes the environment operates on the individual. She may be struck by lightning or burned by fire. When we wish to refer to the operation being performed, we define it strictly in terms of that operation. In the case of aggressive behaviors, kicking, biting, and hitting are operational definitions that describe specific behaviors. We can still group these behaviors under the term *aggressive acts,* but we lose a great deal of specificity and increase the likelihood of error.

Not all terms can be operationally defined, that is, we are unable to observe everything in operation. How do you observe what someone is thinking? There was a time when philosophers actually doubted if thinking existed, but Kant seemed to have solved that philosophical problem. Recently scientists have been able to measure thought processes in action through recordings of alpha and beta waves. In the next decade or two, we may be able to operationally define thinking in terms of machine-recorded events and even discover what a person is thinking. There are many other commonly used words which defy operational definition: *feeling, hate, ego, idea, mind, soul, creative hunch, dream, attitude.* Although scientists studying human behavior are limited to observable behaviors, this is not a denial that unobservable events or factors, such as intervening variables or emotions, do exist. They simply are not the target of empirical study.

But in spite of precise definition of terms, accurate recording devices, careful observation procedures, complete honesty of the investigator, and tight control, many factors can bias the observation process. As Roe (1961) points out in her article, "The Psychology of the Scientist," observations are only as good as the men and women who make them.

How observations are *recorded* is also of critical importance in scientific investigation. Much of the data collected in psychological research involving animal studies have been recorded using cumulative counters. Response data may be charted graphically and studied in detail. An entire chapter of this book will be devoted to methods of recording and charting behaviors. It is the foundation of the scientific method.

In summary, scientists depend on accurate observation of events in the environment in order to gather a body of knowledge. These observations must be of a public nature so there can be agreement among all observers, and they must be repeatable, not single, occurrences. Finally, the events observed must be capable of being operationally defined.

Determinism

If our world was without laws and orderliness, we would submit to utter chaos, close up our laboratories, cross our fingers, and take what comes. But fortunately, this world is filled with order. The job of the scientist is to discover the basic laws of this "orderly" world. Physicists have discovered laws of motion; chemists, laws of chemical structure; physicians, laws of bodily function; biologists, laws of heredity; and psychologists have been searching for laws of behavior.

Recently, W. B. Webb (1962) wrote that psychology in all its diversity is bound by the single, common principle that human behavior is lawful. B. F. Skinner (1956), reflecting upon his early experiments with laboratory animals, said, "Of course, I was working on a basic assumption—that there was order in behavior if I could only discover it." These were the same assumptions that Aristotle, Socrates, Galileo, Newton, Einstein, and other noted scientists made when they began making their observations.

Once laws have been discovered, we can make predictions about events! We can predict that the sun will rise and set at specific times, that water will run downhill, that ice will melt above zero degrees centigrade, and that glass will crack under a specified pressure. Scientists are interested in functional relationships between two or more events. The simplest expression of a law states, "If A then B." There is a functional relationship between A and B, which allows us to predict B from A. Consider situation A is releasing a marble, and situation B is the marble striking the floor. The law states if A (releasing the marble), then B (marble strikes floor). We must add one more factor to this statement—the conditions. The relevant condition in this example is 14.2 lbs./sq. in. of atmospheric pressure. For example, if a marble was dropped in a spaceship on its journey to the moon where these atmospheric conditions do not exist, the marble would remain suspended in midair. A would not be followed by B because of a different set of conditions.

Graham (1951) presented a simple, mathematical equation for describing functional relationships such as the one cited above: $y = f(x)$ under empirical conditions c. In the example above, the marble striking the floor (y) is a function of being released (x) when atmospheric pressure is 14.2 lbs./sq. in. (c). This, of course, is the law of gravity. It is nothing more than a functional relationship between mass and distance. You may not know *why* event y always follows x, but the outcome can always be *predicted*. We can predict y, but x cannot be predicted when y is known.

R–R Laws. This equation is used extensively in the science of psychology; one application is to establish *R–R laws.* The equation here would be interpreted as $R = f(R_2)$ under c. An example of R (response) might be performance in graduate school, and R_2 (response 2) might be grade-point average. Both performance and grade-point average represent the result of student performance, that is, the student's responses. One of the conditions might be the subject matter studied. It could be reasoned that if a student has a high grade-point average in math courses, then she will perform well as a math major in graduate school. This is a simple statement regarding probability. Of course, there will be exceptions due to the wide variety of conditions, such as emotional stability, type of teachers, health, distractions, and so on, many of which we are unable to control.

Another example in the area of communication disorders can be drawn from Van Riper and Erickson's (1969) Predictive Screening Test of Articulation. This was an attempt to establish a functional relationship between a score on an articulation test (R_2) and proficiency of articulation at a later point in time (R_1). Some of the main conditions were the child's age, her enrollment in school, and absence of speech therapy. The authors sought to establish a predictive law that would enable them to determine which children would require speech therapy and which ones would not. Here again, the R–R laws do not tell us *why* some children will articulate correctly at a later date; they only enable us to predict which ones will.

Van Riper (1971) has also presented some evidence to indicate a functional relationship between the occurrence of the schwa vowel in syllabic repetitions (R_2) and development of stuttering (R_1). Johnson (1961) developed the Iowa Disfluency Index in order to enable an examiner to relate severity of stuttering (R_2) and scores made on a speaking task (R_1). There are many other instances of R–R type laws to be found in communication research.

S–R Laws. A far more useful type law is the establishment of a functional relationship between stimulus events (S) and response events (R). This can be written as $R = f(S)$ under c. Environmental (stimuli) events are related to behavioral (response) events. This relationship has sometimes been called an experimental law because it allows us to pinpoint cause and effect. If a response always varies directly with the manipulation of the stimulus, we must conclude the stimulus causes the response. We thereby gain *control* over the response by controlling the stimulus.

For example, suppose we prick the skin of a person with a pin (stimulus). We get a withdrawal response and maybe a verbal remark such as "Ouch!" (response). Do this over and over again (repeated observations), and measure the withdrawal reactions as amount of movement. We can both *predict* that movement will follow the pin prick, and we can *control* the amount of movement depending on whether or not we prick the skin and how deeply the prick penetrates.

Many teachers are interested in S–R laws chiefly because once determined, they allow us to control selected behaviors. Many have reacted against concepts of controlling behavior. But the word *control* does not imply that scientists wish to dominate the world or inflict their will over others. Control, as used here, simply means that the scientist knows how the event comes about. Knowing what causes the event and having control over the conditions, they can bring about the event.

S–R laws have been used extensively in speech therapy. For example, Mowrer, Baker, and Schutz (1968) demonstrated the functional relationship between producing correct /s/ sounds on a criterion test (R) and being rewarded for saying /s/ correctly many times (S) under conditions of using a programmed set of instructions (c). The authors collected over twenty-one thousand observations of /s/ productions made by sixty children over a three-day period. From these data and the results of the ensuing, statistical treatment, we can establish a functional relationship. Reward a child for making correct /s/ sounds and she will produce these sounds correctly on a prescribed task, provided the following conditions are met: a prescribed instructional program is followed; the child has average or above average intelligence; dental structure is adequate; and hearing acuity is within normal limits. Thus, we are not only able to predict the child's performance on the criterion task, but we can "control" her performance as well, i.e., the response is functionally related to, or brought about by, the stimulus.

Again it must be stated there is no guarantee that our predictive or control statements will be 100% correct since when dealing with human behavior, we can never gain perfect control over the conditions, especially those which have influenced the individual prior to the event. Nevertheless, S–R laws have allowed us to make substantial gains in education, leading us from ignorant to functional behaviors. Without them, we would fall prey to superstitious behaviors such as those practiced by "medicine men."

Drawing from a more naturalistic setting, consider one more application of R–R and S–R laws as they relate to the prediction and control of weather. We note many times that when barometric pressure decreases sharply (R_2), it will rain (R_1), provided warm, moist air is present (c). After many observations of this sort, we are able to accurately predict when rain will fall, although we cannot *make* it rain, i.e., we have no control over rain. But when we find out what causes rain, we can formulate an S–R law and literally control the occurrence of rain. It has been found that when the air is seeded with a certain chemical (S), rain will follow (R), providing moisture is present (c). Thus, once having discovered the S–R functional relationship, we are able both to predict and to control the occurrence of rain.

If we seek to modify the behavior of individuals, it is vital that we discover functional relationships between stimulus events and behavioral responses. Until these relationships have been clearly established, we must rely on common sense and hit or miss procedures, which frequently are less than desirable. For example, a teacher who believes a young mind must be disciplined like an underdeveloped muscle will spend a great amount of time drilling worthless facts into the child's head. Another teacher who follows principles of Gestalt psychology will drill very little on details and will present holistic experiences of a naturalistic sort. Similarly, those who feel people who display "bizarre" behaviors are mentally ill will confine them to mental hospitals and treat them with drugs, as though they were in ill health. Parents, acting on the belief that certain personality traits or behaviors are inherited, will respond to their child with hopelessness, as though "fate" has dictated what shall be. It makes a great deal of difference in how we deal with human behavior, whether we adopt a scientific attitude or a nonscientific one.

Parsimony

A third attitude of science is referred to as the law of parsimony. A parsimonious person is one who is exceedingly stingy or frugal. When this term is applied to science, it means the scientist should be very frugal with her use of abstract, complex explanations. One should always look for a simple explanation of phenomena and verify it through experimentation.

William of Occam was one of the first fourteenth century philosophers to employ the law of parsimony when he revolted against the metaphysics of St. Thomas Aquinas. He laid the groundwork for behaviorism by stressing observation as a key factor in analyzing the world. *Occam's Razor* is a term which refers to cutting away beliefs that are metaphysical and unrelated to naturalistic events.

Psychologist-philosopher Lloyd Morgan helped turn nineteenth century psychologists away from their studies of the "minds" of animals toward study of what animals actually do. He advised psychologists not to attribute any higher mental activity to animals than absolutely necessary. This rule became known as Lloyd Morgan's Canon. It illustrates clearly the law of parsimony.

One should not misinterpret this law to mean that the simplest explanation is always the correct one. It merely states we should always look for the simplest explanation. One of Freud's major faults in his explanation of human behavior was that he based his theory on the existence of a complex set of internal mental states or attributes. *Libido, super ego, ego urges,* and the *id* all played a complicated role in Freud's theory. The problem was that these concepts were unobservable and, therefore, untestable. A more parsimonious way of viewing behavior simply states that behavior is affected by its consequences. Complex explanations based upon the existence of illusive egos, ids, and super egos find no company with scientists today.

The wayward soul who pleads "The devil made me do it" may find comfort in his belief, but he is violating the law of parsimony. The speech pathologist who explains stuttering as acting out one's repressed anxieties against his mother who failed to nurse him properly when he was a baby is also infringing on this law. We must be cautious in offering complex explanations for events we do not fully understand.

One of the best illustrations of the violation of parsimony is found in the belief in flying saucers. On June 24, 1947, Ken Arnold, piloting his plane near Mt. Rainier, sighted nine circular objects 25 miles away, flying in a diagonal chain formation. They were slightly smaller than a DC-4. They flew like saucers skipped across the water. The news interpreted this as saucer-shaped and this word caught on. All over the country, people reported seeing saucers over their farms, towns, and cities. Even if those who reported sightings described objects in many different ways, newspaper reports of the sightings always referred to them as flying saucers. In a few weeks, sightings were reported in every state, Canada, Australia, England, and Iran. Then came reports of balls of fire, ice cream cones, flying hub caps, doughnuts, cigar-shaped crafts with rows of lights, and long orange exhaust streams flying through the skies.

A B-25 bomber was sent to investigate the report of a doughnut-shaped craft that dropped lava-like rock on Maury Island near Tacoma, Washington. On the return flight, the plane's left engine caught fire. Two men parachuted to safety but two others perished in the crash. Mr. Arnold said the plane carried a corn-flakes box full of samples of the mysterious lava. The news media suggested the officers were dead long before the crash and mysterious forces caused their death. Later, two Tacoma men confessed to the hoax hoping to sell a story to an adventure magazine.

It was theorized these saucers were spaceships from another world. Stories appeared in numerous magazines and books published by reputable publishing houses. For example, in January 1948, an army pilot reported seeing a white object in the sky and followed it to 18,000 feet. He radioed that he would pursue the object to 20,000 feet, then abandon the chase. He climbed to 30,000 feet, blacked out and crashed before recovering. The news media reported that the flying object killed him. In another example, a suspension bridge was ignited mysteriously in 1947. Mr. Arnold reported the fire was caused by the saucers. His book contains the photograph of a mummified man 14 inches tall discovered in the Rockies in 1932. According to Arnold, this was a tiny space man left from an earlier saucer crash.

True magazine concluded in an article published in the January 1950 issue that during the past 175 years, we have been under close surveillance by living beings from another planet; the frequency and intensity of those surveillances increased during 1948–50. Shortly after this article, Navy Commander Robert McLaughlin theorized the saucers were piloted by Martians small enough to fit into 20-inch disks, propelled by three sets of motors using light radiation.

Frank Scully, who published *Behind the Flying Saucer* in 1951, stated that saucers were flown to the earth from Venus by magnetic propulsion at the speed of light. They were piloted by earthlike people three feet tall. According to Scully, four saucers landed on earth, three have crashed, and the remains including several dozen bodies were being studied in undisclosed government laboratories. The saucers were made of a hard, light metal unknown to our chemists. All dimensions of the saucer were divisible by nine. One ship defied all efforts at penetration, even $35,000 worth of diamond drills. He blamed President Truman for trying to hush up the investigation.

Gerald Heard, who published "Is Another World Watching?" (*Harpers,* 1951) was a sincere and devoted mystic who actually believed everything he wrote. He felt saucers came from Mars. Since only a tough insect could withstand space travel, the saucers were piloted by "super-bees" two-inches long with an IQ superior to man. They were investigating the earth's atomic explosions. A huge mothership circles the earth and smaller saucers are used as scouts. Mars' two satellites are not moons but artificial launching jetties for spaceships. He has half a dozen photographs of saucers; one looks like a garbage can lid thrown into the air.

Now these are *not* simple explanations! Let's look at some facts that provide a much more parsimonious explanation. In 1947 when saucers were first reported, the Navy had been launching huge skyhook balloons used for cosmic-ray research. These giant plastic bags, 100 feet in diameter reaching heights of 100,000 feet, move at 200 MPH in jet streams. At a distance, a balloon loses its three-dimensional spherical shape and appears as a disk. From beneath, instruments hang that could give the impression of a doughnut from below. Through binoculars a curious optical illusion occurs. A globular object resembles a plate. Also, the plastic balloon surface is highly metallic and looks silver in reflected sunlight. At sunset, it can shine in the sky for thirty minutes after darkness sets in. Light reflected from one side may appear as the glow from an engine. The instrument reflection may appear as exhaust. By 1951 the Navy had released 270 skyhooks from various spots in the United States, and some stayed aloft as long as 30 hours. There are many other types of balloons in the sky: weather balloons, radar-target balloons with large aluminum tails, guided missiles, etc. Also, unusual weather conditions foster illusions about objects in the sky. After the Navy's 1952 report, sightings of flying saucers decreased. Today, members of certain occult groups believe the saucers are from outer space. In summary, we see a major violation of the law of parsimony in the flying saucers controversy. Don't set up elaborate explanations for events that might otherwise be explained by simpler facts.

Scientific Manipulation

As we have noted, the discovery of functional relationships between events is of the utmost importance for establishing empirical laws. This is especially true for those laws which indicate causal relationships, since discovery of these relationships allow both prediction and control. If two events appear to be related and you wish to find out if the relationship is one of cause and effect, you must change one event, or condition, and see what happens. This is *scientific manipulation*. We shall see how this procedure was used to investigate the case of Hans, the intelligent horse.

Some years ago a German horse trainer claimed to own a remarkable horse named Hans. It was claimed that Hans could solve mathematical problems by tapping out answers with his hoof. Scientists from many countries came to see Hans perform and were greatly impressed at this animal's ability to perform mathematical computations. His trainer would call out, *"Wieviel ist zwei und sieben?"* Hans would methodically tap out nine and stop. Truly it appeared as though this horse had human talents (violation of the law of parsimony).

Hans, the intelligent horse, was paraded throughout Europe as he continued his amazing performance, adding, subtracting, even dividing and multiplying, until some suspicious investigators changed some conditions of the demonstration. First, one of the scientists asked Hans some mathematical questions which, to the amazement of all, Hans solved with ease. Other scientists also posed questions to Hans, and they were equally amazed with his accuracy. Then one of the scientists placed the horse trainer behind a screen and instructed him to ask Hans a question. *"Wieviel ist nine und sechs?"* Hans did nothing. Again and again questions were asked of Hans, but poor Hans never tapped. Through scientific manipulation what was thought to be an intelligent horse proved to be a unique, perceptive animal. Hans was attending to slight, visual cues, unknowingly provided by those who asked him questions. These cues consisted of facial expression and certain bodily movements which Hans detected. An examiner might nod his head slightly while counting the taps and stop nodding when the correct answer was given. Having found the true explanation for this animal's performance, he was returned to pasture.

There is a Latin phrase often quoted in logistics which states, *Post hoc ergo propter hoc*. Translated literally, it means after this therefore because of this. It refers to a cause-effect relationship that is not true or that has not been scientifically verified. We can find many examples of the *post hoc ergo propter hoc* fallacy, especially when people are ignorant of actual determinants of an event. Many physicians daily prescribe placebos to their patients whose ailments are eliminated by what they, the patients, conceive of as "wonder drugs." They are convinced that the pill was responsible for their recovery. Yet, when put to test by scientific manipulation, any pill reputed to be *the* wonder drug produces the same results.

Let's consider other examples of how falsehoods are exposed through scientific manipulation. Late in the eighteenth century, Dr. Elisha Perkins proposed a theory that certain metals could draw diseases from the body. In 1796, he patented a device consisting of two metal rods each three inches long. One was an alloy of copper, zinc, and gold; the other was an iron-silver-platinum alloy. By drawing the Metallic Tractor over ailing parts of the body, the disease was pulled out. George Washington and his family used them, as did Chief Justice Oliver Elsworth. Perkins' son, Benjamin Perkins, a graduate of Yale, made a fortune selling the Tractors in England. In Copenhagen, Denmark, 12 doctors published a book hailing the wonders of "Perkinism." Perkins published a book containing hundreds of testimonials from doctors, ministers, professors, and congressmen attesting to the benefits of the metal rods. Orthodox medicine simply ignored Perkins and his medical discovery. But finally, one doctor tested a set of nonmetallic rods against the Metallic Tractors. His results showed absolutely no difference between either type of rod with respect to healing or reducing pain. Yet today, you may notice people wearing copper bracelets to ward off arthritic pain.

Electricity was also thought to have magical curative powers. Early in the twentieth century, Dr. Albert Abrams, a noted physician, found he could diagnose illnesses by noting the vibratory rate of sounds produced while tapping on the abdomen. He developed a "dynamizer" machine, an insane jungle of wires powered by electricity. A drop of the patient's blood was placed inside the machine. A healthy person was attached to the machine and the vibrations from the blood of the patient went to the healthy person's spine and were absorbed or amplified. The doctor could then detect these vibrations by tapping. Later he found he could determine the patient's age, sex, and whether he belonged to one of six religious groups. Then he found he could make the same diagnosis from handwriting samples placed inside the machine even after the person's death. He determined that Samuel Johnson, Poe, and Longfellow each had syphilis. Then he invented an "ocilloclast" that produced vibrations that would heal by directing radio waves of the same frequency as the disease at the patient to kill the bacteria. He died in 1923 leaving a $2-million estate, mostly made by leasing ocilloclast machines at $250 each plus $200 for a course in their operation. Purchasers were required to swear they would never open the box. But a group of scientists took it upon themselves to investigate this mysterious instrument. Inside, they found an ohm meter, a rheostat, a condenser, and other electrical components wired together without rhyme or reason. And yet, Upton Sinclair wrote that Abrams' instrument was the most revolutionary discovery of this age. He claimed it had cured over 95% of the 15,000 people who were treated with it.

A doubting AMA doctor sent Abrams a blood sample from a healthy male guinea pig under the name of Miss Bell for diagnosis. The report said she had cancer to the amount of six ohms, infection of left frontal sinus, and a streptococcic infection of her left fallopian tube. Another doctor sent in a blood sample from a Plymouth Rock rooster and the diagnosis was malaria, cancer, diabetes, and two venereal diseases. Abrams' diagnosis failed miserably in every test of scientific manipulation performed by the medical profession. But in spite of the conclusive test results proving the inadequacy of Abrams' methods, Sinclair Lewis insisted the problem was due to the interference from signals sent out by radio broadcasting companies conflicting with those of the dynamizer.

More recently, Dr. Ruth B. Drown used another electronic instrument developed to cure various diseases. She puts a blood sample in her machine, and broadcasts the vibrations that send the healing rays directly to the patient's home! When Tyrone Power and his wife had an auto accident in Italy, they were treated by one of Dr. Drown's machines. Dr. Drown learned about electronics working in an electrical assembly department of the Southern California Edison Company. Ever since 1929, she has practiced radio therapy selling her machines to chiropractors, osteopaths, and naturopaths all over the country. Dr. Drown is a licensed osteopath.

The Dean of the University of Chicago's Biological Sciences Division agreed to test the machine through scientific manipulation. Dr. Drown operated the machine personally with no success. Given blood samples of 10 patients, her diagnoses of the first three were so far off she didn't attempt to diagnose the remaining seven. One of the ten patients suffered from tuberculosis. Dr. Drown's diagnosed a Type IV cancer present in the patient's left breast and which had spread to the ovaries, uterus, pancreas, gall bladder, spleen, and kidney. She said the patient was blind in her right eye and 18 other bodily functions were malfunctioning; also she had a blood pressure of 107/71.

Dr. Drown also made use of radio photography in diagnosing illnesses. Upon close investigation, it was found that the images she thought to be internal organs were nothing more than fog patterns produced by exposing the film to white light before it was adequately fixed. The images were mere artifacts, totally without clinical value.

Examples of the use of scientific manipulation abound in the field of medicine. Looking back only 100 years into the history of surgery, the work of Dr. Ignaz Semmelweis stands out as an excellent illustration of scientific manipulation. He noted that 10% of the women about to give birth to babies in the hospital section served by medical students died of internal infection, whereas less than 1% who were attended by midwives in an adjacent hospital section perished. He adopted obstetrical techniques identical to those used by the midwives; yet, the death rate did not diminish. Through a series of events, Semmelweis concluded that doctors, after making prior examination of cadavers, were introducing infectious material from their hands into the expectant mothers during vaginal examination. To put this to scientific test, he and his students cleansed their hands before each examination. The death rate dropped from 12.34 fatalities to 3.04 per 100 births. He now had an R–R law. He could make a rough prediction about fatality rates, and he suspected why his predictions would come true; yet, he knew little about germ theory.

Then came what seemed to be a setback on October 2, 1847. All of the twelve expectant mothers came down with puerperal fever in spite of the fact that no one with unwashed hands entered the ward. This seemed proof to the unbelieving medical students "the senselessness of his [Semmelweis's] fanatical cleanliness." Nine of the twelve women died within a few days. Semmelweis then discovered that in the first bed of his ward lay a woman with a discharging uterine carcinoma. While the physicians washed their hands before entering, none washed their hands between examining patients on the ward. Hence, a second discovery was made. Infectious material not only could be carried from the dead to the living, but also from one diseased living patient to another healthy one. Yet, strange as it may seem, Semmelweis's conclusions were rejected by his colleagues. It remained for Joseph Lister some 20 years later to convince the medical profession that bacteria transported by hands of examining physicians caused surgical infection.

The above illustration taken from Thorwald's book, *The Century of the Surgeon* (1956), dramatically portrays the infancy of scientific methodology of that time. It also represents a man who through scientific manipulation, though sometimes by accident, was able to formulate S–R type laws, which meant the saving of human lives. Semmelweis, and others like him, represent what Roe (1961) calls the "creative scientist." B. F. Skinner (1956) also fits this role when he attributes much of his success to luck and unforeseen events. It wasn't until his food dispensing apparatus broke down that he discovered the curve of extinction. It would be nice to believe that all scientific manipulation is carefully planned. Often it is not. Walter

Cannon described it with a word coined by Horace Walpole—*serendipity*—the art of finding one thing when looking for another.

But usually scientific manipulation is a purposeful activity, well designed to assist the scientist discover truths. One commonly used manipulative technique found in behavioral psychology is the *reversal method*. Baer (1971) reports a study of a 3½-year-old child who had the habit of clobbering other children in his nursery school group. He would pick up large objects and fling them at whoever was nearby. Observers noted that immediately following such aggressive behaviors, one or more of the teachers would immediately intercede, reason with, reprimand or, in some way, interact with the aggressive child for up to 5 minutes. The functional relationship assumed was an S–R type law; fighting (S) produced teacher attention (R). To test this theory, teachers were instructed to provide attention only to the victim of aggression, while completely ignoring the aggressive child. At the end of a few weeks, the child's aggressive behaviors declined to only 5% of his total interaction with other children, whereas before, aggressive behavior comprised 30 to 40% of the interaction time.

Up to this point, it could have been coincidence that there were fewer objects flying around the room; perhaps the child was just getting adjusted to his environment. To verify that teacher attention following aggression was a cause-effect relationship, the original conditions were resumed, i.e., the child received attention from the teachers following his acts of aggression. This is called *reversal;* and during the next few weeks of these conditions, the aggressive behavior returned to its original 30% level.

A second reversal, during which aggressive behavior was ignored, resulted in reducing these behaviors to the near zero level in only 6 days. The reversal process was repeated two more times, followed by the same results. Thus, through the careful application of scientific manipulation, the aggressive behavior of this young child was successfully brought under control.

There are a wide variety of other means used to manipulate factors which will provide credulity to a theory. Some involve the use of control groups, others use statistical analysis, and still others consist of stringent laboratory controls and meticulous attention to instrumentation. Each has its own set of advantages and disadvantages, but all are aimed toward scientific manipulation.

Two variables are studied in behavioral research: the independent variable, which is manipulated by the experimenter, and the dependent variable, which is always the observable behavior under investigation. The dependent variable is the subject's response, while the experimenter controls, or attempts to control, the relevant, independent variables, which may influence the response. If all variables are held constant and only one independent variable is changed, then change in the dependent variable indicates it is related to the independent variable. This may at first seem quite complicated. An example should help clarify the relationship between the two variables.

Some years ago, I constructed an instructional program to remediate lisping in the speech of young children. The program was given to a number of children who lisped. Each time a child said the /s/ sound correctly, I presented a token. After the session, the child could exchange the tokens for small toys. After three sessions, a criterion test was given. The program worked quite well; in fact, about 80% of the children to whom this program was given passed the criterion test with high scores. Although I could predict success, I was not able to identify the independent variables responsible for the change in articulation. Of course, I had some hunches. Certainly, the instructions I was giving had a lot to do with it and so did the rewards the children earned. But what about the method of delivery? Could my instructions be delivered via tape recording and have the same effect as a live presentation? And what about the child's response? Was it important for children to actually say the sounds and words aloud, or would they learn as much by just listening? These were some of the independent variables that seemed important to study.

There were numerous variables I could have selected as possible independent variables, such as the color of my shirt, the sex of the experimenter, rate of delivering instructions, amount of time allowed for child's response, type of pictures used in the program, and experimenter's attitude. We could go on and on identifying possible independent variables which might influence the single dependent variable. The dependent variable, in this case, was the child's score on the criterion test. It is called *dependent* because it relies on other events (independent variables).

The independent variables are manipulated, one at a time, under carefully controlled conditions. For example, to study the effects of reward, one group of children is given a reward following each correct response, while another group receives no reward. All other aspects of the session are identical. Then the criterion test scores of both groups are compared. If those who received rewards make higher scores on the criterion test than those who do not receive rewards, we can conclude there is a relationship between giving rewards (the independent variable) and high scores received on the criterion test (dependent variable). By this manipulation we should be able to identify almost all the independent variables responsible for change in the dependent variable.

The identification of dependent and independent variables is illustrated in a study by Drash et al. (1970). They identified correct and incorrect vocal response rates as dependent variables in their study of the effects of two types of reinforcement schedules. The authors concluded that incorrect and correct response rates were very sensitive measures which reflected change of independent variables. A large number of similar studies can be found in the literature which report identification of independent variables from observing changes in behaviors.

Criticism of Scientific Method

Through the use of scientific methodology, there can be little doubt of our steadily increasing ability to understand, influence and change human behavior. Purposeful and successful control of human behavior is not a dream; it is a present reality. The introduction of behavioral management techniques, derived from research in psychologists' animal laboratories, has not been warmly received by some educators. Many even reject the notion that the scientific method is a suitable method for the study of human behavior. Several controversial issues summarizing the bulk of these criticisms will be discussed next.

The Issue of Prediction and Control

One of the core arguments against using scientific methodology in the study of human behavior is its use to predict and control events related to human behavior. Basic to this notion is the idea that humans have free wills. It is freedom of choice that distinguishes humans from animals—freedom from prediction, in that humans are novel agents—and freedom from control, in that each individual determines his or her future. Theologian Reinhold Niebuhr violently opposes the notion that science can be used to study human behavior. He said, "In any event, no scientific investigation of past behavior can become the basis of predictions of future behavior." Andrew Hacker reacted similarly when he referred to scientific predictions of human behavior as "the specter of predictable man." Prediction of human behaviors becomes sinister when the National Safety Council issues its estimate of the number of highway deaths that will occur over a given holiday weekend. For some reason, people do not really want to know what will happen in the future. For one thing it smacks of chicanery, or even quackery, and for another, knowing what will happen in the future takes some of the excitement out of life. It rules out the element of chance. What point would there be in watching a football game, a car race, or a boxing match if we could predict the outcome of every play or each event beforehand?

The inference that behavior can be controlled is even more threatening than prediction. Control implies someone, or something else, determines how we will behave. Dogs are taken to obedience schools to bring their behavior under "control." Hitler used his Gestapo to control those who opposed him. The Declaration of Independence was written in an effort to liberate Americans from the unreasonable controls issued by the king of England. Criminals are incarcerated to control or restrain their unlawful behaviors. U. S. soldiers were brainwashed by Chinese Communists in an effort to control their thoughts. In view that so many negative associations accompany the term *control,* you can well understand why many people rebel against educators who speak of controlling student behaviors. Perhaps this explains the popular acceptance of the term *behavior modification.* Society is not yet prepared to accept behavior control as an objective of education.

George Orwell's book, *1984,* is frequently cited as the ultimate realization of what conditions will be like in the future if scientific methods of control are left unchecked. As a counter to the use of external controls imposed by someone else, Carl Rogers, in an article by Rogers and Skinner (1956), proposed that control should come from within. He argued that humans can be taught self-control through a process of self-actualization. Rogers, realizing the power of the products of scientific methodology, stressed concern over *who* the controlling agent should be and to *what* degree this agent should be allowed to control behavior. Most people today feel it is not so much whether or not we *can* control behavior; most educators would agree we can. The issue is whether or not we *should* control behavior and, if so, to what extent? Some contend it is fine to control behaviors of sick people, i.e., psychotics, misfits, derelicts, criminals, and undesirables; but these behavioral controls should not be placed upon "normal" people. They feel controls in the hands of the wrong element of society would eliminate freedom of choice, creating a society that would be a haven for demagogues and dictators.

Thus, you can begin to see the far-reaching ethical and moral issues involved when one speaks of controlling human behavior. The issue is far from being resolved and will doubtless remain one which will generate much controversy for years to come.

The scientific study of man is inappropriate. Humanists are deeply concerned with the dignity and value of humans. Reducing the achievements of humans to nothing more than a set of S–R relationships is dehumanizing. Conceiving of complex humans and their ambitions, their emotions, their sorrows, their empathy, and their courage as merely a set of variables is one of the chief dangers seen in using scientific study methods. Koch (1964) saw the psychologist's scientific treatment of humans "as demeaning as it is simplistic." Humanistic objectives are largely holistic. They concern matters of responsibility to one's self, values, feelings of identification, and the discovery of personal meaning. They are concerned with affective aspects of learning and those qualities which make us human. Humanists rebel against the mechanistic treatment of human behavior, with all its sophisticated, electronic gear to provide precise contingencies. Humans are coerced into producing robot-like responses in an unnaturalistic setting. While humanists do not deny that human behavior can be studied as a science, they are vehement in their feelings that humans should not be subjected to that sort of scrutiny. They particularly oppose operant conditioning experiments conducted in mental institutions which employ extreme, aversive treatments, such as electric shock, intense noise, deprivation of food, or isolation.

A few years ago I wrote to a state mental hospital in the South, asking if I could view some video tapes I heard they had produced. The tapes showed some dramatic changes in behavior of a young boy who had engaged in many self-destructive behaviors. Electric shock was administered, contingent upon self-destructive behaviors. I was denied permission to view these video tapes, as was anyone else. It would be too dangerous for the hospital staff to permit public viewing due to the admonishment they would receive from laypeople with humanistic views against using electric shock on humans. I also recall an instance a few years ago when a federal grant award to some local psychologists was terminated because the experimenters were physically striking children and using loud noise as an aversive stimulus to control self-destructive behaviors. Some benevolent citizens found out about the techniques used and vigorously protested to Washington about the inhumane treatment methods.

Since around 1970, any experiments conducted under the direction of university or college personnel, where human subjects are to be used, must be approved by a special committee set up to review the rights of subjects participating in the project. Several years ago, one congressman in Arizona went so far as to sponsor a bill to outlaw use of behavior modification techniques in the public schools!

In spite of what might seem to us to be extreme legislative measures, humanists, as a whole, are deeply concerned about what scientific study of human behavior might eventually lead to. Behavioral psychologists, on the other hand, claim they are nonhumanistic and lay no claim to support any one set of ethical principles or standards to which humans must conform. They simply follow the dictates of society, and therein lies the problem—who is society?

Some speech pathologists have also voiced a reaction against the use of scientific methodology. Walle (1975) reacted rather strongly against the use of operant conditioning techniques in the treatment of stuttering when he made the following statement: "My personal readings and talks with nonstuttering experts in the main remind me of mad scientists with all their Chi-Squares, electronic cattle probes, various noxious stimuli, time-out devices, computer based programs of approvals and insults." Walle contends that many clinicians do not have any "real feel" for the disorder of stuttering or for the stutterer himself. He feels important issues to be investigated are the stutterers' "real intelligence, the humor, the fine human qualities and frailties." Clearly, Walle is rebelling against what many consider the cold, calculating, dehumanized scientist.

Siegel (1975) was concerned about the lack of the human factor in the application of scientific methodology in speech therapy. Citing several articles stressing the importance of accountability in speech therapy, Siegel points out that there is more to effective speech therapy than just the tabulation of observations. He states, "Wherever we reduce behavior to numerical indexes we trade a loss of richness in detail for the conveniences that accrue to manipulating, averaging and storing numerical data." While not denying the usefulness of scientific methodology in research endeavors, Siegel appears cautious about accepting these same methodologies when providing speech therapy services.

Some years ago, I wrote an article describing how business accountability procedures could be applied to methods used in speech therapy (Mowrer, 1972). I attempted to show how speech clinicians could increase their effectiveness by following procedures similar to those used by businesses in turning out products on assembly lines. Needless to say, this type of article generated much furor among humanists. In reply, Brodwitz (1972) said if the suggested method were followed "it would make us think and act like business men and could rob us of the dignity of belonging to the great community of physicians, psychologists and speech therapists—the community of healers." Brodwitz went on to say that the children will hate therapy sessions, and the clinicians will resent being held accountable to "Big Brother," who will be tabulating their correct responses. He concluded with an appeal to preserve and to return to the dignity of the intimate, personal relationship between patient and client.

It is beyond the scope and purpose of this chapter to present rebuttal arguments toward views which have been presented concerning the humanistic rejection of scientific methodology. It is important that the reader understand that the use of scientific methodology will not be accepted with "open arms" by large sectors of the community. One cannot expect to change old ways and cherished beliefs simply because new procedures are more effective. One has only to look at the history of medicine to discover the overwhelming difficulties scientists experienced in attempting to change protocol of medical procedure. We can expect no easier path in speech therapy.

Emphasis on specific behaviors only. Behavior therapy has been criticized by the Gestalt psychologists as a useful, but limited, approach. Typically, behavior therapies alleviate only one problem, such as aggression, certain verbal behaviors, feeding problems, and the like. They fail to cope with the whole child in a total rehabilitation process. Total case management is seldom considered as a target behavior. Behavior therapists are viewed as "behavior technicians," rather than individuals who desire to treat total aspects of the patient's environment. Behavioral objectives, Gestaltists maintain, deal only with the simplest, most primitive aspects of educational goals. Finally, it is felt that holistic goals do not lend themselves to measurement of specific behaviors.

Inaccuracy of laws of learning. Some educators seriously question the findings of scientific investigation as it pertains to the study of human behavior. McKeachie (1974) presents pertinent data which refute the well-known laws of effect and exercise. The author takes B. F. Skinner to task by presenting research evidence which demonstrates that each point enunciated by Skinner in his book, *The Technology for Teaching,* is "untrue." Beliefs held as laws by many learning theorists hold only for very limited conditions. Skinner's popularity has resulted, according to McKeachie, from the fact that his theory is so simplistic. Teachers are exceedingly eager to grasp at any new, workable method to help them solve educational problems. The teacher's enthusism and energy are more responsible for behavior change produced in their pupils than all the alleged laws of learning, McKeachie asserts.

McKeachie is not alone in his doubts. Both Postman (1947) and Chomsky (1959) point out the circular nature of certain "laws" of learning. For example, consider candy as a stimulus and jumping as a response. If the rate of jumping increases by presenting candy following each act of jumping, candy is said to be a *reinforcer.* Note that candy is now defined as a stimulus that increases the probability that jumping will occur. The reinforcer, candy, cannot be defined independently of the behavioral change (jumping), which it is supposed to explain. Candy holds meaning as a stimulus property only when it is related to the increase of a specific response, in this case, jumping. To define a stimulus in this way is simply a circumlocutious way of saying whatever increases the probability that the behavior will occur will continue to occur in the future.

This problem of defining terminology to suit the law or to make the law "work" is illustrated by Strike (1974). Suppose you wanted a pigeon to walk in circles, and you offer it sunflower seeds each time it walked in a circle. And suppose that after 50 trials, walking in circles has not increased. It would be concluded that sunflower seeds are not reinforcing. Then you switch to corn and circle walking increases. You, therefore, conclude that corn is a reinforcer for circle walking, sunflower seeds are not. But you cannot *predict* which will be a reinforcer until you actually try the sunflower seeds and the corn! A valid, scientific law, such as Boyle's Law, allows one to make predictions about events with great accuracy. Obviously, you cannot test a theory by using an experiment in which the outcome of the experiment is the same as the truth of the theory.

Concluding Remarks

The basic ingredients of the scientific method have been clearly identified. The benefits derived from using this method to predict and to control natural events are well known to everyone. The astronaut's voyage to the moon represents one high point in the culmination of scientific technology. Only recently has this new methodology been applied to the study and control of human behavior. Judging from the many articles and books on the market describing the successful use of behavior modification procedures in school, institution, and home environments, there can be little doubt as to the efficacy of the method and its application to education.

But serious opposition has been voiced from several different sectors, especially the humanist sector, concerning the wholesale adoption of scientific methodology in education, not to mention its introduction into society at large. Some fear the new techniques are too powerful and if placed in the hands of questionable leaders, could destroy what the nation stands for. Others feel that by offering a panacea for our instructional ills, we will be diverted from the important, sociological issues in the education of individuals. Our concerns will only be for those observable behaviors for which we can write acceptable, behavioral objectives. Perhaps due to the spectacular successes reported of modifying heretofore "unmodifiable behaviors," we have lost sight of what an education means.

The few who challenge the theoretical foundation of this new learning theory have made little impact against the growth of the scientific movement in education. After all, science is an unquestioned virtue during these times. Those who argue against it find little company.

The speech clinician, too, is confronted with these issues. To what extent should behavior modification techniques be used? What should our goals be? Who determines which individual should receive speech therapy? These are only a few of the types of questions faced by all educators today. There are many more. The speech clinician who unthinkingly follows an educational "fad," either because some important people recommend it, or because it's the current trend, is not contributing gainfully to the welfare of his clients. Criticism of scientific methodology in education was presented here with the distinct purpose of alerting the reader to contrasting views. While the remaining chapters of the book will emphasize the essentials of applying scientific methodology to speech therapy, I will attempt to maintain an objective attitude concerning the value and the use of the procedures suggested.

BIBLIOGRAPHY

Baer, D. M. Behavior management from pre-schoolers to adults. In J. G. Morrey (Ed.), *Learning and behavior management in teacher training.* Pocatello, Id.: Idaho State University, 1971.

Brodwitz, F. S. Where are we going? *Asha,* 1972, *14,* 346.

Brookshire, R. Speech pathology and the experimental analysis of behavior. *Journal of Speech and Hearing Disorders,* 1967, *32,* 215–227.

Chomsky, N. A review of B. F. Skinner's *Verbal Behavior. Language,* 1959, *35,* 26–58.

Drash, P., Caldwell, L., & Liebowitz, J. Correct and incorrect response rates as basic dependent variables in operant conditioning of speech in non-verbal subjects. *Psychological Aspects of Disability,* 1970, *17,* 16–23.

Graham, C. H. Visual perception. In S. Stevens (Ed.), *Handbook of experimental psychology.* New York: Wiley, 1951, 868–920.

Hewett, F. M. *The emotionally disturbed child in the classroom.* Boston: Allyn & Bacon, 1968.

Holland, A. Some applications of behavioral principles to clinical speech problems. *Journal of Speech and Hearing Disorders,* 1967, *32,* 11–18.

Johnson, W. Measurements of oral reading and speaking rate and disfluency of adult male and female stutterers and nonstutterers. *Journal of Speech and Hearing Disorders,* Monograph Supplement, 1961, *7,* 1–20.

Koch, S. Psychology and emerging conceptions of knowledge as unitary. In T. W. Wann (Ed.), *Behaviorism and phenomenology.* Chicago: The University of Chicago Press, 1964.

Lindsley, O. R. Direct measurement and prosthesis of retarded behavior. *Journal of Education,* 1964, *147,* 62–81.

McKeachie, W. J. The decline and fall of the laws of learning. *Educational Researcher,* 1974, *3,* 7–11.

McReynolds, L. Contingencies and consequences in speech therapy. *Journal of Speech and Hearing Disorders,* 1970, *35,* 12–24.

Mowrer, D. E. Evaluating speech therapy through precision recording. *Journal of Speech and Hearing Disorders,* 1969, *34,* 239–244.

Mowrer, D. E. Accountability and speech therapy. *Asha,* 1972, *14,* 111–115.

Mowrer, D. E., Baker, R., & Schutz, R. Operant procedures in the control of articulation. In H. Sloane & B. MacAulay (Eds.), *Operant procedures in remedial speech and language training.* Boston: Houghton Mifflin, 1968.

Peter, L. J. *Prescriptive teaching.* New York: McGraw-Hill, 1965.

Postman, L. The history and present status of the law of effect. *Psychological Bulletin,* 1947, *44,* 489–563.

Roe, A. The psychology of the scientist. *Science,* 1961, *134,* 456–459.

Rogers, C. R., & Skinner, B. F. Some issues concerning the control of human behavior. *Science,* 1956, *124,* 1057–1066.

Siegel, G. M. The high cost of accountability. *Asha,* 1975, *17,* 796–797.

Skinner, B. F. A case history in scientific method. *American Psychologist,* 1956, *11,* 221–233.

Sloane, H., & MacÁulay, B. *Operant procedures in remedial speech and language training.* Boston: Houghton Mifflin, 1968.

Strike, K. A. On the expressive potential of behavioristic language. *American Educational Research Journal,* 1974, *11,* 103–120.

Thorwald, J. *The century of the surgeon.* New York: Pantheon Books, 1956.

Thorndike, E. L. *Human learning.* Cambridge, Mass.: The M.I.T. Press, 1931.

Thorndike, E.L. *The fundamentals of learning.* New York: Columbia University Press, 1932.

Van Riper, C. *The nature of stuttering.* Englewood Cliffs, N.J.: Prentice-Hall, 1971.

Van Riper, C., & Erickson, R. Apredictive screening test of articulation. *Journal of Speech and Hearing Disorders,* 1969, *34,* 214–219.

Walle, E. L. To stand and be counted. *Journal of Fluency Disorders,* 1975, *1,* 46–48.

Webb, W. B. (Ed.), *The profession of psychology.* New York: Holt, Rinehart & Winston, 1962.

Whaley, D. L., & Surratt, S. L. *Attitudes of science.* Kalamazoo, Mich.: Behaviordelia, 1968.

UNIT 1 STUDY QUESTIONS

1. Describe the essential characteristics of Perennialism, Essentialism, Progressivism, and Social Reconstructivism.
2. Differentiate between structuralism and functionalism as early theories.
3. How does behaviorism differ from Gestalt psychology?
4. What was Thorndike's important contribution to psychology?
5. What major psychological principles did Van Riper draw upon to formulate his procedures of speech therapy?
6. How is Guthrie's model used in speech therapy?
7. What contribution did Hull make to learning theory?
8. What was Skinner's unique contribution to learning theory?
9. How do cognitive theories differ from behavioristic theories?
10. How has learning theory affected speech clinicians in their choice of procedures?
11. Why is observation so important in science?
12. What is the chief difference between R–R and S–R laws?
13. Give some specific examples of the violation of the law of parsimony.
14. Explain the meaning of the Latin phrase, *post hoc ergo propter hoc.*
15. Explain the research technique called the *reversal method.* Why is it used?
16. Differentiate between dependent and independent variables.
17. Why are some educators opposed to the term control when used in education?
18. How have some speech pathologists reacted to the introduction of behaviorism in speech therapy?
19. List an argument against there being laws of learning.
20. What do you think is the most valid argument against the use of behavior modification techniques in the schools?

READING LIST FOR SPECIAL ASSIGNMENT

Berlitz, C. *The Bermuda triangle.* Garden City, N.Y.: Doubleday and Company, Inc., 1974.

Busch, N. You can live to be a hundred, he says. *Saturday Evening Post,* August 11, 1951.

California: The exorcist. *Newsweek,* September 10, 1973, 31.

Corbett, M. D. *How to improve your sight.* New York: Crown Publishers, Inc., 1970.

Critchfield, R. The persistent past, passing the buck to demons. *New Republic,* November 8, 1975, 15–17.

Däniken, E. von. *Gods from outer space.* New York: G. P. Putnam's Sons, 1968.

Däniken, E. von. *Chariots of the gods?* New York: G. P. Putnam's Sons, 1970.

Davies, R. A few kind words for superstition. *Newsweek,* November 20, 1978.

Dawson, J. The heavenly composer. *The people's almanac #2,* 1261–1263.

Drown laboratories submerged in pseudo-science. *Journal of the American Medical Association,* March 1941, 888.

Fort, C. *Wild talents.* New York: Garland Publishers, Inc., 1932.

Fort, C. *The book of the damned.* New York: Garland Publishers, Inc., 1975.

Fort, C. *New Lands.* New York: Garland Publishers, Inc., 1975.

Galton, L. Improve your eyesight without glasses. *Coronet,* October 1955, 170–173.

Hubbard, L. R. *Dianetics: The modern science of mental healing.* Los Angeles: The Church of Scientology of California Publications Organizations U.S., 1950.

Huxley, A. A case of ESP, PK, and psi. *Life,* January 11, 1954.

Huxley, A. Facts and fetishes. *Esquire,* September 1956.

Keyhoe, D. *The flying saucers are real.* New York: Fawcett Publications, 1950.

King, S. V. *Pyramid energy handbook.* New York: Warner Books, Inc., 1977.

Kleeman, R. H. Beware of medical frauds. *Saturday Evening Post,* August 11, 1951.

The long road to sainthood. *Time,* July 7, 1980.

Mensedleck, B. M. Positive lady. *Time,* April 5, 1937.

Morse, A. D. Don't fall for food fads. *Woman's Home Companion,* December 1951.

Oberg, J. E. Astronauts and UFOs—the whole story. *Space World,* 1977, N-2-158, 4–28.

Payne-Gasposchkin, C. *Proceedings of the American Philosophical Society,* October 1952, *96.*

Pferffer, Dr. The city with the golden garbage. *Collier's,* May 31, 1952.

Price, G. Cranks and prophets. *Catholic World,* October 1930.

Rhine, J. B. An investigation of a "mind-reading" horse. *Journal of Abnormal and Social Psychology,* 1929, *23,* 449.

Rhine, J. B. Second report on Lady, the "mind-reading" horse. *Journal of Abnormal and Social Psychology,* 1929, *24,* 287.

Riddick, T. Dowsing is nonsense. *Harper's,* July 1951.

Riddick, T. Dowsing: An unorthodox method of locating underground water supplies or an interesting facet of the human mind. *Proceedings of the American Philosophical Society,* October 1952, *96.*

Russell, B. In the company of cranks. *Saturday Review of Literature,* August 11, 1956, 7.

Smith, H. A. *Low man on the totem pole.* Philadelphia: Blakiston Publishing Co., 1941.

Smith, K., & Cannon, H. A methodological refinement in the study of "ESP" and negative findings. *Science,* July 23, 1954.

Standen, A. *Science is a sacred cow.* New York: Dutton Publishing Co., 1950.

Tromp, S. W. *The religion of a modern scientist.* Leiden: A. W. Sijthoff, 1947.

Velikovsky, I. *Worlds in collision.* Garden City, N. Y.: Doubleday Publishing Co., 1950.

Velikovsky, I. Answer to my critics. *Harper's,* June 1951.

Whiton, L. C. Under the power of the gran gadu. *Natural History,* March 1972, 14–21.

Wood, R. W. *How to tell the birds from the flowers.* Alexandria, Va.: Dover Publications, Inc., 1959.

Unit 2

Observing, Recording, and Assessing Speech Behaviors

Objectives

The objectives of this unit are to help you (1) identify and describe relevant speech behaviors, (2) compute, record and display behavioral data graphically, and (3) interpret and use these data to improve speech therapy. You will learn how to observe and evaluate your client's behavior as well as your own.

Suggested Assignments

Carefully study chapters 3 and 4. First, skim through the text so you will be familiar with the material to be presented in class. Many new concepts will be presented such as: recognizing differences between percentage and rate computations, using the logarithmic graph, and determining floor, ceiling and aim points on the logarithmic graph. The computations required in this assignment require a working knowledge of addition, subtraction, multiplication, and division. The use of various graphing techniques and computations involved will be discussed in class.

Two assignments are included at the end of this unit. A session on the tape cassette accompanies each assignment. Assignment 1 is designed to help you identify instances of correct and incorrect speech responses.

Assignment 2 provides you with practical experience using Boone and Prescott's system for evaluating the effectiveness of speech therapy sessions. Answer keys follow these assignments.

Finally, a list of 27 study questions is provided, following these assignments, to assist you in reviewing the important information presented in chapters 3 and 4.

3

Observation in Speech Pathology

It was pointed out in chapter 2 that observation was one of the four fundamental attitudes of a science. Observation is the beginning step in science. Through systematic observation techniques, humans were able to break away from metaphysical theory and establish empirical laws of the physical universe. And so it is with the study of human behavior. Observation of behavior plays a major role toward our understanding of why humans behave the way they do. Yet, *how* we observe, *what* we observe, *where* we observe, and *when* we observe, and what we *do* with the observations is, as you will discover, a very complex process. An entire book could be written on the topic of observation procedures in speech therapy. In fact, Johnson, Darley, and Spriestersbach (1963) and Darley (1964) did just that! These two books discuss just one phase of observation used in diagnostic procedures. I will attempt to condense into this chapter the important material from two areas in speech pathology where observation plays a key role. First we will consider the kinds of observations made to predict the course of speech development; then the kinds of observations made for diagnosis of speech problems will be presented.

Why We Observe

People observe events for many different reasons. You may observe a sunset purely for aesthetic purposes, or you may observe the redness of the sunset in the belief

60

that this coloration may predict tomorrow's weather. A scientist may observe flaming gases escaping the sun to determine the amount of radiation that will be transmitted to the earth. A home owner observes the path of the sun in order to aim his solar heating unit properly. The Boy Scout, by observing a small beam of light, adjusts his magnifying glass for maximum heat concentration from the sun. Each individual, in his own way, makes different observations of the same object for different reasons. Some use special instruments; some observe at certain times and under certain conditions.

We also have different reasons for observing communication behaviors. We may observe them with the intent of *predicting* what future speech behaviors will be like. Several articulation tests have been designed to enable us to predict which children will no longer misarticulate sounds at a future time and which ones will likely continue to misarticulate sounds if speech therapy is not provided. In the area of language development, investigators are seeking to identify certain features of language present in the child's daily speech patterns which might be indicators of future language skills.

Not only do we observe for purposes of prediction, but also to determine *cause* of the behavior. Oftentimes by eliminating the causal factors associated with the behavior, treatment procedures may be unnecessary. Through careful observation, we may discover the cause of hypernasality to be insufficient velar tissue. This being the case, it would be useless to practice blowing type exercises as a treatment for the hypernasality.

We may observe to discover and to identify factors which serve to *maintain* the behavior. It would be unwise to provide therapy in one situation for the correction of a speech problem when conditions outside that situation are supportive of the problem. Unfortunately, clinicians spend too little time in efforts to discover environmental conditions that serve to maintain certain behaviors.

Finally, we observe in order to assess the *effect* our therapy has on the speech behaviors. This process has recently received a great deal of attention from behavior therapists. There has been an attempt to standardize observation and recording procedures among both teachers and researchers.

The common factor to all reasons for observing is an appropriate and accurate description of the behaviors in question. If our basic procedures for describing behaviors are faulty, then it follows that our predictions about behavior, our ability to identify maintaining or causal factors, and our assessment of the effects of therapy will also be faulty. It is important that speech clinicians develop precise skills in the accurate description and evaluation of communication behaviors.

Basic Description and Evaluation Procedures

In describing communication problems, the speech clinician observes both *structural* and *behavioral* factors exhibited by the individual. Structural factors refer to dentition, shape of palatal arch, size of nasal cavity, vocal tract, and other physical dimensions imperative to speech production. Observations of physical dimensions are objective descriptions, frequently verified by measurement using precision instruments. Many times observation of the speech-producing structures provide the clinician with clues as to the cause of the communication problem. They are also made to determine results of some intervention or changes which occur due to maturation. For example, anatomical features of velopharyngeal relationships are assessed using X-ray film taken before and after surgery in order to determine the success of the surgical procedure. Production of speech is dependent upon physiological and neurological systems. Accurate descriptions of relevant elements of each system should be provided by the speech clinician before effective treatment of a communication problem can be provided. Discussion of the anatomical features speech clinicians should be familiar with is presented in a variety of texts on this subject and, subsequently, will not be presented here.

Behavioral descriptions are equally important, not only because they may be related to etiological factors, but also because they assist the clinician in planning therapy. There are two types: (1) descriptions of what the behavior *is,* and (2) descriptions of the *effect* the behavior has upon the listener.

Behavior implies movement, quite unlike the static features of an anatomical structure. In the case of communicative behavior, we observe muscular changes of the rib cage, the laryngeal tract, and the oral structure, which in turn moves air molecules in ways that can be measured. Descriptions of these changes can be measured and can also be very complex depending on what kinds of observations are made. The speech scientist, or speech physiologist, may wish to describe what muscle groups were involved in the behavior. Such a description might include a spectographic analysis of the sound frequency and intensity changes in the speech signal. You can appreciate how difficult and cumbersome it would be if clinicians described speech behavior in such complex terms.

But there is another way to describe speech behavior that is more practical. The behavior may be described in terms of its effects on the listener, that is, what the behavior *does,* as opposed to what the behavior *is.* I recall a student in one of my classes a few years ago who questioned my description of how /f/ was produced. I described movement of the airstream as flowing centrally through a narrow passageway formed by the upper front teeth and lower lip. The student said she produced /f/ by directing the airstream laterally to the right. Although the behavior (direction of airstream) differed from my description of the airstream position, the effects of the behavior were the same. Everyone described her sound production and my sound both as /f/ sounds. From one point of view, her behavior could be evaluated as incorrect, but from another point of view, the effects of the behavior were judged as correct.

We can describe what disfluent speech is by counting the number of syllabic repetitions, or we can describe the effects these repetitions have on the listeners. Upon hearing a portion of disfluent speech, the listener may describe her reaction. Thus, you may describe a behavior in terms of someone else's behavioral evaluation. Voice problems are frequently described in this manner. Suppose a certain voice quality is described as hoarse. This evaluation is an effect of something that happens to anatomical features, intensity of the sound, action of the vocal cords, and the like.

There are a number of associated features about behavior which also can be described. These would include how rapidly behavior occurs, its latency, accuracy of response, and response amplitude. Lewis (1963) lists seven behavioral measures which are commonly used to describe and evaluate behaviors. He maintains that we must be as specific and accurate as possible in our descriptions. Some of these descriptive measures are used by speech clinicians, some by audiologists, and others by laboratory researchers.

Techniques for Describing Behavior

Simple enumeration. This is the simplest type of behavioral measure. The purpose is to determine whether or not a behavior occurred. The behavior may be tied to a time base of say, 1 minute. The clinician simply counts the number of times the behavior occurs during 1 minute. A description of the behavior is that it occurred two times in 1 minute. Of course, you would also have to identify what behavior you were enumerating. Saying /s/ sounds, pointing to a picture, or asking a question might be the target behavior.

Number of correct responses. Having defined what constitutes a correct response, each behavior is evaluated accordingly. The total number of correct responses produced during a test containing a certain number of items is tabulated. A correct response count is frequently used as a measure of competence in articulation, where numerous presentations of a single sound are included in a test.

Amplitude of response. Precision instruments are usually employed to measure the intensity of the behavior. Diaphragmatic movement during speech production or the amount of nasal emission present can also be accurately measured. Usually, the practicing speech clinician will not need to observe amplitude of response.

Response rate. This is a very common measure used by many speech clinicians. It is simply a count of the number of responses that occur over a given period of time. As we will soon see, the response rate per minute will be very useful datum to have when we graphically display behavior change. Observations of behavior rates are tied directly to a time scale. A stutterer's rate of speech, in terms of syllables per minute, is a measure frequently employed to describe the stutterer's speech.

Latency of response. Two pieces of information are required to determine latency: (1) the onset of the stimulus, and (2) the beginning of the response. The time between these two events is a measure of latency. This is not a common measure used by speech clinicians since it requires precise timing. Yet, evidence shows that it may be a very important observation we should be making when assessing behavior in the therapy session. Usually, the faster an individual is able to respond, the better he has mastered the task. This holds true for the young child who is learning new articulatory skills, as well as for the aphasic patient learning word order sequences. Usually, the aphasic, whose latency is short, has better command over his speech than the individual whose speech is marked by long latencies.

Threshold. This is a common term to speech clinicians since it is used extensively in audiology. *Threshold* is that point where the stimulus is recognized 50% of the time. A lower threshold is the lowest value given to the stimulus, whereas the upper threshold is the highest value. In audiology, the lower threshold for frequency is about 30 Hz, and the upper threshold is about 20,000 Hz. A difference threshold is that point when the subject recognizes two stimuli as different 50% of the time. This measure might be used in sound discrimination tests.

Rating scales. For behaviors that cannot be measured quantitatively, rating scales are used. The quality of behavior is judged according to some characteristic. For example, the speech of stutterers may be rated on a 1:5 scale, from mild to severe. Speech intelligibility can be scored on a rating scale, as can voice quality. Some use a −2 : +2 rating scale to make judgments about voice quality. Frequently, anxiety producing speech situations can be identified by asking the individual to rate these situations. His rating scores serve as the behavior we describe.

Reducing Errors of Observation

An accurate evaluation of behavior is not always as simple as it might appear. In discussing administration of articulation tests, Winitz (1969) observed four major sources of variance which might bias description of articulatory behaviors: (1) subject variance, (2) experimenter variance, (3) instrument variance, and (4) interaction of subject with experimenter variance. Winitz emphasized that we cannot assume a person's evaluation is accurate unless some controls, or constraints, are placed on the observation process. Diedrich and Gerber (1974) report that speech clinicians who made judgments about the articulatory responses of their cases upon termination of therapy frequently differed with the descriptions of the same articulation responses provided by other speech clinicians. Shriberg (1972) found that when speech clinicians he tested evaluated tape recorded samples of /s/ sounds, they were in agreement only about 69.7% of the time, while interjudge agreement for /r/ was 79.1%. Clase (1976), regarding ethical implications of speech screening in the schools, points out that perhaps speech clinicians are too quick to evaluate some children's speech as constituting a problem; perhaps they are too critical in their evaluation. Also, clinicians find it difficult to agree whether a certain speech sample represents stuttering or just normal disfluency.

There are effective ways of reducing errors of description. Johnson and Harris (1968) suggest several techniques which can be employed to increase reliability. Usually, a second observer is assigned to record simultaneously with the regular observer. If both observers are describing their observations as correct and incorrect behaviors, then the number of trials on which they agree are totaled. From this, a percentage of agreement can be determined. Figure 3–1 illustrates how this tabulation is accomplished.

Suppose observations are made during certain time intervals and the observers are to describe the number of times a behavior occurs each period. Again, the number of times the observers agree can be totaled and divided by the total number of time periods to produce a percentage of agreement. Oftentimes, a speech clinician may wish to know how many times a child vocalizes over certain time periods. Observation periods are scheduled for 5 minutes each day for a week, and two observers make independent judgments regarding the number of times vocalization

Trials	Observer A	Observer B	Agreement
1	correct	incorrect	0
2	correct	correct	1
3	incorrect	incorrect	1
4	incorrect	incorrect	1
5	correct	correct	1
6	incorrect	correct	0
7	correct	correct	1
8	correct	correct	1
9	incorrect	incorrect	1
10	incorrect	correct	0
11	correct	correct	1
12	correct	correct	1

Total times of agreement 9

Total agreement (9) divided by number of trials (12) equal percent of agreement (75%).

FIGURE 3–1. Computation Of Percent Of Agreement Of Two Observers

occurred. A simple, statistical procedure to compare these data would be to compute a correlation coefficient. The raw data are presented in Figure 3–2.

It might surprise you to discover that in this example, there is a perfect correlation (1.00) between the two observers. This means the relationship between the two sets of numbers is always the same, although in each instance, the observers never agree as to the number of vocalizations. The percentage of agreement for each of the five observational periods is obviously zero. Descriptions of behavior become even more complicated when observations are submitted to statistical treatment.

Johnston and Harris (1968) provide techniques for training observers to be reliable in their descriptions and evaluations of the same events. They suggest that when explicit behavioral criteria are used and careful on-the-job supervision is provided, nonprofessional personnel can be trained to describe behavior with great

Day	Observer A # Vocalizations	Observer B # Vocalizations
1	4	8
2	6	10
3	8	12
4	10	14
5	12	16

FIGURE 3–2. Record Of The Number Of Observed Vocalizations By Two Observers Over A Five-Day Period

accuracy. Usually, no more than five to ten sessions are required to train individuals how to accurately describe behavior. It is advisable to start with observations of gross behaviors, gradually moving to observations of smaller components. Observers begin by writing down in long hand informal descriptions of the target behavior, which includes antecedent events. From this point, specific behaviors are recorded. Several behaviors can be described at once, using a coding system. Periodic checks are made of the observer's accuracy until the desired degree of reliability is acquired.

The behavior to be described must meet certain requirements. First, it must be a behavior that can be described in the same way by more than one person. You may recall in chapter two that we stated a science deals with observations that are "public." This means they can be identified by everyone, not just one person. People who claim to have "visions," or to see colors emanating from individuals, are unable to put these experiences to scientific test since they are "private" observations. Since the private observer is the only person who can observe the event, we are unable to verify the observation.

Our vocabulary is filled with vague terminology, which we use to describe behavior. For example, we frequently refer to a *nice* boy, a *good* girl, a *friendly* person, a *jovial* man, a *charming* woman. We talk about a person's *good* attitude, an *excellent* sense of humor or, by contrast, a *negative* attitude or inability to get along with others. Modern terminology applied to large classes of behaviors are equally vague. It's difficult to define the behaviors of a person who has "got it together," or who is "doing his thing." Speech clinicians usually refrain from using vague terms in describing attributes of speech, but occasionally, when describing voice, fluency, and language problems, ambiguous descriptions frequently are used.

When describing behaviors, be sure to use terms that refer to specific behaviors with a definite beginning and ending. For example, syllables have beginnings (releasers) and endings (arrestors). A syllable released through the nasopharynx has a beginning and ending and so does an uttered word, an eye blink, a lip tremor, a verbal statement, and a belch. All have beginnings and endings. Observers must agree when a behavior has occurred by noting its onset and termination. If we are unable to place limits on behavioral definitions, we can expect no uniformity of observations.

Finally, it is important that the behavior is repeatable. If it is not repeatable, it cannot be changed. Also, the behavior should occur frequently. We are familiar with the "sometimes stutterer," who is perfectly fluent during the interview, but complains of stuttering on rare occasions. Although the behavior can be described adequately enough, it occurs so infrequently that it is difficult to manipulate.

Observation in the Prediction of Communication Disorders

Predicting what communicative behavior will be like at some future time implies that there is lawfulness in speech development. Given certain conditions at time *A,* we should be able to predict events at time *B,* providing there is a functional relationship between the two. Weather forecasts follow this same principle. If conditions at time *A* consist of warm, moist air, a sudden drop in barometric pressure, and an approaching cold air mass, the meteorologist is usually able to predict thundershowers 6 to 10 hours in advance at time *B*. He has observed the functional relationship between these two events many times before. The extent to which he knows all of the relevant conditions will determine how accurate his prediction will be.

Siegel (1975) points out there have been many attempts to identify variables which would enable us to predict whether or not a child would require speech therapy. Referring especially to the study of language disorders, Siegel concluded that these attempts have been unsuccessful. The factors that lead to communication difficulties appear to be too complex and are subject to numerous influences. Perhaps researchers are observing irrelevant events. In the sections which follow, we shall examine the factors investigators have been observing in their attempts to pinpoint predictor variables.

Predictors of Articulation Skills

It has been well documented that many children with faulty articulation at age 6 are able to articulate correctly a few years later (Roe & Milisen, 1942). But of the group of 6 year olds, which of them will retain all, or part, of their original, faulty articulation? If we could make this prediction accurately, we could provide intensive speech therapy to those children most likely to continue faulty articulation and reduce, or eliminate, aid to those who predictively would achieve correct articulation without therapy.

An early investigation of factors identifying children who would continue misarticulating sounds was made by Carter and Buck (1958). They tested 175 first-grade children who had articulation problems when they first entered school, and again, upon completion of first grade. They concluded that children who were able to correctly imitate the clinician's nonsense syllable production 75% of the time when first tested would most likely articulate sounds correctly during final testing. Therefore, ability to correctly imitate the misarticulated sound was the variable observed for prediction.

Several other variables were identified by Steer and Drexler (1960). Selecting 93 kindergarten children who misarticulated at least one sound, the authors administered several tests at the beginning of the school year and then evaluated articulation skill at the end of the year. They found that the more errors a child had at the original time of testing, the more likely he would misarticulate sounds at the end of the school year. Other factors contributing to this condition were number of errors in the final position of words, number of sound omissions in the final position of words, and errors on /f/ and /l/. Two variables observed, intelligence and social quotient, were not found to be related to articulation outcome.

Farquhar (1961) administered a series of tests at the beginning of the school year to 100 kindergarten children—50 classified as mild and 50 as having severe articulation problems. An articulation test was given again at the end of the school year. Her results support those found by Carter and Buck (1958). Among the "mild" group, ability to imitate the defective sound correctly in words was significant, while in the severe group, the ability to correctly imitate the incorrect sound correctly, both in words and in nonsense syllables, was the determining, predictive factor. Auditory discrimination test scores did not have predictive value.

Van Riper and Erickson (1969) constructed and standardized the Predictive Screening Test of Articulation (PSTA), designed to identify those children in the first grade who would require speech therapy. In designing the test, they compiled a pool of some 500 items which seemed to have prognostic value including the following: samples of articulation behavior; phonemic synthesis and analysis ability; auditory discrimination; motor coordination; jaw and tongue mobility; and a variety of other imitative- and error-recognition behaviors. From this group, 111 items were selected as most predictable of future articulation skills. Following a 2-year test program, 47 items were found which differentiated between individuals who would retain articulation errors and those who would not. While the authors felt this instrument was not a perfect predictor, it was considered a first step toward accurate prediction of future articulation skills. The types of observations made by Van Riper and Erickson for their PSTA test were very similar to those identified by investigators some 10 years previously. The 47 items included in the PSTA sampled children's ability to correctly initiate stimulus words, isolated phonemes, nonsense syllables, words in a sentence, plus ability to recognize a misarticulated /r/ and clap hands in response to a demonstrated rhythm pattern.

We can apply the predictive formula presented in chapter two, $R_1 = f(R_2)$ under c, to examples such as the PSTA. R_1 would be the child's performance on an articulation test administered in the third grade. R_2 is his score on the 47-item test and the conditions are that this test be administered to the child during the first 10 weeks of first grade. If this relationship holds, then the child who produces 34 or less correct responses (R_2) would probably continue to misarticulate sounds at least until the third grade (R_1). By establishing functional relationships between two sets of behaviors, we are able to predict one by observing another. Barrett and Welsh (1975) conducted a follow-up study of the PSTA to reevaluate its effectiveness as a predictive test. They identified 502 first graders who scored 34 or higher on the PSTA. Three years later, 371 of the original group were tested in third grade. They found the PSTA 90% accurate in identifying children in first grade who would not require therapy.

Arndt, Elbert, and Shelton (1971) used observations of a child's early articulation improvement during therapy as a measure to predict later articulation improvement. Although baseline scores, i.e., scores obtained before therapy was started and mean final scores (scores obtained when therapy was completed) did not hold predictive value, the *predictor scores* did. A predictor score was defined as a measure obtained by subtracting the number of correct responses on the Spontaneous Production Task, administered after a specified lesson, from the mean baseline score. Observations of how well children progress early in therapy seemed to be good predictors of success in therapy.

Prediction in Stuttering

Research investigations which attempt to differentiate stutterers who develop fluent speech from those who do not are, surprisingly, few in number in view of the wealth of literature about stuttering. Yet, those who have investigated predictive elements have uncovered some interesting points. Stromsta (1965) observed spectrograms of disfluencies and concluded those speakers who showed anomalies in coarticulation failed to "outgrow" their stuttering, whereas those children who exhibited normal junction formats had become fluent within the 10 year observation period. Van Riper (1971) confirmed Stromsta's findings through his own observations of subjects and suggested that the use of the schwa vowel in syllabic repetitions might be a reliable predictor of whether or not a child will continue to stutter. It has also been suggested that a fairly reliable prediction can be made on the basis of the age of the stutterer. If we observe stuttering in the speech of a child who is 12 years old or older, it is likely he will continue to stutter. At the present time, there is no research evidence which would allow us to make predictions about stuttering based on the 12-year-old age criterion. It is strictly a clinical observation.

Johnson et al. (1963) hypothesized that adaptation might have predictive value of a stutterer's potential to improve fluency in conjunction with speech therapy. But it was not until Prins and McQuiston (1964) empirically tested this hypothesis, and later Lanyon (1965), that it was concluded adaptation scores hold no predictive value for fluent speaking. An additional study by Prins (1968) confirmed this finding.

Several studies have been conducted to determine if the stutterer can predict when speech difficulty will occur. Most adult stutterers, when asked to signal when they anticipate stuttering during oral readings, are able to do so with remarkable accuracy (Van Riper, 1936). Young stutterers, however, are noticeably poor at predicting when they will stutter. At age 8 to 10, they could only predict stuttering with 38% accuracy (Bloodstein, 1960). Exactly what stimuli the stutterer is reacting to that allows him to make predictions about his fluency is unknown. It would be interesting to find out whether one's ability to predict occasions of stuttering has any utility in predicting future success in therapy. One of the more thorough attempts to determine whether or not a child would continue to stutter in the future was made by Cooper (1973). His observation that two out of every three stutterers encountered by school speech clinicians attain fluent speech without the aid of therapy lead him to investigate nine factors persistent stutterers seemed to have in common: family history of stuttering, stuttering severity, duration of stuttering, type of initial disfluency, sex of the stutterer, parental attitudes, stutterer's attitudes, gradual improvement, and distinctive features of the stuttering moment. Cooper constructed a questionnaire to determine the predictive value of these factors. Based upon an individual's score on this questionnaire, he hypothesized the clinician could predict whether an individual would continue to stutter or if spontaneous recovery was more likely. Unfortunately, Cooper presented no data to validate his instrument, nor did he present information that would assist the clinician in interpreting results. Van Riper (1971) constructed some guidelines for differentiating normal from abnormal disfluencies, but as in the case of Cooper's questionnaire, they amount to nothing more than clinical "hunches."

Prediction in Language Development

As in the case of stuttering, speech clinicians have done little to identify predictive variables for language development. Some studies have attempted to discover relationships between language skills and other factors, such as discrimination ability, certain home background variables, stress, and word position. No reliable predictive measures have been found. With increased emphasis on language problems in the schools, much more activity in this area is expected. As Siegel (1975) points out,

"I think our problems with prediction derive, at least in part, from the fact that verbal skills are complex and evolving, and subject to numerous influences." Siegel may have identified an important reason why we have so few adequate, predictive language tests. We simply do not agree on a definition of language. Perhaps the term *language* is too broad for any meaningful kind of observation. We must use precise definitions of behavior when we set out to observe it.

There are some indications which might provide valuable, predictive information about language development. One is the amount of echolalia in the child's speech. Van Riper (1963) points out that echolalia in a child's speech is normal at one stage of development but is seldom observed after 2½ years of age. If it is present after that age, one might suspect language skills will not develop satisfactorily. The amount of stereotyped utterances in a speech sample may also be an indicator of language delay. On the other hand, the use of novel sentence constructions may be a good predictor of language development.

A number of other factors have been investigated which hold prediction potential but, as yet, no one has attempted to link these factors with predicting language acquisition. The most extensively used measures of assessing verbal output are mean length of response (MLR) and the number of different words (NDW). According to Shriner and Sherman (1967), MLR had a higher correlation with scale values of language development than any other variables studied.

Lee (1966) developed a language measure involving structural analysis of the child's language, based upon a theoretical hierarchy of developmental sentence types (DST). Four levels of structural complexity are identified, each of increasing linguistic complexity: the two-word combination, the noun phrase, constructions, and sentences. Another language measure, evaluated by Shriner (1967), the length complexity index (LC), consists of a combination of the MLR and structural complexity score. He concluded that initial results indicate that the LC index was the best single predictor of language development of children 5 years of age or younger. But until the LC index can be refined, the MLR appears to be a highly satisfactory measure.

All of the above language measures were evaluated by Sharf (1972). He reported that language development patterns were so erratic among the 13 children he studied, no valid conclusions could be reached regarding at what age a child should reach a certain proficiency of language skill. Some children showed little change in months; others would make sudden, large gains. There was considerable agreement among scores obtained by children on the MLR, NDW, LC, and DST language measures regarding general rate of language development, i.e., they all seemed to be related to language growth. At present, we are far from an accurate identification of variables which can be related to predicting success in language acquisition. As Siegel (1975) suggested, perhaps we are looking at a class of verbal behaviors which is too vague and too large for systematic study.

Prediction in Voice Disorders

The same problems which exist in the study of language exist in the area of voice disorders; no valid predictive measures have been developed. There are data, for example, to show that vocal abuse and misuse can lead to hyperfunctional voice problems, particularly vocal nodules. But given a group of children who abuse their voices through frequent yelling and screaming, it is impossible, at present, to predict which of the children will develop voice problems. We are fairly confident in our analysis of the cause of the disorder, but we are unable to predict its occurrence.

Sharp (1963) made an unusual attempt to relate certain vocal characteristics to mental disorders. He asked judges to evaluate certain vocal characteristics of several tape-recorded speech samples and to attempt to identify speakers who might have emotional conflicts. The judges could not reach agreement on who was, or was not, suffering from emotional conflict on the basis of voice characteristics. If such a relationship between vocal characteristics and emotional disorders could be found, the vocal characteristics might be used as early, predictive signs indicating treatment needs.

Although not concerned directly with voice disorders, Lubker and Morris (1968) used prediction in estimating the amount of velopharyngeal opening from viewing single-exposure, still X-ray films. They found accurate predictions can be made, providing one seeks only to rank order individuals in terms of amount of opening.

Factors leading to success in learning esophageal speech following laryngectomy have been studied by several investigators. One early study by Robe et al. (1956) represents a major research attempt to identify factors relating to success or failure in learning esophageal speech. They found that successful laryngeal speakers had narrow fields of surgery.

A few years later, Shames et al. (1963) identified several factors useful as predictors of speech proficiency with alaryngeal patients. Biographical, medical, personality, social communication, and speech training variables were studied in some 153 alaryngeal patients. The factors they found to be important to achieving speech proficiency were age at the time of operation, amount of education, intact strap and cricopharyngeal muscles, length of time between surgery and being understood, presurgical knowledge of resulting voice problems, and number of speech lessons. Several personality variables, measured by the Edwards Personal Preference Schedule, also seemed to be related to whether or not there was success in learning esophageal speech. It is surprising that no one has taken the step to test these variables as reliable predictors, especially since they have been known for almost two decades.

Prediction in Aphasia

A substantial amount of research has been conducted regarding prediction of speech improvement among aphasic patients. Four factors are useful in estimating a patient's communicative potential: psychological, situational, physiological, and linguistic factors.

Among important psychological factors, Eisenson (1949) found the patient's general health and strength to be a good predictor of success in speech therapy. Also, the younger the patient, the faster the recovery with the exception of head injury cases (Sands et al., 1969). Even handedness seems to be a good predictor (Smith, 1971); and the amount of motor speech impairment is an important factor, according to Keenan and Brassell (1974).

Predictive, situational factors involve the length of time from the onset of the aphasia to the beginning of speech therapy (Vignola, 1964). The amount of the patient's prior education, as well as the type of home environment to which the patient returns, is a decisive factor in recovery (Buck, 1968; Smith, 1971).

Important psychological variables include observations of the patient's willingness to attempt speech, his level of aspiration, his ability to be independent, and his anxiety state (Eisenson, 1949; Keenan, 1970).

Finally, several linguistic variables appear to be related to the amount of future improvement. Many clinicians note that patients whose initial language impairment is mild, or moderate, have a greater chance for speech recovery. Initial listening and talking performance and speech stimulatability are among variables Keenan and Brassell (1974) found that are important predictors for aphasia. The patient's recognition and correction of his own errors have been found to be an important indicator of future success (Vignola, 1964; Keenan, 1970).

Attempts to predict future speech behaviors are at an infant stage of development, as you might guess from the publication dates of the literature about prediction. Not only are there very few standardized prediction instruments, but in some areas, only clinical hunches exist with regard to what factors might be helpful in predicting speech behavior. One reason for this may be that there are many combinations of variables which could be responsible for future speech development. Identification of these combinations could be, in some cases, an almost impossible task due to a wide variety of environmental and hereditary factors.

Another discouraging element in the area of prediction is the lack of any systematic, investigative effort. Studies of prediction require longitudinal investigations, which require long-term planning of from 2 to 10 years. Little help can be expected from research efforts of students in training, since their research commitment is usually a brief one. Nevertheless, there is still considerable interest in predictive research. We can look forward to an increasing number of tests designed to assist the clinician in making predictive statements about the course of communication disorders. Presently, predictive tests fall into two distinct categories: (1) those that predict future speech behavior when no therapy is provided, and (2) predictions about what changes will occur in speech behaviors following therapy. A wide assortment of variables have been observed in making predictive statements about speech behavior. The current problem is identifying those variables which have predictive value and devising valid, standardized tests that will allow the clinician to make accurate, predictive statements about future speech behavior.

Observation in
the Diagnosis of
Communication Disorders

When we make predictions, we observe behaviors and events that tell us something about what behaviors will be like in the *future*. Diagnostic information, on the other hand, consists of observations of the individual's *past* which caused the behavior. Just as we look for functional relationships between two or more events when predicting behavior, we also search for these functional relationships when seeking to pinpoint the cause of behaviors. In order to explain a behavior, something more than observing and describing similar events must occur. The antecedent conditions necessary for the behavior to occur must be known, as well as the antecedent conditions which will prevent the behavior. The relationships between the communicative disorder and the events which determine the disorders are established through diagnosis.

The causes of behavior can be classified into two general categories of events: physiological and environmental. Physiological events include hereditary factors, physiological structures, native intelligence—in short, the physiological and biological properties of the person. These factors play an important part as causes for many communication disorders, especially those involving aphasia, cerebral palsy, and cleft palate. Congenital defects, diseases, surgery, and injuries are among important factors which can lead to impaired speech.

A large number of environmental factors have also been identified as the cause of many communication disorders. An individual's history of reinforcement and punishment, important consequences for establishing and maintaining certain speech behaviors, also, the type of stimuli presented to the child, both verbal and nonverbal, help determine the course of speech development. If, for example, a young child lisps and her parents delight in her misarticulation, the rewards for lisping may strengthen and maintain the behavior for many years, diverting what might have been a transitionary speech development process. The cause of continued lisping, in this case, may be parental reinforcement. Identification of environmental determinants as causal factors is frequently difficult since we rely more on conjecture and hypothesis than upon empirical evidence. While there can be little doubt about the cause of hypernasality in one case, drawing conclusions about the effect of parental reward for lisping as a causal factor becomes speculative.

The functional relationship established through diagnosis is called an S-R law, as opposed to the R-R type law, which only allows us to predict behavior. S-R laws permit us to both predict and control behaviors. If we have observed the relationship between hypernasality and insufficient velopharyngeal closure, then we can predict hypernasal speech and follow surgical removal of the velum. We can predict certain aphasic symptoms if certain areas of the brain are impaired. But in addition to prediction, we achieve a large element of control through discovery of determinants of speech problems. A pharyngeal flap operation may eliminate hypernasality, orthodontic work may correct certain misarticulations, or removal of vocal nodes may result in improved voice quality. If environmental factors are responsible for the observed behaviors, then by manipulating these factors, we may be able to modify the behaviors. Assuming the cause of lisping behavior was positive attention by the parents, contingent upon lisping behavior, then removing the reward for lisping and providing reward following correct /s/ production should result in correction of the lisping problem. In this way, we are able to control behavior by treating the cause of the behavior.

The chief reason speech clinicians diagnose speech problems is to aid us in planning a remedial treatment program. We may be only one member of a diagnostic team involved in total evaluation of the individual, or we may be solely responsible for diagnosis. In any case, we observe the symptoms and gather as much relevant information as possible to enable us to hypothesize about the cause of the problem. Schultz (1973) views the ideal diagnostic process as one in which hypotheses are formulated based on the cause of the problem, careful examination of the data from the case history, objective and semiobjective tests, plus informal observations. From these data the clinician selects tentative hypotheses and rejects others until probable causal factors are identified. When the clinician is satisfied a valid hypothesis has been reached, she is in the position to make some predictive statements about the possible outcome of the disorder (with and without therapy), as well as formulate a remedial plan for changing the behavior. Schultz advocates diagnosis should not be simply a post hoc observation, occurring once before remedial action. Diagnosis should be "on line," or a continuing process, conducted throughout remediation. This concept of diagnosis is slightly different from the traditional, initial battery of tests given before therapy begins. Schultz feels an "on-line" evaluation holds many advantages over the one time post hoc evaluation.

Types of Observations Made in Diagnosis

Gathering information needed to predict the outcome of speech behaviors depends solely on observation. This also holds true for the process of diagnosis. While many of the factors analyzed are similar, diagnosis implies a much more thorough investigation into past events. Diagnosis relies heavily on a wide variety of tests, many of which have standardized norms. An accurate diagnosis also depends on the observations of those in other disciplines, such as medicine, education, social work, psychology, and the like.

One of the first steps in making a diagnosis is to collect information about the individual's past history. The *case history* is usually obtained either from the individual himself or from a close associate like a parent, wife or husband, or close relative. It includes events occurring prior, during, and shortly after birth which might have a bearing on later speech development. Developmental milestones such as age of sitting, walking, talking are recorded, as are other relevant, physical growth patterns. Medical information, such as types of illnesses or deformities, medical treatment, handicapping conditions, dentition, and other pertinent information is included. Relevant data regarding psychological factors, emotional stability, mental health, school performance, and social development are also considered. Results from intelligence tests, sociograms, and manual dexterity tests are sometimes secured from evaluators in other areas. A detailed speech history usually includes a review of the individual's speech development from birth to the present.

The *speech examination* comprises the second part of the diagnostic process. Typically, this includes an oral examination, plus the administration of a variety of tests, depending upon the problem. Objective test instruments with established norms are often preferred measures because they yield data that are usually more valid and reliable than other measures. Semiobjective tests include those measures which have not been statistically validated. They may be locally devised tests or may depend solely upon the clinician's skill in interpreting the results. Finally, the clinician utilizes informal observations of the individual's behavior under various conditions to assess the nature of the communicative problem. These observations may consist of informal conversation with the individual, exploratory therapy, play activities, and the like, depending on the age of the individual and the type of problem. To assist the clinician in compiling these observations, numerous case history and speech examination forms have been provided, each following the general outline listed above. Dickson and Jann (1974) compiled a four-page case history form. West, Ansberry, and Carr (1957) devote an entire chapter to case study and evaluation, as do most other texts in speech pathology. As was mentioned before, there are several textbooks written solely about diagnostic procedures used for each type of communicative disorder.

A review of diagnostic procedures and tests available for each type of communication disorder lies far beyond the scope of this chapter. For example, in the area of language disorders alone, McConnell et al. (1974) list 11 developmental language scales, 5 comprehensive test batteries, and 34 different tests to assess expressive language behavior, not to mention special case history and informal observational techniques to be used. The Clinical and Educational Materials (1972) section of *Asha* lists some 65 standardized diagnostic tests applicable to individuals who have communication problems—a "brief review of a few of the tests currently on the market," according to the editor.

It is evident that speech clinicians view the diagnostic process as a fundamental and important activity related to the treatment of communication disorders. The basis for the diagnostic process emanated from the medical profession. This medical model implies (1) a strong reliance on the logic and goals of the traditional medical diagnostic process; (2) treatment should be directed toward elimination of the causal factors, rather than attention to the "symptoms;" and (3) individuals with behavior problems should be treated as "ill" in the same sense as patients who have physical ailments.

Etiology, diagnosis, and prognosis form the basis of the doctor's prescriptive program. The patient who complains of stomach cramps, which were unsuccessfully treated with anti-acid pills, visits the doctor's office. The doctor may begin his diagnosis by taking a brief case history to search for causes and to eliminate certain possibilities. He may probe the stomach area for tender spots, or X-ray the patient's digestive tract to better pinpoint the cause. Once the illness is properly diagnosed, remedial steps are taken, either in the form of prescriptive medication, diet, or perhaps, surgery. Thus, the patient's cramps disappear. There are many valid and reliable S–R type laws in medicine; but treating symptoms with no knowledge of causal factors would be unscientific and, most probably, harmful.

The medical model, an outgrowth of the scientific methods of the sixteenth and seventeenth centuries, was quickly adapted by Freud (1920) to the treatment of behavioral problems. Freud, a physician, followed medical diagnosis to its completion by identifying causes of behavior residing in what he identified as the *id,* the *ego,* and the *super-ego.* Psychoanalysis was a procedure that would allow the physician to uncover the true causes responsible for bizarre, behavioral symptoms. Unfortunately for Freud's theory, the independent variables he selected as causal agents were not publically observable and, hence, were not subject to objective testing. Generally, most psychologists today no longer consider Freud's theories as valid.

Nevertheless, Freud's impact on psychiatrists and educators alike has had a strong influence on how behavior problems are treated.

Diagnostic procedures were practically unheard of before the twentieth century. With the advent of Wechsler and Binet's attempts to measure individual differences, diagnostic techniques were gradually introduced in the schools through the intelligence testing movement of the 1920s. It was expected that diagnosis would also play an important role in speech pathology, especially since there is a close relationship between it and the medical profession. It is, therefore, not surprising to find strong emphasis on diagnostic procedures in speech pathology.

Recently, the medical model has come under strong criticism from some psychologists (Sarbin, 1967; Szasz, 1960; Ullmann & Krasner, 1969). Clinical psychologists who used a series of assessment techniques, including projective tests and questionnaires aimed at providing diagnostic labels, found the resultant information lacked clinical utility, predictive validity, or even reliability. There has been a gradual shift away from attempts to evaluate personality traits toward the use of behavioral observations of specific situations which include the individual's special environment (Kanfer & Phillips, 1970). The shift is away from the medical-psychiatric model toward the social-psychological model.

One of the chief criticisms of the medical model stems from its failure to apply relevant principles about conditions that produce, maintain, and modify social behavior (Mischel, 1968). Many diagnostic tests are of little use for making practical, clinical decisions. Meehl (1960) surveyed therapists who worked with behavioral disorders and observed that only 17% found prior testing of any value in their treatment. Sloane and MacAulay (1968) maintain that speech clinicians would be better off using a behavioral analysis of the speech problem itself in planning a remedial program, rather than viewing the speech as a "symptom" of some underlying difficulty.

In contrast to the traditional, medical-diagnosis approach, many behavioral psychologists prefer the term *behavioral diagnosis*. This type of diagnosis pinpoints specific behaviors that are targets for change, identifies conditions which maintain the undesirable behavior, and indicates the most practical means for producing desired changes. Some behaviorists rely solely on operant conditioning as the etiological basis for behavior problems (Ferster, 1965). They seek functional relationships which will allow them to effectively treat behavioral problems. Such a search for relevant, functional relationships prompted Kanfer and Saslow (1969) to construct a behavioral analysis guide for conducting an interview and recording the case history. It includes a wide range of specific data necessary for a clinical-functional analysis: historical, social, cognitive, biological factors, as well as directly observed behavior. The seven categories studied are

1. Analysis of problem situations—A description of the target behavior(s) needing change.
2. Clarification of the problem—People and circumstances which maintain problem behaviors.
3. Motivational analysis—A description of the hierarchy of people, events, and objects that serve as reinforcers to the individual.

4. Developmental analysis—A study of the individual's biological equipment, his sociocultural development and behavioral progress.
5. Analysis of self-control—Methods and degrees of self-control in daily life.
6. Analysis of social relationships—Examination of the interpersonal relationships in the individual's environment.
7. Analysis of social, cultural, physical environment—The individual's behavior is compared with norms in his community.

The case history presented above enables the clinician to amass important data about an individual which would be very useful in selecting a treatment strategy. Standardized, diagnostic tests are rarely relevant in devising behavior therapy strategies. While many standard diagnostic tests provide some basis for assessing the nature and the extent of the problem in the test situation, they usually provide little information about the individual's functioning in his environment. Johnston and Harris (1968) point out that labeling a language disorder in terms of etiology contributes little toward planning a treatment program.

Some behaviorists have almost totally ignored traditional, diagnostic procedures. Their initial observations consist only of "baseline," or base-rate, measures of the behaviors in terms of frequency of occurrence over a period of time. They view problem behavior simply as an outcome of the same functional process that effects all behavior, with the reinforcement history as the primary etiological element. The focus is on the symptoms, not some internal, mediating process. By altering reinforcement patterns, problematic behavior can be, and is, manipulated with little attention given to traditional, diagnostic procedures. Salzinger (1968) notes that it is the current fashion among some behaviorists to ignore the individual's reinforcement history altogether.

The influence of new trends in diagnostic procedures is evidenced in Turton's (1973) presentation in articulation testing. While advising the clinician to rule out contributing etiological variables by screening for a hearing loss, intellectual deficits, and emotional and social problems, he stresses the importance of "behavioral evaluation." This evaluation should begin with a series of tests to assess the child's articulation competencies and to assist in planning a therapy strategy. Once therapy is initiated, he suggests intrasession, as well as intersession, measures be taken as part of the ongoing, behavioral evaluation. This is similar to the recommendation Schultz (1973) made concerning an "on-line" evaluation.

Ryan (1974) constructed two stuttering evaluation forms, one for adults and one for children, in which the stutterer is asked to speak in a variety of situations from counting to conversation. Each requires approximately 40 minutes to administer. The purpose of these tests is to determine if the individual needs speech therapy, to identify specific speaking situations which are difficult, and to serve as pre- and post-therapy measures of fluency. Following the evaluation, a base rate of fluency is taken to evaluate reading, monologue, and conversational speech. This approach to the diagnostic evaluation of stuttering is typical of ones used by many behaviorists. Ryan's descriptive approach is in sharp contrast to the kinds of information sought by those who were searching for etiological factors. The Iowa Scale of Attitude Toward Stuttering and the stutterers' self-ratings of reactions to speech situations

(Ammons & Johnson, 1944) are typical of some of the earlier tests designed to investigate a stutterer's attitude and feelings. A growing number of speech clinicians are focusing upon sociological factors that appear to maintain stuttering and less upon trying to discover etiological factors through time-consuming, diagnostic procedures.

In spite of recent criticism of traditional diagnostic methods and the medical model, it would be extremely unwise for the speech pathologist to overlook their proper place in our profession. Our profession is not one which deals strictly with behavior. Speech is dependent upon a well-functioning, neurological and physiological system. These systems simply cannot be ignored. Treatment of a disorder without regard to all etiological factors sounds more like an art than a science. In fact, Kanfer and Phillips (1970) suggest many behaviorists are as much artists as they are scientists when it comes to making decisions about which responses should be considered as target responses, which treatment method should be selected, and when treatment procedures should be changed. We cannot afford the risk of overlooking some key element in an individual's case history which, if known or corrected, might save needless hours of therapy.

I think the important point to be learned from the behaviorists in psychology is that we have overlooked much important information about the individual which can greatly aid therapeutic planning. Those observations suggested by Kanfer and Saslow (1969) in their behavioral diagnosis scheme would seem to be a very necessary part of the clinician's assessment program. The second thing we should learn from the behaviorists is the value of daily, therapeutic assessment as part of an ongoing, diagnostic-evaluative procedure. This area has been greatly neglected by speech clinicians. This topic will be discussed in detail in chapter 4.

We can expect continued activity in the area of prediction, especially during the age of accountability. We can no longer afford the luxury of correcting speech problems which will disappear in a few years. As predictive measures improve, we will move closer to becoming a science. Diagnostic procedures are currently undergoing change; hopefully this change will enable the speech clinician to select and to design more effective therapeutic strategies than before.

Basic to our discussion in this chapter has been the process of careful observation. Perhaps you can now begin to understand the complexity of the observation technique; understand why it is the basis of the scientific method. It is through careful and systematic observation that R–R and S–R laws are yielded. So far, we have considered the role of observation in prediction and diagnosis. We shall now consider what part observation plays in assessment during the therapeutic process.

BIBLIOGRAPHY

Ammons, R., & Johnson, W. Studies in the psychology of stuttering: XVIII. The construction and application of a test of attitude toward stuttering. *Journal of Speech Disorders,* 1944, *9,* 39–49.

Arndt, W., Elbert, M., & Shelton, R. Prediction of articulation involvement with therapy from early lesson sound production task scores. *Journal of Speech and Hearing Research,* 1971, *14,* 149–153.

Barrett, J. C., & Welsh, J. W. Predictive articulation screening. *Language, Speech, and Hearing Services in the Schools,* 1975, *6,* 91–95.

Bloodstein, O. The development of stuttering: I. Changes in nine basic features. *Journal of Speech and Hearing Disorders,* 1960, *25,* 219–237.

Buck, M. *Dysphasia.* Englewood Cliffs, N.J.: Prentice-Hall, 1968.

Carter, E. T., & Buck, M. W. Prognostic testing for functional articulation disorders among children in the first grade. *Journal of Speech and Hearing Disorders,* 1958, *23,* 124–133.

Clase, J. M. Ethical implications of screening. *Language, Speech, and Hearing Services in the Schools,* 1976, *7,* 50–56.

Clinical and educational materials. *Asha,* 1972, *14,* 618–620.

Cooper, E. B. The development of a stuttering chronicity prediction checklist: A preliminary report. *Journal of Speech and Hearing Disorders,* 1973, *38,* 215–223.

Darley, F. L. *Diagnosis and appraisal of communication disorders.* Englewood Cliffs, N.J.: Prentice-Hall, 1964.

Dickson, S., & Jann, G. R. Diagnostic principles and procedures. In S. Dickson (Ed.), *Communication disorders, remedial principles and practices.* Glenview, Ill.: Scott, Foresman, 1974.

Diedrich, W. M., & Gerber, A. J. Analyses and management of articulation learning. ASHA Shortcourse. *Asha,* 1974, *16,* 568.

Eisenson, J. Prognostic factors related to language rehabilitation in aphasic patients. *Journal of Speech and Hearing Disorders,* 1949, *14,* 262–264.

Farquhar, M. Prognostic value of imitative and auditory discrimination tests. *Journal of Speech and Hearing Disorders,* 1961, *26,* 342–347.

Ferster, C. B. Classification of behavioral pathology. In L. Krasner & L. Ullman (Eds.), *Research in behavior modification: New developments and implications.* New York: Holt, Rinehart & Winston, 1965.

Freud, S. *A general introduction to psychoanalysis.* New York: Boni & Liveright, 1920.

Johnson, W., Darley, F. L., & Spriestersback, D. C. *Diagnostic methods in speech pathology.* New York: Harper & Row, 1963.

Johnston, M. K., & Harris, F. R. Observation and recording of verbal behavior. In H. Sloane & B. MacAulay (Eds.), *Operant procedures in remedial speech and language training.* Boston: Houghton Mifflin, 1968.

Kanfer, F. H., & Phillips, J. S. *Learning foundations of behavior therapy.* New York: John Wiley & Sons, 1970.

Kanfer, F. H., & Saslow, G. Behavioral diagnosis. In C. Franks (Ed.), *Behavior therapy: Appraisal and status.* New York: McGraw-Hill, 1969.

Keenan, J. S. Some prognostic factors in aphasic rehabilitation. Audiotape, Veterans Administration Hospital, Atlanta, 1970.

Keenan, J. S., & Brassell, E. G. A study of factors related to prognosis for individual aphasic patients. *Journal of Speech and Hearing Disorders,* 1974, *39,* 257–269.

Lanyon, R. L. The relationship of adaptation and consistency to improvement in stuttering therapy. *Journal of Speech and Hearing Research,* 1965, *8,* 263–269.

Lee, L. Developmental sentence types: A method for comparing normal and deviant syntactic development. *Journal of Speech and Hearing Disorders,* 1966, *31,* 311–330.

Lewis, D. J. *Scientific principles of psychology.* Englewood Cliffs, N.J.: Prentice-Hall, 1963.

Lubker, J. F., & Morris, H. L. Predicting cinefluorographic measures of velopharyngeal opening from lateral still x-ray films. *Journal of Speech and Hearing Research,* 1968, *11,* 747–753.

McConnell, F., Love, R. J., & Clark, B. S. Language remediation in children. In S. Dickson (Ed.), *Communication disorders: Remedial principles and practices.* Glenview, Ill.: Scott, Foresman, 1974.

Meehl, P. E. The cognitive activity of the clinician. *American Psychologist,* 1960, *15,* 19–27.

Mischel, W. *Personality and assessment.* New York: John Wiley & Sons, 1968.

Prins, D. Pre-therapy adaptation of stuttering and its relation to speech measures of therapy progress. *Journal of Speech and Hearing Research,* 1968, *11,* 740–746.

Prins, D., & McQuiston, B. Differential analysis of pre-therapy adaptation in stutterers and its relation to selected indices of therapy progress. *Asha,* 1964, *6,* 401.

Robe, E. J., Moore, P., Andrews, A. H., Jr., & Hollinger, P. H. A study of the role of certain factors in the development of speech after laryngectomy, I. Type of operation. *Laryngoscope,* 1956, *66,* 173–186.

Roe, V., & Milisen, R. The effect of maturation upon defective articulation in elementary grades. *Journal of Speech Disorders,* 1942, *7,* 37–50.

Ryan, B. *Programmed therapy for stuttering in children and adults.* Springfield, Ill.: Charles C Thomas, 1974.

Salzinger, K. *Behavior therapy models of abnormal behavior.* Paper presented at the Biometrics Research Workshop on Objective Indicators of Psychopathology. Tuxedo, N.Y., February 1968.

Sands, E., Sarno, M. T., & Shankweiler, D. Long-term assessment of language function in aphasia due to stroke. *Archives of Physical Medical Rehabilitation,* 1969, *50,* 202–206.

Sarbin, T. R. On the futility of the proposition that some people be labeled "mentally ill." *Journal of Consulting Psychology,* 1967, *31,* 447–453.

Schultz, M. The bases of speech pathology and audiology: Evaluation as the resolution of uncertainty. *Journal of Speech and Hearing Disorders,* 1973, *38,* 147–155.

Shames, G. H., Font, J., & Matthews, J. Factors related to speech proficiency of the laryngectomized. *Journal of Speech and Hearing Disorders,* 1963, *28,* 273–287.

Sharf, D. Some relationships between measures of early language development. *Journal of Speech and Hearing Disorders*, 1972, *37*, 64–74.

Sharp, F. A. Judgments of psychosis from vocal cues. *Journal of Speech and Hearing Disorders*, 1963, *28*, 371–374.

Shriberg, L. Articulation judgments: Some perceptual considerations. *Journal of Speech and Hearing Research*, 1972, *15*, 876–882.

Shriner, T. H. A comparison of selected measures with psychological scale values of language development. *Journal of Speech and Hearing Research*, 1967, *10*, 828–835.

Shriner, T. H., & Sherman, D. An equation for assessing language development. *Journal of Speech and Hearing Research*, 1967, *10*, 41–48.

Siegel, G. M. The use of language tests. *Language, Speech, and Hearing Services in the Schools*, 1975, *6*, 211–217.

Sloane, H., & MacAulay, B. Teaching and environmental control of verbal behavior. In H. Sloane & B. MacAulay (Eds.), *Operant procedures in remedial speech and language disorders*. Boston: Houghton Mifflin, 1968.

Smith, A. Objective indices of severity of chronic aphasia in stroke patients. *Journal of Speech and Hearing Disorders*, 1971, *36*, 167–207.

Steer, M. D., & Drexler, H. G. Predicting later articulation ability from kindergarten tests. *Journal of Speech and Hearing Disorders*, 1960, *25*, 391–397.

Stromsta, C. A spectrographic study of disfluencies labeled as stuttering by parents. *De Therapia Vocis Et Loquellae*, 1965, *I*, 317–320.

Szasz, T. S. The myth of mental illness. *American Psychologist*, 1960, *15*, 113–118.

Turton, L. J. Diagnostic implications of articulation testing. In W. D. Wolfe & D. J. Goulding (Eds.). *Articulation and learning*. Springfield, Ill.: Charles C Thomas, 1973.

Ullman, L. P., & Krasner, L. A. *A psychological approach to abnormal behavior*. Englewood Cliffs, N.J.: Prentice-Hall, 1969.

Van Riper, C. Study of the thoracic breathing of stutterers during expectancy and occurrence of stuttering spasm. *Journal of Speech Disorders*, 1936, *1*, 61–72.

Van Riper, C. *Speech correction: Principles and methods*. Englewood Cliffs, N.J.: Prentice-Hall, 4th ed., 1963.

Van Riper, C. *The nature of stuttering*. Englewood Cliffs, N.J.: Prentice-Hall, 1971.

Van Riper, C., & Erickson, R. A predictive screening test of articulation. *Journal of Speech and Hearing Disorders*, 1969, *34*, 214–219.

Vignola, L. A. Evolution of aphasia and language rehabilitation: A retrospective exploratory study. *Cortex*, 1964, *1*, 344–367.

West, R., Ansberry, M., & Carr, A. *The rehabilitation of speech*. New York: Harper & Row, 3rd ed., 1957.

Winitz, H. *Articulatory acquisition and behavior*. New York: Appleton-Century-Crofts, 1969.

4

Recording and Assessing Behaviors

Anyone who is an avid sports fan is well versed in the performance of many of the players he or she watches. This awareness of player performance is increased as one views the TV screen where batting averages, passes received, yardage run, and the like are flashed on the screen. What the spectator does not know is the extent to which the behavioral data of each player is analyzed. An example of a behavioral scoring system some coaches use to analyze baseball player performance is shown in Figure 4–1. This information enables the coach to reconstruct and to analyze the performance of each team member. Football coaches use similar forms and record data from viewing slow motion movie film. Coaches of hockey, badminton, tennis, basketball, and many other sports employ similar techniques enabling them to carefully analyze behavior. Not only is post-game performance analyzed, but also coaches keep accurate records of performance during the game. Based on these records, substitution of players is made and specific plays are recommended during the course of the game. The spectator's knowledge of the coach's scrutiny of each player is limited to performance averages, yet, there are great quantities of data kept about each player's performance.

Keeping data of the player's performance is the coach's way of assessing each individual. He will use these data to achieve goals during future practice sessions.

FIGURE 4–1. Record Used To Analyze Baseball Player Performance

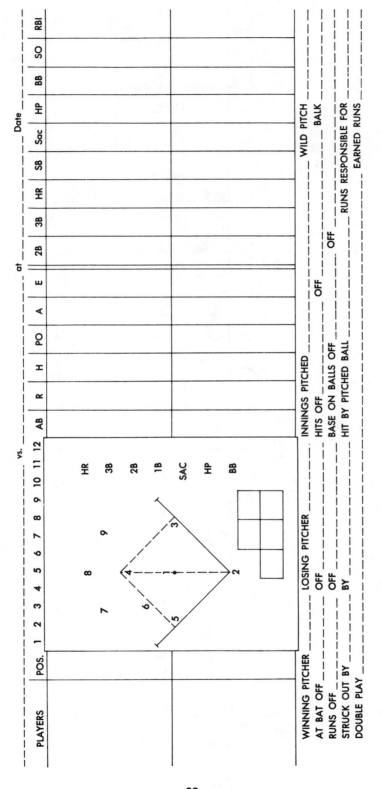

INDIVIDUAL RECORD OF STATISTICS

TEAM: _____

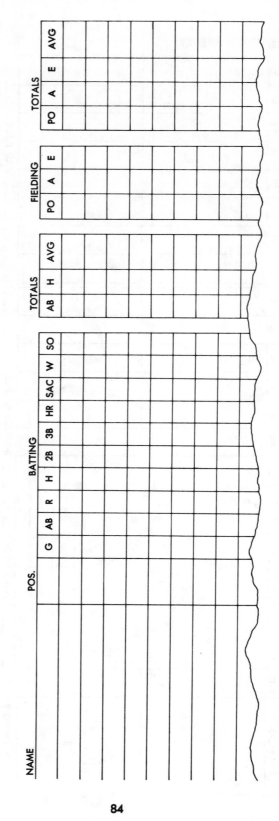

NAME	POS.	BATTING										TOTALS			FIELDING			TOTALS			
		G	AB	R	H	2B	3B	HR	SAC	W	SO	AB	H	AVG	PO	A	E	PO	A	E	AVG

The quarterback who consistently overthrows the football will be given practice on accuracy throws. The base runner who is from 1 to 3 seconds slower than his teammates running to first base will be assigned daily running exercises. The basketball player who frequently misses foul shots will receive more instructive training in this skill. Past player performance becomes a prescription for future instruction. It may also be indicative of the quality of prior instruction and may alter the coach's teaching strategy. Of course, other variables are also important, such as physical condition of the player, his motivational state, his cooperation with other players, etc.

Speech pathologists have much to learn from the way behavioral assessments are made in athletics as well as from the coach's scientific approach to behavioral analysis. Anyone who has achieved excellence in athletics knows that practice is only one of the ingredients of success. A coach's careful analysis of the performance, plus his corrective feedback, are vital if improvement is to occur. Speech clinicians are engaged in this same sort of activity. We establish goals, provide instruction, analyze behavior, and give corrective feedback in order to obtain behavioral change. Obviously, our final objectives are different from those in athletics, but the process is strikingly similar.

While behavioral assessment procedures have been used for some time by other disciplines, the concept is relatively new in speech pathology. Turton (1973) notes that most speech clinicians administer a diagnostic test before initiating therapy but make no effort to measure progress during the therapy period until therapy is terminated. During therapy, clinicians make only subjective evaluations. These evaluations are important, of course, but the criticism of most traditional techniques is that they do not yield sufficient information to be of any use. Most of us are familiar with thermometer charts and space rocket progress indicators which reflect an individual's achievement during therapy. A typical charting of this type of progress indicator appears in Figure 4–2 (see Van Riper, 1963, p. 287).

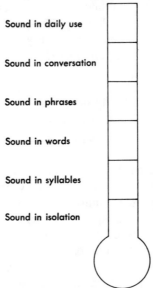

FIGURE 4–2. Thermometer-Type Articulation Progress Chart

In addition to this type of progress chart, many clinicians keep anecedotal records of a child's progress in terms of a written evaluation, such as "He was able to produce /k/ in all positions," or "Voice quality was much improved today." Clinicians may be aware that progress is or is not being made, but without an accurate knowledge of increase or decrease in the frequency of the correct response, it is impossible to evaluate the effectiveness of specific therapy procedures.

We are not only concerned with assessing behaviors of our cases, we are also concerned with the performance of clinicians. For over two decades, The American Speech and Hearing Association has attempted to evaluate the proficiency of practicing clinicians. Upon meeting academic requirements, passing a speech and hearing pathology test, and successfully completing a year of supervised work, the applicant is entitled to a certificate of clinical competency, which indicates the recipient is qualified to work in the field of speech pathology or audiology. Many states are considering legislation which will legalize this qualification process. The student clinician is also assessed during the training period with regard to academic performance and to clinical skills. Each professor, or clinical supervisor, has a personal, evaluative "yardstick" which includes observations of a wide variety of student behaviors. Assessment of performance, whether that performance is the clinician's or the patient's, has been a common practice in speech pathology and audiology.

There have been, and will continue to be, attempts to improve the quality of assessment procedures. There has been a considerable interest in improving assessment procedures in the past 10 to 15 years, not only in speech pathology, but also in all fields of psychology from counseling to animal experimentation. White and Haring's (1976) text, written to assist classroom teachers to improve instruction, presents detailed information about effective assessment procedures. Menges (1975) reviews current literature relating to assessment procedures used by professionals in teaching, engineering, medicine, and law. Assessment in the treatment of behavioral disorders has been a key factor in planning therapeutic strategies (Mischel, 1968). We shall examine the role assessment plays in psychology in terms of the behavior of both the patient and the speech pathologist.

Assessing
Behaviors
of the Case

The main purpose of assessment is to determine if the behaviors of the individual are *changing*. We also want to find out *why* they are changing. By establishing functional relationships between stimulus conditions (therapeutic procedures) and changes in response characteristics (speech behaviors), we can establish S–R laws. These laws will allow us to both control and to predict behavior. Without careful assessment, we are unable to determine precisely what instructional procedures are best suited to control behavior.

Objectivity is extremely important in making assessments of behavior. This requires the precise definition of the behavior under observation as stated in chapter 3;

the behavior should be publicly observable, have a definite beginning and ending, and should be repeatable. Anyone should be able to *count* each occasion of the behavior. Fortunately, most of the behaviors we deal with in speech therapy are observable and countable.

The conscientious speech clinician will probably observe almost every occasion of the target response that occurs during therapy. It would be ideal if all of these observations could be recorded and analyzed. But for the most part, this would be a very time-consuming task, too burdensome for most clinicians. Instead, many clinicians prefer to *probe* behavior by taking a sample of the behavior during therapy. This enables the clinician to make an accurate inference about the remainder of the individual's behavior. One special probe device, a *criterion test,* reflects the objectives of the particular lesson. In an /s/ articulation instructional program, Mowrer, Baker, and Schutz (1968) used criterion tests as probes following approximately each 100 responses. Irwin and Griffith (1973) used pre- and posttraining probes of 20 training words to test mastery of articulation skills. Obtaining periodic samples of behavior during therapy is a common practice found in most all types of programmed therapy, as well as in research studies involving therapy (Diedrich, 1971; Elbert et al., 1967). Data from these samples are used to determine the effectiveness of the procedures and when to introduce new materials or skills.

If possible, it is wise to make a permanent record of the behavior probes. The use of an audio, or in some cases, a videotape recorder is the best means of recording behavior since it allows the clinician to check performance at a later time or recheck questionable responses. A hand counter is an effective means of recording responses as they occur. I have used the cumulation of a series of lights as a method of recording the occurrence of responses. Such a device is shown in Figure 4–3. Usually an *X*

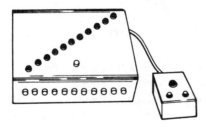

FIGURE 4–3. Reinforcement Display Panel

or a check mark indicates correct responses and a zero indicates incorrect responses when pencil and paper techniques are used to record behavioral data. In some cases, the child can be taught to record her own correct and incorrect responses. Some clinicians suggest children be taught to use wrist counters to simplify tabulation of responses. Stopwatches are often used to record precise time samples of behaviors. Sometimes teacher's aides, volunteer observers, or parents are asked to help the clinician record behaviors.

We must be consistent in the way we assess the child's behavior. If you reward the child occasionally for correct responses but other times you do not, the performances may differ because of inconsistent rewards, not because of instructional variables. Also, try to be consistent in the number of samples taken. A probe of three responses might present a much different picture than would a probe of 30 responses. Be sure to take enough samples to be representative of the behaviors you are evaluating.

What Calculations Tell You

There are two ways data can be presented once it is collected: (1) as a percentage, or (2) as rate. Calculating the percentage of correct and incorrect responses would, at first, seem to be the easiest procedure to assess most speech behavior observations. The chief advantage of percentages is that they equalize different sample sizes and are easy to calculate.

It is convenient to use percentages to compare Probe A in which 28 correct and five incorrect responses were counted with Probe B in which 68 correct responses were counted along with 18 incorrect ones. From the calculation shown in Example 1, it is clear that Probe A resulted in more correct responses in terms of *percent correct* than Probe B. Thus, we are able to compare two behavior samples equally even though the number of opportunities for total behaviors differ greatly.

Example 1

To find the percentage of correct responses in Probe A:

$28 + 5 = 33$ Total responses

$28 \div 33 = 85\%$ Percent correct

To find the percentage of correct responses in Probe B:

$68 + 18 = 86$ Total responses

$68 \div 86 = 79\%$ Percent correct

A percentage statement reflects two behaviors: the proportion of both correct and incorrect behaviors. Making a statement about a child's correct percentage also says something about her error percentage. Percentages are used when we want to find out about the *accuracy* of an individual's performance, that is, how the number of correct responses compare to the number of incorrect responses. But accuracy is only one dimension which can show improvement of a behavior—it is not always the most important way of showing this improvement. For example, a stutterer may be fluent on 100% of the words spoken, but if we consider his rate of speaking, we may find that he is speaking very slowly. When asked to read faster, fluency may drop to 70%. Percentages tell us nothing about the speed or number of responses sampled. In high school, as a seat-warmer for the school basketball team, I had the highest percentage of baskets scored—100%! No other team member came near that mark; yet, the coach rarely put me in the game longer than three minutes. Based upon such an excellent scoring record, why do you think he was so reluctant about putting me in the game? He knew how I acquired such an accuracy record. You see, I only shot the ball once, and fortunately, it went through the basket. Had I shot another time and missed, my average would have fallen to

50%. One more miss would have reduced my average to 33⅓%, far below that of every other team member. The coach knew my accuracy record during practice periods was pretty bad.

You can understand now that if your assessment of a child's behavior includes only a few responses, sampled only from the speech therapy setting, you would not get an accurate picture of her performance. Also, if two percentages, one representing a large number of responses, the other representing a very small number of responses, are compared, the conclusions drawn from the comparisons may be very inaccurate. But if the conditions under which samples gathered are similar and the sizes of the samples are similar, then percentage comparisons constitute an effective means of treating data, providing you are interested only in response accuracy.

The second means we have of assessing behavior is to calculate rate of response. Rate of behaviors allows us to compare behaviors taken over different *time* periods. If, for example, Bill produced 80 correct responses during a 5-minute session and 40 correct responses during a 3-minute session, calculating the average rate of responding per minute allows us to compare the two observations. These computations are shown in Example 2. Session 1 yielded the highest number of correct

Example 2

To calculate rate of response:

$$80 \div 5 = 16 \qquad \text{Correct RPM session 1}$$
$$40 \div 3 = 13.3 \qquad \text{Correct RPM session 2}$$

responses per minute. Rate gives us information that percentage does not reveal. From rate figures we can calculate the number of responses per unit of time. If the correct and incorrect rates per minute are both known, then an accuracy statement can also be made about the data using percentage. Consider the child whose correct response rate is 8.5 per minute and whose incorrect rate is 2.3 per minute. The percentages of correct and incorrect calculations are shown in Example 3.

Example 3

To find percent of correct and incorrect responses:

$$8.5 + 2.3 = 10.8 \qquad \text{Total RPM}$$
$$8.5 \div 10.8 = 79\% \qquad \text{Percent correct RPM}$$
$$2.3 \div 10.8 = 21\% \qquad \text{Percent incorrect RPM}$$

Thus, we are able to calculate both amount and accuracy from statements about rate of response. It was once felt accuracy was the only important factor in therapy sessions. Percentage statements were best suited for this purpose. But there is an increasing amount of evidence to indicate that rate of response, that is, how many responses an individual makes, may be a better indicator of a person's ability to maintain, generalize, and apply the skill outside the therapy setting. In most all situations, rate of behavior provides us with more information, imposes fewer constraints, and takes no more effort to calculate than percent correct or incorrect alone. The same cautions about selecting samples for percentage calculations also hold for sampling behavior rates. Rate samples should be taken under similar conditions and for similar time lengths if they are to be compared.

Charting Behaviors

Progress charts: There are numerous types of behavior charts that display a permanent record of the individual's behavior. Colored stars are often used on charts to indicate a child's successes. Each time the child reaches an objective or produces a certain number of correct responses, a colored star is added behind her name. Accumulating stars seem to provide effective motivation to children but tell us little about the child's daily achievement.

"Rocket to the moon" and "thermometer" charts are similar to star charts and portray how far the child has progressed toward some therapy goal. These charts are fun to make and add to the decor of the therapy room. Children strive hard to move their rockets ahead. Bar or line charts can be equally motivating. The clinician should use these devices as incentive builders; but for assessment purposes, there are other charts which will provide much more precise information about behavior change.

Recording time: In order to accurately assess the individual behaviors and relate these behaviors to therapy procedures, we need to record data from the behavior probe of each child for every session. There are two ways to record the passage of time on a chart. One is to record results from each therapy session; the other uses calendar days (see Figure 4–4).

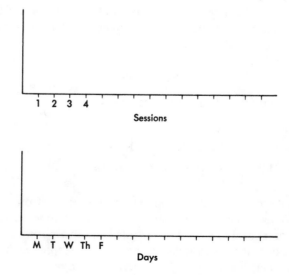

FIGURE 4-4. Ordinance Showing Sessions And Days

Recording data for each session would be economical since many clinicians contact cases only two or three times weekly. Each session would show data. But the problem with using only session times is that you are unable to see the effects absences from therapy sessions have upon response rate and accuracy. By recording calendar days, we obtain a much better picture of the child's overall rate of development. We can also easily compare the performance of two different individuals over the same time period by laying one chart over the other. If sessions were used instead of calendar days, a child receiving therapy once a week could not be compared equally with the one who received therapy three times a week. Calendar days provide us with valuable information about the effects of passage of time upon behavior and is the preferred method of recording behavioral data.

The percentage chart: Percentage charts are simple to construct and easy to read. Both correct and incorrect percentages can be recorded on equal interval graph paper, which is inexpensive and available in most stationery shops. Figure 4–5 illustrates a percentage graph using calendar days as intervals. As was mentioned previously, this type of chart is useful when you wish to record information about the child's response accuracy, but it tells us nothing about his rate of responding.

Charting raw data: Sometimes the clinician may wish to record the actual *number* of responses, rather than record an average or percentage. For example, Shelton et al. (1967) used a raw data chart similar to the one shown in Figure 4–6 to display the number of correct responses on a speech production task. A total of 30 items

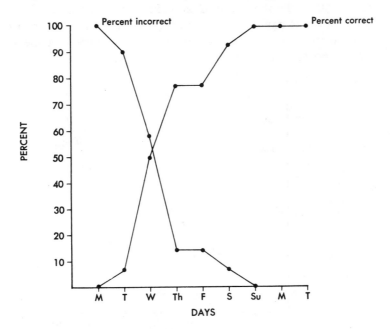

*FIGURE 4–5. Percent Chart Showing Percent Correct And
Incorrect Using Calendar Days*

was presented. Each point shows the number of items produced correctly during each testing session. The points are connected to indicate the trend of the child's progress.

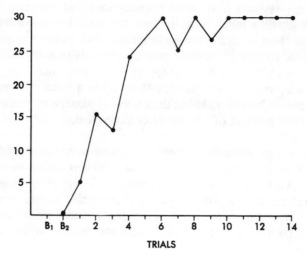

FIGURE 4–6. Chart Of Correct Responses Per Session

Skinner (1959) took the raw data from his animal experimentation and recorded these data cumulatively. That is, if 40 responses were recorded on the first day, 38 on the second, 50 on the third, and 62 on the fourth day, then the points on the graph would be shown as day one, 40; day two, 78; day three, 128; and day four, 190. Such a cumulative record is shown in Figure 4–7. Note that the line never descends. If no responses are made, the line is horizontal.

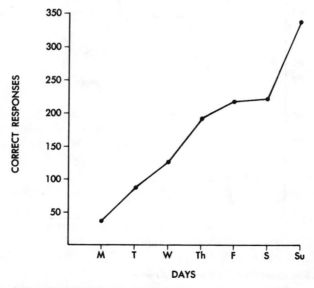

FIGURE 4–7. Cumulative Record Of Correct Responses

The plateau between days 5 and 6 reflect that no responses were produced. A steep incline like the one between days 6 and 7 indicates high rates of response. By relating the slope of the line to the introduction of variables like instruction, shock, reward, and the like, one can determine the effects these variables have upon response rates. Cumulative record graphs are encountered widely in research reports written by behavioral psychologists, especially those written during the 1960s. They have seldom been used by speech clinicians as a method for charting speech behaviors.

The rate chart shown as equal intervals: Rates of behavior are usually recorded in terms of the average number of responses occurring in 1 minute. Rates can just as easily be computed on a per second or per hour basis, but per minute figures are more practical to use as a measure of speech behaviors. Rates may be plotted on an equal interval graph as shown in Figure 4–8 using either calendar days or

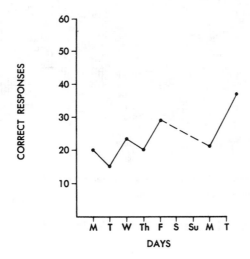

FIGURE 4–8. *Correct Responses Plotted On An Equal Interval Graph*

sessions as a time basis. In this case, a dotted line separates the 2 days over the weekend during which no data were taken. This is called an equal interval graph because the ordinate is divided into equal intervals just as a ruler is divided into equal intervals. The distance from 10 to 20 is exactly the same as the distance from 50 to 60 since both are separated by 10.

A Universal Behavior Graph was designed by Johnson (1970) to overcome some of the limitations found in making one's own graph paper or using the common graph paper available in most stationery shops. Johnson's linear equal interval graph has the following features: (1) it allows for a variety of labels on the ordinate, such as a number, rate, or percentage; (2) the numbering system on the ordinate can vary greatly using a multiplicative factor and/or additive factor; (3) there is room for a large number of intervals on the abscissa; and (4) it is simple and quick to use.

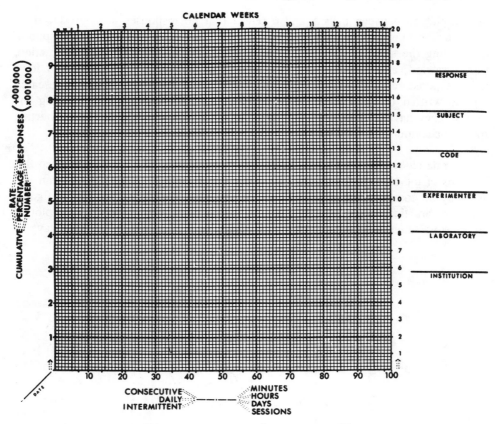

FIGURE 4–9. A Universal Behavior Graph (Reprinted By Permission Of
James Johnston, University Of Florida)

This graph is reproduced in Figure 4–9. It can also be used to record data cumulatively if desired.

The rate chart shown as a ratio: The frequency of behaviors can be plotted on a different type of chart which uses ratios on the ordinates rather than equal intervals. The data presented on the chart shown in Figure 4–8 are now plotted on the ratio chart in Figure 4–10. These data now appear quite different when plotted on a ratio chart. Ratio charts show the amount of *proportional* change. Notice that the distance between 10 and 20 is much greater than the distance from 50 to 60, although there are 10 points between each. But consider that 20 is twice as much as 10, whereas 60 is certainly not twice the value of 50. That is why the proportional difference between 10 and 20 is greater than the difference between 50 and 60. Equal interval and ratio charts are shown in Figure 4–11, which illustrates the differences between these two types of charts. When a response is doubled, the ratio chart always represents this fact with a line that is the same distance between the two points. Therefore, we would assume that the proportional increase is the same in all of the following situations: 2 to 4, 9 to 18, 32 to 64, 800 to 1,600. A proportional representation will show that each increase is the same. Each set of numbers

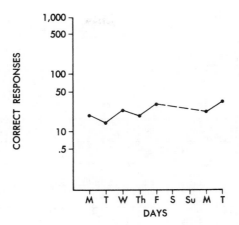

FIGURE 4–10. Correct Responses Plotted On An Equal Proportional Graph

represents the same proportion of increase, which is a 100% increase. An equal interval graph would display different amounts of increases for each group; a very small increase from 2 to 4, but a very large increase from 800 to 1,600, although in both instances, the ratio is the same.

The ratio graph is used in many fields of science. The ordinate increases logarithmically to show proportional changes. It appears that most things in nature change proportionately. The standard audiogram uses a logarithmic ratio for the measurement of increments in hearing acuity because of the way we perceive increase of intensity. Only recently have educators seen the advantages of using such a graph to chart progress in the behavior of children. O. R. Lindsley (1964), one of the first psychologists to use logarithmic charting, developed the Standard Behavior Chart (see Figure 4–12) as a means of standardizing behavior measurement. Mowrer (1969a) later showed how a similar logarithmic chart could be used to record speech behaviors. Diedrich (1971) also illustrated how logarithmic charting could be used advantageously by speech pathologists. Diedrich (1973) developed a booklet, a 16 mm film, and a tape recording to teach speech clinicians how to use logarithmic charting to record speech behaviors. These charting procedures were used by Johnson (1975) to record daily instances of vocal abuse by children being

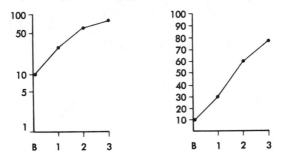

FIGURE 4–11. Comparison Between Interval And Proportional
            Graphing Of The Same Data

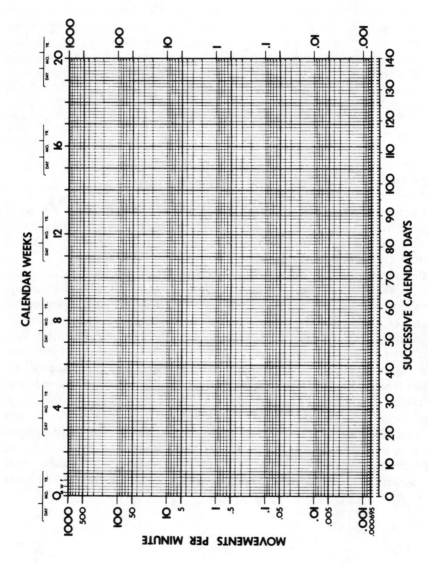

FIGURE 4-12. Standard Behavior Chart (Reprinted By Permission Of O. R. Lindsley, Available From Behavior Research Co., Box 2251, Kansas City, Kansas 66103)

96

treated for voice disorders. Ryan (1974) used logarithmic charting procedures to graph data from stutterers.

The complexity of the logarithmic chart, such as the one developed by Lindsley, may discourage the speech clinician from using it. It would seem easier to simply record "percent correct" on an equal interval graph. There are some instances where this is possible, but if we are interested in improving our instructional techniques through assessment procedures, we need more precise behavioral measurements. White and Haring (1976) point out that use of logarithmic charting is the foundation of exceptional teaching. Charted data allow us to determine what the teacher does, or should do, to help the child acquire new skills.

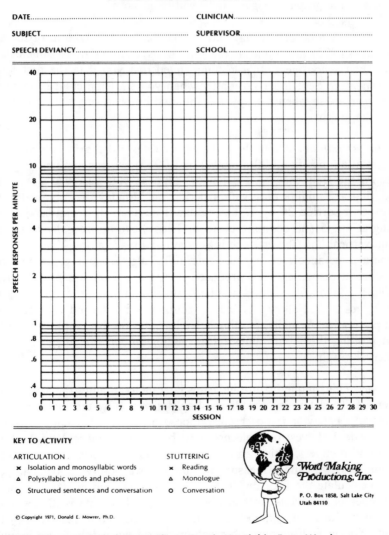

FIGURE 4–12B. *Mowrer's 2-Cycle Logarithmic Graph (Available From Word Making Productions, Box 15038, Salt Lake City, Utah 84115)*

There are several other advantages of using logarithmic charting. A wide range of behaviors can be recorded. Behaviors which occur as seldom as once in a 1,000 minutes (once in 16½ hours) to those which occur as frequently as 1,000 times a minute can be documented on this chart. Several different behavior rates from the same individual can be recorded simultaneously on the same chart; also, changes in rates of each behavior can be compared. The length of time taken to sample a behavior, as well as the total number of responses possible if limits are placed on size of sampled behavior, can be calculated from the floor and ceiling of the chart. Projected target dates for behavioral increments and decrements can be noted and assessed in light of the individual's performance.

To aid the reader in learning to use logarithmic graphs, detailed descriptions of each feature of the graph in Figure 4–12 will be given next.

Calendar days. A total of 140 days are marked across the bottom of the abscissa, while the weeks (20) are found at the top abscissa line. This is sufficient time to record one half school year. It is recommended that you date the first Sunday as the first Sunday in September no matter when you start the child in therapy. This allows us to establish when therapy was initiated by observing the position of first entries on the graph.

Movements per minute. Along the ordinate are rates of behavior which occur from .001 per minute (once in 1,000 minutes) to 1,000 times per minute.

To record the frequency of a behavior, suppose you observed 24 correct /s/ sounds during a 3-minute observation period on Monday. To obtain the average rate of response, divide 24 by 3. The resultant number, 8, is plotted on the graph by starting at line 5 and counting up to 8. Then move horizontally to the right to the second vertical line (the first one is Sunday) and place a dot. You may also wish to plot the average incorrect response rate, following the same procedure. Suppose only 2 incorrect responses were produced during the 3-minute probe. Dividing 3 into 2 yields .6⅔ or .7 in round numbers. Begin counting at .5 on the graph and move up 2 lines to .7. Follow this line horizontally to the second vertical line (Monday) and place an *x*. Actually, plotting behavior rates on this graph is no more difficult than plotting threshold values on an audiogram or percentage figures on an equal interval graph.

Record floor. This unique feature indicates how many minutes the sample behavior was observed. To determine the floor, simply divide 1 by the number of minutes the individual's behavior is observed. Suppose a person's behavior is observed 3 minutes. Divide 1 (lowest possible non-zero behavior frequency) by 3 to get .3⅓ or .3 in round numbers. This means if the individual's rate is not at least .3, or 1 every 3 minutes, we cannot measure it. Suppose we observe a behavior over 20 minutes; to calculate the floor divide 1 by 20. The dividend is .05. This means the lowest number of behaviors we can observe during 1 minute is .05, which is the same as 1 behavior in 20 minutes. It would be impossible to record .01 behaviors per minute during a 20-minute observation period since this figure would mean the behavior occurred once in 100 minutes. Consequently, when we know where the floor is located on the logarithmic graph, and we know how long the behavior was observed. The floor is represented by a dotted horizontal line (see Figure 4–13). Remember, to calculate the floor, always divide the observation time into 1. If you observed no correct behaviors during a 3-minute observation probe, record a question mark just below the record floor. This allows for the possibility that correct behaviors may be occurring at other times of the day when you are not observing. If you observed behavior 24 hours a day and no correct behaviors were observed, then there would be no floor and a true 0 score could be recorded.

Record ceiling. If only a certain number of behaviors are observed during a fixed period of time, then a ceiling is established. For example, if a test containing 30 items is administered and 5 minutes are allowed to administer the test, then the record ceiling would be 30 divided by 5, or an average of 6 responses per minute. We would place a dotted horizontal line at 6. This would represent the most responses the person could average per minute. If 7 responses were produced per minute, this would mean 35 responses were produced during the 5-minute testing period which, of course, would be impossible. A record ceiling merely indicates a limit was placed on both the amount of responses allowed and the amount of time to produce them.

Acceleration and deceleration targets. A dot is used to record behavior rates we want to increase, while an *x* is used for behavior rates we want to decrease. When daily observations are made, the dots and *x*'s are connected with lines. They are not connected if days intervene when no assessments are made. Therefore, use dots to indicate correct responses, *x*'s for incorrect responses.

The aim. The aim is the *goal* of the instructional program. We should have some idea of how many correct responses the individual should be making at some future date. The symbol for the desired correct response rate per minute is an upward pointing arrow with a line through it, ⩱. A downward arrow with a line through it, ⩲, is the symbol for the target of deceleration.

Phase-change lines. Each time a change is made in the instructional program, a vertical line is drawn ¼ day before the day line on which we record the results of the first assessment of the new program goal or task. For example, if you change from using pictorial stimuli to evoke speech to spontaneous speaking situations, you would want to indicate this change since it may affect both performance and aims.

Notes. The clinician can make notes directly on the chart, adding important information about the behaviors or instructional materials.

White and Haring (1976) have prepared a useful calculator which is suitable for Standard Behavior Charts like the one in Figure 4–12. A rate finder is illustrated in Figure 4–14. These calculators make plotting very simple and save calculation time.

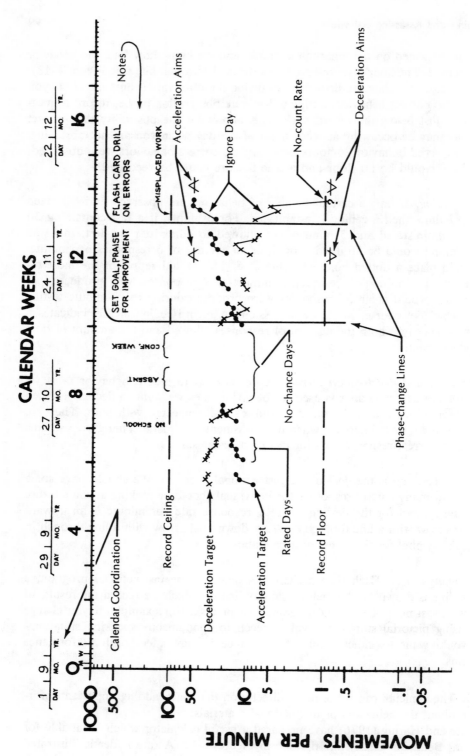

FIGURE 4-13. Data Which Can Be Plotted On A Six-Cycle Chart
(Reprinted By Permission Of Charles E. Merrill)

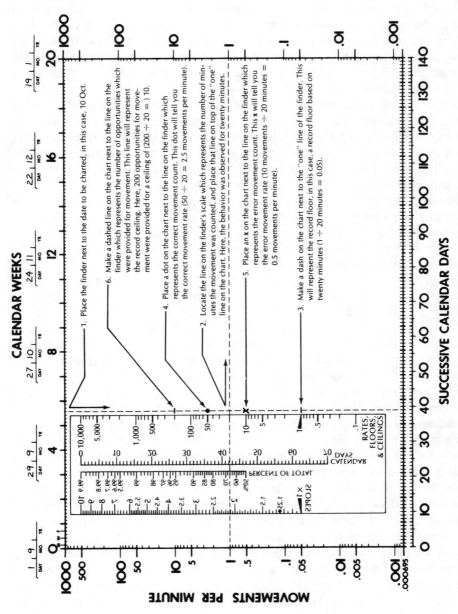

FIGURE 4–14. *Rate Finder For A Six-Cycle Graph (Reprinted By Permission of Charles E. Merrill)*

101

Calculator *A* is used to plot correct and incorrect rates. Place the rate finder next to the day line you wish to plot and align it so that the number of minutes the sample was observed lines up with the number 1 on the ordinate of the graph. In this case, the behavior was observed for 20 minutes. Make a dash next to the number 1 on the rate finder. This represents the floor. Place a dot next to the total number of correct responses made in the 20-minute session. Place an *x* beside the total number of incorrect responses produced. Using this calculator, there is no need to make divisions or find rate per minute.

Calculator *B* gives the percent of correct responses. Simply place 50% beside the incorrect rate and read off the correct percentage where it lines up with the percentage number on the calculator scale. In this case, 83% of the responses were correct. Subtracting this figure from 100% reveals 17% of the responses were incorrect. If incorrect responses are higher, then conversely, the upper percentage figure will represent the percentage of incorrect responses.

White and Haring (1976) also suggest a method of using data plotted on this chart which will enable the teacher to evaluate progress and to make corrective changes in teaching strategies. First, an aim rate is set using the symbol A to represent correct response rate. Suppose we select the 30-item test of /s/ words, the spontaneous production task (SPT) devised by Elbert et al. (1967) or a similar type test and allow the child 1½ minutes to say the items. The floor, in this case, would be set at .7 (1.0 ÷ 1.5 = .66). Suppose the child says two of the 30 items correctly. His starting place would be at 1.3 (2.0 ÷ 1.5 = 1.3). The aim, or goal, is to say all 30 words in 1½ minutes, or 20 in 1 minute (30 ÷ 1.5 = 20). We can anticipate when the child should attain this goal in the future, say 3 weeks from now, and place the A symbol at line 20 on the vertical ordinate and 21 lines from the starting point along the abscissa. These have been plotted on the chart in Figure 4–16. A line is then drawn from the starting point to the aim. This represents the minimum celeration line. Ideally, the child's score on each of the probe tests given at the conclusion of each day's therapy should be on, or above, the minimum celeration line. Figure 4–16 shows the progress a child made during 10 therapy sessions. Note that only once did his performance drop below the celeration line. White and Haring suggest if three consecutive performances drop below the line, changes should be made in therapy plans or a new celeration slope should be drawn.

The value of drawing celeration slope lines is that we have objective evidence of whether or not our therapy is effective. The slope line sets daily behavioral goals for us to achieve; they also hold us accountable for our work. Of course, much depends on where we set our aims. If our aims are too low, we may expect too little from our therapy efforts; if they are too high, we may constantly be disappointed. White and Haring suggest several techniques which help the teacher set realistic aims. One way is to base improvement rates upon past improvement rates of the child's peers. Check the child's improvement rates in other areas of learning if classroom teachers are charting his performance. Only through experience gained from making trials and errors in setting aim points and slope lines can one arrive at realistic criteria for establishing these anticipated levels of performance.

Up to this point, we have discussed plotting correct responses. Deceleration aims for wrong responses can also be set and slope lines drawn for them as well. The

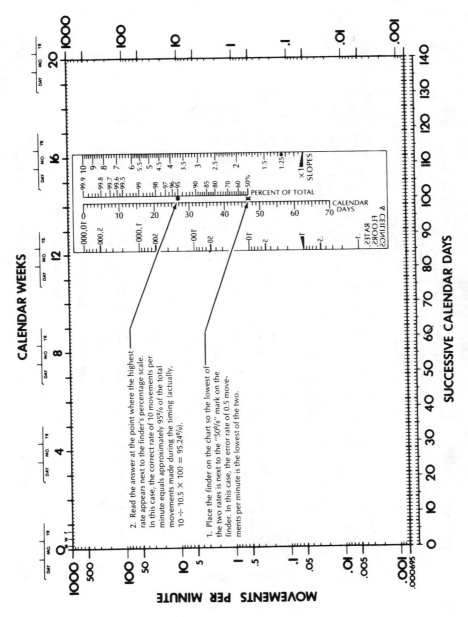

FIGURE 4–15. *Using The Rate Finder To Determine Percentage Of Response*
(*Reprinted By Permission Of Charles E. Merrill*)

103

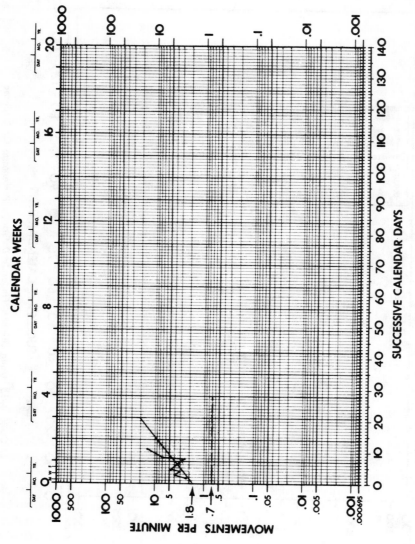

FIGURE 4–16. Minimum Celeration Line And Performance Of The Child On
The Probe Test During 10 Therapy Sessions

same things that apply to acceleration behaviors also apply to behaviors we wish to decelerate.

A great deal more could be written about the use of the Standard Behavior Chart. The material in this chapter serves only to introduce the reader to the procedures and benefits which can be derived from charting observations on a logarithmic graph. I predict an increased use of these charting procedures by classroom teachers, especially those in special education where precision teaching techniques are used. The speech clinician will need to understand the use of precision charting techniques so she can be conversant with other teachers who use these procedures with children who attend speech classes.

Mastery of the charting procedures demands considerable effort in order to learn how to use them effectively. They also require time for analysis, but accountability movements in education are creating a demand for precision recording procedures. There was a time when the speech clinician could satisfy her supervisor with an attendance sheet of her case enrollment, along with her promise to "do my best." Today, this pledge is no longer accepted by knowledgeable educators. Precision assessment techniques are being developed and used in all areas of education. We in speech pathology can only benefit from this expansion. Those who do not possess the skills for using effective assessment techniques may find it difficult to obtain or keep jobs in systems geared up for precision teaching. It remains the schools' primary responsibility to provide students with skills in those areas through courses and workshop presentations.

Assessing
Behaviors
of Clinicians

The American Speech and Hearing Association (ASHA) is vitally concerned about the quality of services offered by speech clinicians. ASHA (1973) has adopted an assessment procedure to evaluate all speech clinicians and audiologists who wish to be certified by that organization. An assessment is made of the speech clinician's professional training in terms of (1) accumulation of 60 semester hours of coursework pertaining to speech, language, and hearing; (2) completion of 300 clock hours of supervised, clinical practicum with individuals who have communication disorders; (3) completion of 9 months as a full-time speech clinician under supervision of an approved certified ASHA member; (4) obtaining a passing grade on a national examination in speech pathology (Perkins et al., 1970); and (5) application for membership in ASHA. Similar requirements are necessary for certification as an audiologist. In addition, members are expected to abide by a professional Code of Ethics, established by the organization.

These assessments are helpful in screening out unqualified, poorly trained, and even unscrupulous individuals from the profession. Several states now have licensure laws that require speech clinicians and audiologists meet stringent requirements before they can provide services. Many other states are considering such legislation.

It is probable that within 10 years, almost all states will have adopted legal assessment procedures for speech clinicians and audiologists.

The assessment procedures used by ASHA and state governments were not designed to assist the speech clinician to improve his skills or even to help him diagnose communication problems. There is no provision or attempt to rank speech clinicians on a proficiency scale. Either one meets all of the qualifications or the applicant is rejected.

Most clinical supervisors have some criteria which they use to assess speech clinicians. Frequently these criteria include (1) personality factors, such as ability to take criticism, poise, neatness, attitude, and maturity; (2) skills in administering therapy; (3) ability in managing therapy sessions, such as punctuality, conferring with parents, motivating children, organizing therapy materials, and establishing rapport; and (4) academic knowledge as displayed by resourcefulness in solving problems or application of clinical procedures. Some supervisors have developed rating scales which include the above criteria. The resulting score is used to evaluate the clinician's performance and abilities.

Unfortunately, subjective measures such as the ones listed above may be interpreted in many different ways, depending on the ability of the supervisor who makes the evaluations. Also, there are no data to show that there is any relationship between high scores on the evaluation sheets and the remediation of communication problems. For example, a clinician may be untidy, surly to her supervisor, unorthodox in her therapy method, prepare poor lesson plans, and yet, be more productive in terms of remediating communication problems than other clinicians.

An interest in the clinical supervision and assessment procedures used by supervisors in college and university clinics developed during the early 1960s (Anderson, 1974a). Halfond (1964) observed that "One outstanding lack in training is in the supervisory aspect of the clinical practicum." He urged that we give clinical supervision greater attention and offered some suggestions regarding the use of student-parent-supervisor conferences in the evaluation process. Van Ríper (1965) also warned that supervision was a neglected area and should be considered as important as college teaching and research.

Assessment of public school speech clinicians through supervision also has left much to be desired. In a report by Black et al. (1961), 33% of school clinicians polled reported their immediate supervisor never observed their therapy. Another 51% indicated that their superiors visited them only one to three times a year. For the most part, supervisors did not view their role as being an evaluator of the clinicians—this implies that practicing clinicians do not need to be assessed. They have already been assessed during their university training, or by an agency or organization. If we were confident the assessment was a standardized one, or was directly related to ability to remediate communication disorders, and if we could assume there will be no further breakthroughs in the area, then, perhaps, we could agree that practicing speech clinicians do not require further assessment. But this seems highly improbable. Van Hattum (1966) identified five basic issues facing public school clinicians. Two of the five dealt directly with inadequacies in clinical skills: (1) training was not appropriate for the tasks with which he is confronted; and (2) some of the training received was inadequate. Among Van Hattum's recommendations was that there should be more observation of public school therapy by university personnel, and supervision of student clinicians should be improved.

The early and mid-1960s saw publications bring the need for better supervision into focus and prompted several suggestions for how to assess the therapeutic process. Up until this time, subjective evaluations were used, but these methods were not much better than educated guesses. Mowrer, Baker, and Owen (1968) analyzed therapy sessions of seven public school clinicians and found that the clinicians outtalked the children at a ratio of 10:1 and that 40% of the clinicians' verbal statements were unrelated to the goal of changing the speech skills of their cases. Children in the therapy sessions produced a mean of 2.56 target responses per minute. It was suggested that the children's low response rate, along with the large amount of irrelevant conversation, was responsible for poor correction rates among speech clinicians.

In a follow-up article, Mowrer (1969b) identified behaviors of clinicians and children associated with activities that produced low-target response rates and those behaviors associated with high-target response rates. These are presented in Figure 4–17. Behaviors associated with high- and low-accuracy ratios are listed in Figure 4–18. It was suggested that two variables are important to look at when assessing a speech therapy session. One consists of the number of target responses emitted by the case during the therapy session; the other is the number of correct

Behaviors Associated With Low RR

    A. Clinicians' Behaviors

        1. Talking about subjects which were unrelated to evoking the target response (social interchanges, homework assignments, game instructions, etc.).

        2. Re-instructing children who failed to repeat all the words of sentence model.

        3. Ignoring children who were silent.

    B. Children's Behaviors

        1. Talking about subjects unrelated to the target response (social interchange).

        2. Watching others perform motor tasks such as those performed in game and playing activities.

        3. Listening to various auditory stimuli (others responding, word discrimination).

        4. Performing motor tasks which were unrelated to producing the target response (drawing cards, opening easter eggs, cutting and pasting, etc.).

Behaviors Related To High RR

    A. Clinicians' Behaviors

        1. Presenting picture cues containing the target sound.

        2. Presenting auditory cues containing the target sound.

    B. Children's Behaviors

        1. Replying to the teacher's instructions to name or repeat a word or phrase containing the target sound.

FIGURE 4–17. Behaviors Associated With Low And High Response Rates

Clinician Behaviors Related To High RAR

   Recognition of a correct response when that response was correct.

Clinician Behaviors Related To Low RAR

   A. Providing verbal praise ("Good") following an incorrect response.

   B. Presenting tasks beyond the child's skill level.

   C. Ignoring a correct response.

FIGURE 4–18. Behaviors Associated With Low And High Accuracy Rates

responses in relation to the number of wrong responses. Two therapy sessions (X_1 and X_2) were observed from five public school clinicians. The response rates in an adjusted 20-minute therapy session involving three children each were plotted along the abscissa. Ratio was plotted on the ordinate (see Figure 4-19). In session X_1 for clinician C, the children produced 158 target responses during the 20-minute period. For every seven correct responses produced, one was incorrect, so the accuracy ratio was 7:1. A session representing a high response rate and a high accuracy ratio is illustrated by session X_1 of clinician D. In this case, 568 target responses were produced at a rate of 34 correct to 1 incorrect.

   As shown in Figure 4–19, clinicians A, C, and E seemed to be making very little progress with their cases, while clinicians B and D experienced considerable success with changing articulation skills. Clinicians B and D presented many verbal cues, answered correct responses with verbal praise, and discriminated accurately between correct and incorrect responses. Inspection of the performance of clinicians A and E revealed a preponderance of activities which were incompatible with target sound production, inaccurate response recognition, and the presentation of tasks which appeared too difficult for the children to master.

   Two tasks are important for the speech clinician to perform if she is to bring about rapid changes in certain speech behaviors: (1) she needs to provide effective

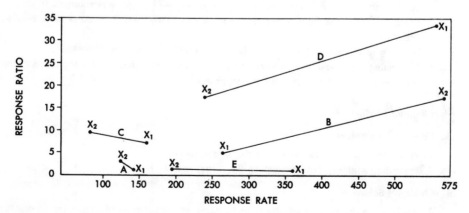

FIGURE 4–19. Response Rate And Ratio Of Two Sessions (X_1 And X_2)
      Of Five Clinicians (A,B,C,D,E)

cues to evoke the desired sound; and (2) correct and incorrect responses must be identified for the child. The clinician's skill and efficiency in performing these tasks is reflected in two measures: response rate and response accuracy. These are objective measures, easily observed and devoid of subjective evaluation. A limitation of this assessment procedure is that it looks at only one phase of the therapy process. Factors such as planning for the session, evaluating progress toward specific goals, conference skills, dealing with special problems, and the like are not considered.

Boone and Prescott (1972) present another approach to the assessment of the clinician's therapy skills. Their system allows the clinician to evaluate his own performance through video and audiotape replay of sections of therapy sessions. The clinician selects for analysis a 5-minute sample of therapy from a 20-minute recording. After listening to the selection, the clinician replays the 5-minute sample and classifies each spoken response according to 1 of 10 categories. These categories and their definitions are listed in Figure 4–20.

Category Number		
1	Explain, Describe	Clinician describes and explains the specific goals or procedures of the session.
2	Model, Instruction	Clinician specifies client behavior by direct modeling or by specific request.
3	Good Evaluative	Clinician evaluates client response and indicates a verbal or non-verbal approval.
4	Bad Evaluative	Clinician evaluates client response as incorrect and gives a verbal or nonverbal disapproval.
5	Neutral-Social	Clinician engages in behavior which is not therapy-goal oriented.
6	Correct Response	Client makes a response which is correct for clinician instruction or model.
7	Incorrect Response	Client makes incorrect response to clinician instruction or model.
8	Inappropriate-Social	Client makes response which is not appropriate for session goals.
9	Good Self-Evaluative	Client indicates awareness of his own correct response.
10	Bad Self-Evaluative	Client indicates awareness of his own incorrect response.

FIGURE 4–20. Boone & Prescott's Assessment Categories Of A Therapy Session
(Reprinted By Permission Of D. Boone, University of Arizona)

The first five categories describe the clinician's verbal behaviors, while the second five describe the responses of the case. The typical therapy session would involve first a statement by the clinician, followed by a response from the child and another response from the clinician, another response from the child and so on. The following dialogue has been scored for you according to this system:

Category	Speaker	Dialogue
5, 1	Clinician	It's good to see you again today, Pat. Are you ready to work on your sounds?"
6	Case	"Yep."
2	Clinician	"All right then, keep your tongue back and say, key."
6	Case	"Key."
3, 2	Clinician	"Right, try it again."
6	Case	"Key."
3, 2	Clinician	"Good, now say, coo."
7	Case	"Too."
4, 2	Clinician	"Nope, you let your tongue come to the front."
8	Case	"Did you see the fire yesterday?"
6, 8	Case	"Coo. That fire was good, wasn't it?"

There will be occasions when it is difficult to assign one of the 10 categories to an utterance, but for the most part, these categories can be used to adequately represent much of the therapy dialogue. Having scored a therapy session, these scores are then placed on a scoring form. The form for the above session is shown in Figure 4–21. The assessments recorded on this chart enable the evaluator to make the following statements regarding percentage of each category:

1. The clinician explained and modeled 31% of the time (6% + 25%).
2. The clinician let the case know he was correct 13% of the time.
3. The clinician let the case know he was wrong 6% of the time.
4. The clinician engaged in social talk 6% of the time.
5. The clinician made 56% of the total comments.
6. The case was correct 25% of the time.
7. The case was wrong 6% of the time.
8. Thirteen percent of the case's responses were not related to therapy goals.
9. The case recognized good responses 0% of the time.
10. The case recognized bad responses 0% of the time.

Finally, the supervisor or clinician can weigh each score in the categories and evaluate the session on a scale of good (10) to poor (1).

This system provides an objective means of assessing behaviors of both the clinician and the case during the therapy session. Boone and Prescott (1972) report that after 3 years experience using this system, they have found that speech clinicians who obtain good results in therapy follow certain patterns, such as 2, 6, 3, and 2, 7, 4. If categories 5 and 8 occupy much time, steps should be taken to reduce extraneous talk.

The practicality of this assessment system was reported by Butler (1974) in an article describing how he used it to evaluate his therapy. He suggested this system

Category Counts	16		Category Counts	16	
Category	No. of Events	% of Total	Category	No. of Events	% of Total
1	1	6	6	4	25
2	4	25	7	1	6
3	2	13	8	2	13
4	1	6	9	0	0
5	1	6	10	0	0
Clinician Total	9	56	Client Total	7	44

Sequence Counts

Sequence	No. of Events
6/3	2
7/4	1
8/1, 2	0

Ratio Scoring	Category		No. of Events		Percent
Correct Response	$\dfrac{6}{6+7}$	=	$\dfrac{4}{4+1}$	=	0.80
Incorrect Response	$\dfrac{7}{6+7}$	=	$\dfrac{1}{4+1}$	=	0.20
Good Eval. Ratio	$\dfrac{6/3}{6}$	=	$\dfrac{2}{4}$	=	0.50
Bad Eval. Ratio	$\dfrac{7/4}{7}$	=	$\dfrac{1}{1}$	=	1.00
Inappro. Response	$\dfrac{8}{6+7+8}$	=	$\dfrac{2}{4+1+2}$	=	0.29
Direct Control	$\dfrac{8/1,2}{8}$	=	$\dfrac{0}{2}$	=	0.00
Socialization	5 + 8	= 1(6%) + 2(13%) =			0.29

Therapy Evaluation	No									Yes
A Good Session	1	— 2	— 3	— 4	— 5	— 6	—⑦	— 8	— 9	
Clinician Effective	1	— 2	— 3	— 4	— 5	— 6	— 7	—⑧	— 9	
Client Effective Progress	1	— 2	— 3	— 4	— 5	— 6	—⑦	— 8	— 9	

FIGURE 4–21. Speech Scoring Form Of Sample Case

could be used by administrators as objective criteria for assessing the performance of clinicians. The appendix of Butler's article contains Boone and Prescott's quick analysis scoring form.

The 10 category analysis system developed by Boone and Prescott was expanded to a 17 category system by Prescott and Tesauro (1974) for use in assessing therapy with aurally handicapped children. Interaction of both parents and clinicians working with children can be analyzed with this system. A scoring system similar to that developed by Boone and Prescott is also used. The description of each category is presented in Figure 4–22.

Category	Description
1—Explain/Describe	Clinician describes, explains, or provides a model for the parent.
2—Input	Clinician or parent provides the child with language input not requiring a response.
3—Clarification	Clinician or parent asks for or gives clarification of a behavior.
4—Auditory Stimulus	Clinician or parent elicits the child's behavior by providing instruction or a direct auditory stimulus.
5—Manual Stimulus	Clinician or parent elicits the child's behavior by providing instruction or a direct manual stimulus.
6—Combined Oral-Manual Stimulus	Clinician or parent elicits the child's behavior by providing instruction or combined auditory and manual stimulus.
7—Good Evaluative	Clinician or parent evaluates the child's response and indicates approval.
8—Bad Evaluative	Clinician or parent evaluates the child's response and indicates disapproval.
9—Neutral Social	Clinician, parent, or child engages in behavior not oriented to session goals.
10—Nonverbal Correct	Child makes a nonverbal response which is correct for the stimulus.
11—Oral Correct	Child makes an oral response which is correct for the stimulus.
12—Manual Correct	Child makes a manual response which is correct for the stimulus.
13—Oral-Manual Correct	Child makes a combined oral and manual response which is correct for the stimulus.
14—Other Correct	Child spontaneously vocalizes in a manner not specifically related to a stimulus from the clinician or the parent.
15—Incorrect	Child makes incorrect response to an instruction or stimulus from the clinician or the parent.
16—Good Self-Evaluative	Child or parent indicates awareness of his own correct behavior.
17—Bad Self-Evaluative	Child or parent indicates awareness of his own incorrect behavior.

FIGURE 4–22. *Seventeen Categories For Describing Events In A Parent-Child-Clinician Therapy Session (Reprinted By Permission Of P. Tesauro, University Of Denver)*

Category totals are computed and percentages of each category are determined for each individual. There are also certain sequences which are scored, like a sequence of 1/2 immediately followed by 6 or 7 followed by 3 or 4. From these data, nine ratios are calculated. These include correct response ratio, incorrect response ratio, reinforcement control ratio, etc. These ratios provide clinicians and parents with objective, quantified information about their interactions with cases.

Boone and Prescott's (1972) 10 category system of therapy assessment is, according to a nationwide survey of college and university speech clinics (Schubert & Aitchison, 1975), one of the best-known and widely used procedures in use. A total of 51½% of the supervisors surveyed knew of the system, and 30% used it in their clinics. Forty-seven percent used some other system, and 26% used no such system. A further modification of the Boone-Prescott Interaction Analysis System was presented by Culatta and Seltzer (1976). They employed a 12 category system to evaluate supervisors' attempts to teach and to advise student speech clinicians. Culatta and Seltzer identified six categories for measuring supervisor's behavior and six for measuring clinician's behavior. Using 5-minute segments of supervisor-clinician interaction, the authors not only recorded each response in one of the 12 categories, but also kept track of how much time was spent by the respondent talking on the category subject. The 12 categories are listed in Figure 4–23.

From this system, it was concluded that supervisors (1) provide very few evaluative comments to the clinicians; (2) probably talk too much; and (3) do not behave the way they say they do. The additional information provided by recording amount of speaking time in each category appeared to be well justified and would appear to strengthen the Boone-Prescott model. After studying Culatta et al.'s (1975) article about confusion among supervisors, with regard to the vague definitions supervisors provide for behaviors they assess in trainees, it seems vitally important that empirical assessment measures be developed. As Anderson (1974b) points out, there is no justifiable excuse for not making explicit those behaviors required for successful intervention.

Two fairly recent techniques designed to assess events in the therapy situation are Schubert's (1974) ABC System and Shriberg et al.'s (1975) W-PACC System. The Analysis of Behavior of Clinicians (ABC) considers 12 categories of both clinician's and client's behaviors. Eight categories are listed for the clinician, three for the client, and one category is shared jointly (see Figure 4–24). Data are recorded at 3-second intervals. A number representing category items from the 12 category list of statements or activities at the end of each 3-second interval is placed on a record sheet. In this way, one is able to determine the amount of time spent on an activity. This feature of accounting for time spent on activities is an advantage over several other systems of therapy assessment. The number of instances that categories occur are then totaled and percentages determined. The data are graphed for analysis by the clinician or the supervisor. Targets for change are as follows:

1. Increase occurrences of Category 9
2. Decrease occurrences of Category 8
3. Decrease occurrences of Category 12

Such a graph of one clinician's therapy session showing analysis of 10 5-minute therapy segments over a 2½-month period is shown in Figure 4–25.

Schubert's ABC System was compared with the system developed by Boone and Prescott using a sample of eight undergraduate speech clinicians conducting speech therapy during three therapy sessions (Schubert & Glick, 1974). The conclusions reached were that although there was a significant difference between the total number of behaviors recorded, the Boone-Prescott system yielding some 891 more behaviors than the ABC System, both systems provided essentially the same information, especially when the session followed the stimulus-response-reinforcement paradigm. But in instances where there was prolonged occurrence of one category, as would be the case if the clinician told a story, the ABC System would record a large number of behaviors (one for each 3-second period), while the Boone-Prescott system would list only one occurrence of that category, regardless of the time factor

Category	Title	Definition	Category	Title	Definition
1	Good Evaluation	Supervisor evaluates observed behavior or verbal report of trainee and gives verbal or nonverbal approval.	Example:	Supervisor:	Pittsburgh sure is a beautiful city in the fall.
			7	Good Self-Evaluation	Clinician provides a positive statement about his own behavior or strategy.
Example:	Supervisor:	You did a good job in reinforcing the correct production of the X sound.	Example:	Clinician:	Sitting on the floor was a really good idea with this child.
2	Bad Evaluation	Supervisor evaluates observed behavior or verbal report of trainee and gives verbal or nonverbal disapproval.	8	Bad Self-Evaluation	Clinician provides a negative statement about his own behavior or strategy.
Example:	Supervisor:	You made a mistake by not reinforcing correct productions of the X sound.	Example:	Clinician:	Boy, it was dumb to sit on the floor with this child.
3	Question	Any interrogative statement made by the supervisor relevant to the client being discussed.	9	Question	Any interrogative statement made by the clinician relevant to the client being discussed.
Example:	Supervisor:	Why did you choose candy as a reinforcer?	Example:	Clinician:	Do you think I should sit on the floor with this child?
4	Strategy	Any statement by the supervisor given to the clinician for future therapeutic intervention.	10	Strategy	Any statement or suggestion made by the clinician for future therapeutic intervention or justification of past therapeutic intervention.
Example:	Supervisor:	I think you will probably keep his attention longer if you give him a piece of candy for a correct response.	Example:	Clinician:	I think in the next session he would pay more attention if I positioned him so that we maintained better eye contact.
5	Observation/ Information	Provision by the supervisor of any relevant comment pertinent to the therapeutic interaction that is not evaluating, questioning, or providing strategy.	11	Observation/ Information	Any statement made by the clinician relevant to the therapeutic interaction that is not evaluating, questioning, or suggesting strategy.
Example:	Supervisor:	It appeared that when you sat on the floor the child gave you more correct responses.	Example:	Clinician:	I notice that when he looks at me he can follow directions better.
6	Irrelevant	Any statement or question made by the supervisor which has no direct relationship to the supervisory process.	12	Irrelevant	Any statement or question made by the clinician which has no direct relationship to the supervisory process.
			Example:	Clinician:	It sure looks like the Steelers are going to win the Super Bowl.

FIGURE 4–23. Twelve Categories Designed To Rate Clinician Behavior In Therapy Sessions (Reprinted By Permission Of R. Culatta, University Of Kentucky)

involved. Thus, for therapy sessions that are poorly planned and executed, the ABC System apparently provides more helpful information regarding time spent on certain activities.

	Category	Definition
Clinician Behavior	1. OBSERVING AND MODIFYING LESSON APPROPRIATELY	Using response or action of the client to adjust goals and/or strategies
	2. INSTRUCTION AND DEMONSTRATION	Process of giving instruction or demonstrating the procedures to be used
	3. AUDITORY AND/OR VISUAL STIMULATION	Questions, cues, and models intended to elicit a response
	4. AUDITORY AND/OR VISUAL POSITIVE REINFORCEMENT OF CLIENT'S CORRECT RESPONSE	Process of giving any positive response to correct client response
	5. AUDITORY AND/OR VISUAL NEGATIVE REINFORCEMENT OF CLIENT'S INCORRECT RESPONSE	Process of giving any negative response to an incorrect client response
	6. AUDITORY AND/OR VISUAL POSITIVE REINFORCEMENT OF CLIENT'S INCORRECT RESPONSE	Process of giving any positive response to an incorrect client response
	7. CLINICIAN RELATING IRRELEVANT INFORMATION AND/OR ASKING IRRELEVANT QUESTIONS	Talking and/or responding in a manner unrelated to changing speech patterns
	8. USING AUTHORITY OR DEMONSTRATING DISAPPROVAL	Changing social behavior for unacceptable to acceptable behavior
Client Behavior	9. CLIENT RESPONDS CORRECTLY	Client responds appropriately, meets expected level
	10. CLIENT RESPONDS INCORRECTLY	Client apparently tries to repond appropriately but response is below expected level
	11. CLIENT RELATING IRRELEVANT INFORMATION AND/OR ASKING IRRELEVANT QUESTIONS	Talking and/or responding in a manner unrelated to changing speech patterns
	12. SILENCE	Absence of verbal and relevant motor behavior

FIGURE 4–24. The ABC System Categories (Reprinted By Permission Of G. Schubert, University Of North Dakota)

The Wisconsin Procedure for Appraisal of Clinical Competence (W-PACC), developed by Shriberg et al. (1975), contains 10 items to evaluate interpersonal skills, 28 items to evaluate professional-technical skills, and 10 additional items which summarize personal qualities, such as appearance, punctuality, and the like. The professional-technical skills include developing and planning, teaching, assessment, and reporting. As the authors point out, the 38 test items included strongly resemble the criteria which have been used by many supervisors in training institutions. For example, one item under interpersonal skills is listed as, "accepts, emphasizes, shows genuine concern for the client as a person and understands the client's problems, needs and stresses." The student clinician is assessed on a 1 to 10 point scale from, "Specific direction from supervisor, does not alter unsatisfactory performance and inability to make changes," which is scored as only 1 point, to, "Demonstrates independence by taking initiative, makes changes when appropriate, and is effective,"

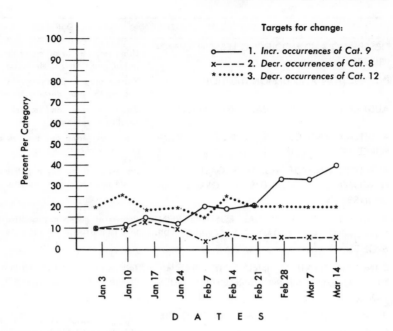

FIGURE 4–25. ABC System Analysis Of 10 Therapy Sessions (Reprinted By Permission Of G. Schubert, University Of North Dakota)

which can earn from 8 to 10 points. Percentage scores are obtained for Level I, II, III, and IV type clinicians. "Product scores" can also be obtained for grading purposes. Four studies using the W-PACC at the University of Wisconsin were conducted, sampling from seven to nine supervisors during a 2-year period. Reliability and validity data were collected for the 10 item interpersonal skills and 28 item professional-technical skills. The rating of the supervisors tended to be relatively stable. Reliability data were considered adequate to excellent. Content, construct, and criterion validity were investigated. For the most part, the 38 evaluation items were approved as being valid measures of clinical ability by "a group" of experienced supervisors. The decision that there is a relationship between job performance or competency and supervisor's judgment about clinical skills is a weak one, as Shriberg et al. point out. This relationship, for the present time, is an assumed one.

One basic difference between the W-PACC and similar evaluative instruments is that efforts have been made to obtain reliability and validity data about the W-PACC. This represents a significant advance in the development of a clinical assessment instrument. But one of the major drawbacks of this type of instrument is that the evaluations are almost entirely subjective. They are not bound to specific, well-defined events such as those found in the Boone-Prescott instrument. Two supervisors who have different philosophies about how speech therapy should be conducted may view the same session but obtain different scores. Once the problems of inter-supervisor and job-competency relationships to test items can be resolved, we should have available an effective assessment instrument, not only suitable to *evaluate* clinician effectiveness, but also to *predict* effectiveness. Of course, the greatest value is that we should be able to control effectiveness by manipulating relevant variables necessary for success in the therapy process. Judging from the current interest in assessment procedures (Pannbaker, 1975), I believe we can look forward to the development of more effective assessment instruments in the near future.

Criteria
for Evaluating
Assessment Instruments

A variety of instruments related to assessment of the therapy process have been presented. These include both objective and subjective assessments of individuals who receive therapy, clinicians who provide therapy, and supervisors who train clinicians. Attempts have been made to validate some instruments, while others serve only as general guidelines for assessment. We will need to develop more precise and reliable techniques of observation as well as standardized recording procedures before we can advance into a science of assessment. It is alarming to me that speech clinicians have not yet standardized a form to record speech responses (Mowrer, 1969a). Imagine the confusion which would exist in audiology if a standard logarithmic scale (audiogram) was not used to record responses to auditory signals.

Herbert and Attridge (1975) presented an excellent set of guidelines for those who wish to develop and to use observation systems. They felt observation of subjects in natural or unmanipulated settings is probably one of the most useful techniques for collecting data. Instruments for systematic observation promise to become some of the most useful new tools researchers and practitioners alike will have in their work. Much of the work done so far to solve methodological problems of observation is far from adequate. The purpose of these guidelines is to assist those who wish to develop or to use observational instruments to establish criteria for observational systems and manuals. Three types of criteria identified by Herbert and Attridge were:

Identifying criteria. These criteria help the user select the correct instrument to suit his purpose. The instrument should have a title, which represents the purpose for which it is used. A Predictive Screening Test of Articulation and the Wisconsin Procedure for Appraisal of Clinical Competence are appropriate titles, while the Klens-Voltz, Flanders Quick Analysis Scoring, or Roth-Parks Interaction Analysis identify the authors but tell us nothing about the intended use. A statement of purpose should accompany the instrument, as well as the underlying rationale or theoretical support. The behaviors to be observed should be clearly specified, as should the applications for which the instrument is to be used. Situations in which the instrument should not be used should also be stated.

Validity criteria. The instrument should accurately and clearly measure events it claims to assess; the observable events must be capable of being observed by any trained observer, either directly through his own senses, or with the aid of equipment. Observations should not be subject to the observer's own performances, bias, expectations, needs, or feelings. The measure should be applicable in all situations for which it is intended if generalizations from the instrument are to be meaningful. The instrument must be reliable in that it produces the same results in similar instances and must be valid in that it measures what it proports to measure.

Criteria of practicality. The instrument must be easy to use and not abnormally time-consuming. The items must be relevant to the purpose of the instrument. Codes must be simple, easy to use and remember, and not depend on special jargon. Qualifications and any necessary training of observers should be carefully spelled out. Data collection and recording procedures must accompany the instrument, as well as procedures for analyzing the data.

The development of valid and reliable assessment instruments is a complicated, arduous task, but so was the development of assessment instruments in every field of science. Only recently have methods of science been applied to the educational process. It is not surprising that we have yet to develop sophisticated means of assessment in speech pathology. In a recent report of an investigation team that scrutinized hundreds of Office of Education grant reports, the investigators stated "not a single evaluation report was found which could be accepted at face value " (Report on Education Research, 1976). The process of assessing human behaviors, nevertheless, has received a great deal of attention within the last decade. I think we can look forward to increased precision in assessing behaviors as teachers gain skills in this area and as researchers refine present techniques and develop new ones.

It appears that almost no one is safe from assessment! The only remaining groups that have so far avoided assessment are the academic professors in the university training centers and those who administer the affairs of ASHA. I would predict from the work being done in other professional fields that methods will soon be developed to assess members of these groups as well (Baird, 1974; Doyle & Whitely, 1974; Heath & Nielson, 1974).

BIBLIOGRAPHY

American Speech and Hearing Association. Requirements for the certificate of clinical competence. Washington D.C.: *ASHA Directory,* 1973.

Anderson, J. L. Supervision: The neglected component of our profession. In L. J. Tuton (Ed.), *Proceedings of a workshop on supervision in speech pathology.* Ann Arbor, Mich.: University of Michigan, 1974a.

Anderson, J. L. Supervision of school speech, hearing, and language program—an emerging role. *Asha,* 1974b, *16,* 7–11.

Baird, L. L. The practical utility of measures of college environments. *Review of Educational Research,* 1974, *44,* 307–329.

Black, M. E., Miller, A. E., Anderson, J. L., & Coates, N. H. III. Supervision of speech and hearing programs. *Journal of Speech and Hearing Disorders,* Monograph Supplement 8, 1961, 22–32.

Boone, D. R., & Prescott, T. E. Content and sequence analysis of speech and hearing therapy. *Asha,* 1972, *14,* 58–62.

Butler, K. W. Videotaped self-confrontation. *Language Speech and Hearing Services in Schools,* 1974, *5,* 162–170.

Culatta, R., Colucci, S., & Wiggins, E. *Communication between supervisors and clinical trainees.* Unpublished manuscript, University of Kentucky, 1975.

Culatta, R., & Seltzer, H. Content and sequence analysis of the supervisory session. *Asha,* 1976, *18,* 8–12.

Diedrich, W. M. Procedures for counting and charting a target phoneme. *Language Speech and Hearing Services in Schools,* 1971, *55,* 2, 18–32.

Diedrich, W. M. *Charting speech behavior.* Lawrence, Kan.: University of Kansas Bureau of Publication, 1973.

Doyle, K. O., & Whitely, S. E. Student ratings as criteria for effective teaching. *American Educational Research Journal,* 1974, *11,* 259–274.

Elbert, M., Shelton, R. L., & Arndt, W. B. A task for evaluation of articulation change I. Development of methodology. *Journal of Speech and Hearing Research,* 1967, *10,* 281–288.

Halfond, M. Clinical supervision—stepchild in training. *Asha,* 1964, *6,* 441–444.

Heath, R. W., & Neilson, M. H. The research basis for performance-based teacher education. *Review of Educational Research,* 1974, *44,* 463–484.

Herbert, J., & Attridge, C. A guide for developers and users of observation systems and manuals. *American Educational Research Journal,* 1975, *12,* 1–20.

Irwin, J. V., & Griffith, F. A. A theoretical and operational analysis of the paired stimuli technique. In W. D. Wolfe & D. J. Goulding (Ed.), *Articulation and learning.* Springfield, Ill.: Charles C Thomas, 1973.

Johnson, J. M. A universal behavior graph paper. *Journal of Applied Behavioral Analysis,* 1970, *3,* 271–272.

Johnson, T. S. *A precision approach to hyper-functional voice disorders.* Logan, Utah: Utah State University, 1975.

Lindsley, O. R. Direct measurement and prosthesis of retarded children. *Journal of Education,* 1964, *147,* 62–81.

Menges, R. J. Assessing readiness for professional practice. *Review of Educational Research,* 1975, *45,* 173–207.

Mischel, W. *Personality and assessment.* New York: John Wiley & Sons, 1968.

Mowrer, D. E. Evaluating speech therapy through precision recording. *Journal of Speech and Hearing Disorders,* 1969a, *34,* 239–244.

Mowrer, D. E. *Modification of speech behavior: Ideas and strategies for students.* Tempe, Ariz.: Arizona State University, 1969b.

Mowrer, D. E., Baker, R. L., & Owen, C. Verbal content analysis of speech therapy session. *Asha,* 1968, *10,* 398.

Mowrer, D. E., Baker, R. L., & Schutz, R. E. Operant procedures in the control of articulation. In H. Sloane & B. MacAulay (Eds.), *Operant procedures in remedial speech and language training.* Boston: Houghton Mifflin, 1968.

Pannbacker, M. Bibliography for supervision. *Asha,* 1975, *17,* 105–106.

Perkins, W., Shelton, R., Studebaker, G., & Goldstein, R. The national examinations in speech pathology and audiology: Philosophy and operation. *Asha,* 1970, *12,* 175–181.

Prescott, T. E., & Tesauro, P. A. A method for quantification and description of clinical interaction with aurally handicapped children. *Journal of Speech and Hearing Disorders,* 1974, *39,* 235–243.

Report on education research. How to tell when to trust an evaluation report. Washington, D.C.: Education News Services Division of Capital Publications, 1976, *8,* 4.

Ryan, B. *Programmed therapy for stuttering in children and adults.* Springfield, Ill.: Charles C Thomas, 1974.

Schriberg, L. D., Filley, F. S., Hayes, D. M., Kivmiatkowski, J., Schatz, J. A., Simmons, K. M., & Smith, M. E. The Wisconsin procedures for appraisal of clinical competence (W-PACC): Model and data. *Asha,* 1975, *17,* 158–165.

Schubert, G. W. *The analysis of behavior of clinicians (ABC) system.* Grand Forks, N.D.: University of North Dakota, 1974.

Schubert, G. W., & Aitchison, C. J. A profile of clinical supervisors in college and university speech and hearing programs. *Asha,* 1975, *17,* 440–447.

Schubert, G. W., & Glick, A. M. A comparison of two methods of recording and analyzing student clinician-client interaction. *Acta Symbolica,* 1974, *5,* 39–55.

Shelton, R. L., Elbert, M., & Arndt, W. B. A task for evaluation of articulation change. *Journal of Speech and Hearing Research,* 1967, *10,* 578–585.

Skinner, B. F. *Cumulative record.* New York: Appleton-Century-Crofts, 1959.

Turton, L. Diagnostic implications of articulation testing. In W. D. Wolfe & D. J. Goulding (Eds.), *Articulation and learning.* Springfield, Ill.: Charles C Thomas, 1973.

Van Hattum, R. The defensive speech clinicians in the schools. *Journal of Speech and Hearing Disorders,* 1966, *31,* 234–240.

Van Riper, C. *Speech correction: Principles and methods,* 3rd ed. Englewood Cliffs, N.J.: Prentice-Hall, 1963.

Van Riper, C. *Supervision of clinical practice. Asha,* 1965, *7,* 75–77.

White, O. R., & Haring, N. G. *Exceptional teaching.* Columbus: Charles E. Merrill, 1976.

Assignment 1
Evaluating Speech Responses

Overview

One of the most important tasks the pathologist performs is providing accurate feedback concerning the accuracy of a client's response. In a sense, the client must rely upon the pathologist's judgment regarding whether or not a response is correct until the client is able to make this judgment independently. If the pathologist provides incorrect feedback, then it will be difficult for the client to make accurate judgments about his or her own performance

Five exercises are presented to help you gain practice in making judgments about the accuracy of different types of client's responses. Two tasks involve making judgments of isolated /ɝ/ and /ɝ/-like sounds and the use of correct /ɝ/ or /ɚ/ sounds in connected speech. The third task consists of counting disfluent utterances in the speech of a client who stutters. A fourth task involves identifying and counting occasions of inflectional pitch change in the speech of a boy. In the last section, you will be asked to discriminate between a child's 1–2 word utterances and utterances containing 3 or more words.

Objective: To discriminate between various types of correct and incorrect speech responses.

Materials: Tape Assignment 1, Selections A–E.

Description of the Session: The next five selections will help you develop skills in identifying instances of correct and incorrect responses. Selections A and B consist of /ɝ/ and /ɚ/ distortions produced by several children. You will be asked to discriminate between correct and incorrect productions as they occur in isolation and in words. Selection C is designed to help you identify instances of disfluent speech. Selection D deals with pitch inflection, and in Selection E, you will receive practice discriminating between two different lengths of child utterances.

These discrimination skills are extremely important, for without accurate identification of correct and incorrect responses, the data we collect are not representative of behavioral samples. As a consequence, the conclusions derived from data are not reliable. The selections in this assignment will introduce you to the types of skills required in behavior therapy.

Procedure: The procedures to be followed differ among the various taped selections; therefore, the procedures you are to follow will be listed separately after each selection.

SELECTION A

When your goal is to evoke a target sound by shaping (successive approximation), it is important to identify slight improvements in responses as the child approximates the target response. This strategy is especially important when attempting to teach /ɝ/.

In this first selection you will hear children produce two /ɝ/ attempts in rapid succession. The children will produce 30 pairs of /ɝ/s. You are to judge *(a)* whether the second attempt sounds closer to /ɝ/ than the first attempt; *(b)* whether the second attempt sounds the same as or no closer to /ɝ/ than the first attempt; or *(c)* if the second attempt sounds more unlike /ɝ/ than the first attempt. The second attempt is always to be judged in comparison to the previous attempt. Check B on the tables below when the second attempt was *better* than the first; S, when both attempts were the *same;* and W, when the second attempt was *worse*.

The ability to make accurate sound discrimination judgments is an important skill speech pathologists must possess in order to successfully shape behavior. Table 1–1 is a sample score sheet marked for you. As you listen to this selection, you will mark the score sheet in Table 1–2, as directed on the tape.

Play Assignment 1, Selection A now.

Table 1–1. *Sample score sheet.*

	B	S	W
1	X		
2			X
3	X		
4		X	

Now, check your evaluations in Table 1–2 with those found in the Answer Key, Table 1–7. Circle each of your evaluations that are in disagreement with the evaluations in the key. Count the number of circles. If you have three or less evaluations circled, you are in agreement with the Answer Key 90% or better; that's very good. If you count four or more circles, you may wish to replay Selection A on the tape, as you watch the answer sheet.

Table 1–2. *Score sheet for evaluating pairs of /ɝ/ sounds.*

	B	S	W		B	S	W		B	S	W
1				11				21			
2				12				22			
3				13				23			
4				14				24			
5				15				25			
6				16				26			
7				17				27			
8				18				28			
9				19				29			
10				20				30			

SELECTION B

In this selection 30 words are presented, all of which contain /ɝ/ or /r/ sounds. Some of the children will pronounce the /ɝ/ or /r/ sounds correctly; some will not. A few /ɝ/ and /r/ attempts will be difficult to categorize as either correct or incorrect. The scoring system you are to use in evaluating these /ɝ/ and /r/ sounds will be as follows: Check *G* column, representing *good,* if you judge the sound as correct. Check the *C* column, for *close,* if you think the sound is not good enough to be placed in the good column, yet not sufficiently incorrect to be placed in the wrong column. Place a check in the *W* column if you think the sound is an unacceptable (wrong) /ɝ/ or /r/ production. Note that some items are starred; this indicates that there was considerable disagreement on these items as evaluated by 50 other speech pathologists. Find Table 1–3 on the following page.

Play Assignment 1, Selection B and check the appropriate columns in Table 1–3, for each word.

When you have finished listening to the tape and have filled in the evaluations in Table 1–3, check your answers with those in Table 1–8 in the Answer Key. If you missed five or more items, replay this selection again.

Table 1–3. *Score sheet for evaluating /ɜ·/ and /r/ productions in words.*

Word	G	C	W	Word	G	C	W
1 run				16 her			
* 2 rope				17 stir			
3 race				18 fur			
4 red				19 dirt			
5 ring				20 her			
6 run				21 fair			
* 7 radio				*22 stairs			
8 ride				23 care			
9 rip				24 tear			
10 write				*25 bear			
*11 car				*26 steer			
12 star				*27 fear			
13 far				28 tear			
14 bar				29 rear			
15 tar				30 dear			

SELECTION C

One would think that it would be a relatively simple job to evaluate sounds as being correct or incorrect; but as you can see, sometimes it is very difficult to place certain sounds in distinct categories. Much depends upon our past experience in judging sounds as well as upon our perceptual abilities. In the next selection, we have an even more difficult task: judging the occurrences of disfluency. Before systematic attempts can be made to change the frequency of the behavior, pinpointing the behavior we wish to decrease is necessary. Yet, it is almost impossible for authorities to agree upon occurrences of disfluency. In the next selection, you will hear many disfluent utterances. You will only be able to recognize audible events as possible occasions of disfluency. A videotape might make it possible to recognize more disfluencies, but frequently we must analyze data from audio information alone. You are to follow the script in Table 1–4 and underline the words or parts of words that indicate disfluent behavior. The first sentence has been marked for you.

Play Assignment 1, Selection C and listen to the following sample items that have been marked for you.

When you have finished underlining the words, check Table 1–9 in the Answer Key.

Table 1–4. *Script of Selection C to be evaluated.*

Sample:

The first <u>ti</u>me I went <u>ca</u>mping was a <u>te</u>rrible experience.

We took a tent, a couple of sleeping bags, and enough food to last two days. Our first problem was getting to the campsite. We selected a remote area about thirty-five miles off the highway. I'll bet that road hadn't been used for fifty years. About five miles in, we hit a hole too big for our Volkswagen to cross. One back wheel lifted off the ground and there we were, stuck. We finally rocked the car loose, but from then on we heard a strange noise in the rear end. Something must have been bent out of shape. After a few more miles of bumpy and washed-out roads, the car began to heat up. We checked the engine and found the fan belt had broken. We had no spare and were too far in to turn back.

SELECTION D

Occasionally, it is important to modify certain pitch characteristics in the speech of children. In the next selection, you will hear a fourth grade boy talking about a balloon. He has a tendency to alter the pitch of certain vowels. The result is a melodic sing-song speech pattern that may interfere with communication. Listen to this brief sample and underline the vowels that contain this unique pitch pattern. These are the behaviors that you would want to decrease. Follow the script in Table 1–5 and underline each vowel in which you recognize a pitch change. You may wish to play this selection several times to verify your markings before you check your answers.

Play Assignment 1, Selection D.

Table 1–5. *Script of Selection D.*

Once upon a time there was a boy that had a balloon an he blowed it up and he blowed it up until it bust and he wonder what should he do with a balloon that bust.

Check your answers with those found in the Answer Key, in Table 1–10.

SELECTION E

Some children need to increase their mean length of utterance. In this next selection, you will hear a dialogue between an adult and a preschool child. You are to count the number of utterances that contain three or more different words, as well as the utterances that contain two or less different words. For example: If the child said, "the, uh, um, the, um, red," this response would be counted as two words, *the* and *red*, even though the word *the* was repeated. The utterance, "He, uh he goes, he goes somewhere," would be counted as a three-word utterance (three different words). Place a check in the appropriate column in Table 1–6 as you listen to this selection.

Play Assignment 1, Selection E now.

Table 1–6. *Number of 1–2 word and 3 or more utterances.*

	Total	
1–2 word utterances		
3 + word utterances		

Check your totals with those found in the Answer Key in Table 1–11. The child made 22 replies to the adult. If you had difficulty with this selection, play the tape again.

You may have found that you did not agree with the answers for certain tasks. Most of the judgments we make about speech are dependent upon perceptions and are subject to error. The best we can do is attempt to standardize our judgments by making comparisons with the perceptions of others who have had training in this area. This is an accepted procedure used in research studies to establish validity of judgments. Even then, we rarely obtain 100% agreement. When you must make rapid judgments in daily therapy sessions, you cannot compare your judgments with others. Our ability to make rapid and accurate judgments about speech behaviors should improve with practice and training when feedback by more experienced pathologists is provided. The practice obtained in scoring the five selections on this tape will help you realize how difficult and how important it is to be able to make accurate judgments about speech behaviors.

Answer Key

SELECTION A

Table 1–7. *Evaluation of paired /ɝ/ sounds.*

	B	S	W		B	S	W		B	S	W
1	X			11	X			21	X		
2	X			12		X		22			X
3		X		13	X			23		X	
4		X		14		X		24		X	
5	X			15		X		25		X	
6		X		16		X		26		X	
7			X	17			X	27	X		
8		X		18		X		28		X	
9		X		19		X		29		X	
10	X			20		X		30		X	

SELECTION B

Table 1–8. *Evaluation of words containing /ɝ/ and /r/.*

Word	G	C	W	Word	G	C	W
1 run	X			16 her	X		
* 2 rope		X		17 stir			X
3 race			X	18 fur			X
4 red	X			19 dirt	X		
5 ring			X	20 her			X
6 run			X	21 fair	X		
* 7 radio	X			*22 stairs		X	
8 ride			X	23 care	X		
9 rip			X	24 tear	X		
10 write	X			*25 bear		X	
*11 car			X	*26 steer		X	
12 star	X			*27 fear		X	
13 far			X	28 tear	X		
14 bar			X	29 rear	X		
15 tar	X			30 dear			X

SELECTION C

Table 1–9. *Script of Selection C showing location of disfluent words.*

We took a tent, a couple of sleeping bags, and enough food to last two days. Our first

problem was getting to the campsite. We selected a remote area about thirty-five miles

off the highway. I'll bet that road hadn't been used for fifty years. About five miles in,

we hit a hole too big for our Volkswagen to cross. One back wheel lifted off the ground and there we were, stuck. We finally rocked the car loose, but from then on we heard a strange noise in the rear end. Something must have been bent out of shape. After a few more miles of bumpy and washed-out roads, the car began to heat up. We checked the engine and found the fan belt had broken. We had no spare and were too far in to turn back.

SELECTION D

Table 1–10. *Script of Selection D showing location of vowel pitch inflection.*

Once upon a time there was a boy that had a balloon an he blowed it up and he blowed it up until it bust and he wonder what should he do with a balloon that bust.

SELECTION E

Table 1–11. *Number of 1–2 word and 3 or more word utterances for Selection E.*

	Total
1-2 word utterance	16
3 + word utterance	6

Assignment 2

Methods of Analyzing
Therapy Procedures

Overview

One method of analyzing a therapy session is presented: the Boone-Prescott 10-Category System.

A 5-minute therapy session is used to illustrate the use of this sytem. A script of the session is provided to assist you in assigning ratings to each segment. In the Boone-Prescott system, statements made by the client and pathologists are assigned categories. You will receive practice scoring responses and analyzing the content of the session.

Objective: To provide practice using an analysis system, designed to evaluate therapy sessions.

Materials: Assignment 2.

Suggested Readings: Boone and Prescott (1972), pp. 58–62.

Description of the Session: Part of a therapy session will be presented in this exercise. You will analyze it using Boone-Prescott's 10-Category System. The session involves a pathologist working with a 5-year-old girl who omits many medial consonants. The pathologist uses the behavior therapy format in attempting to help the child articulate consonants rapidly in medial positions.

Procedure: In this section, portions of a therapy session will be presented to provide you with an opportunity to score statements made by both client and pathologist, according to Boone-Prescott's 10-Category System.

SELECTION A

Your task in this selection will be to analyze and evaluate a 5-minute sample of articulation therapy using the Boone and Prescott 10-Category System.

First, we will review the 10 categories of this system. The following 5 categories describe statements made by the pathologist:

Category 1   Explain or describe.

This category is used when specific goals or certain procedures are explained to the client. A specific client response is usually not expected. Good examples would be:

"Today we're going to play a new game that will help you with your speech."
"Let's start to work now."
"Well, you have to hold the spinner like this."
"We're going to learn how to say our /r/ sound today."
"Let's listen to how you sound on the tape recorder."

Category 2   Model or instruction.

When the client is asked to perform a certain task related to speech or when a model of the correct behavior is presented, Category 2 is assigned. In most all cases, a speech-related response is anticipated following a category or statement.

"Say /s/."
"Stick out your tongue and blow like this."
"Try it once more."
"He *is* going."
"Say it again."
"Can you talk a little louder so I can hear you better?"
"Don't be afraid to say it; come on, let's try it."

Category 3   Good evaluative.

Any response indicating approval of a response is given a Category 3 rating. Sometimes approval is given nonverbally, like a smile or a nod of one's head. These signals cannot be detected from audio samples. The only way you could accurately record instances of nonverbal approval is by observing videotaped or live sessions. Auditory responses of Category 3 might consist of the following:

"Good."   "Gee, that's swell, Tommy."
"That's it."   "You're doing fine."
"Much better."   "Right."
"Uh-huh."

Category 4   Bad evaluative.

Responses indicating incorrect responses are rated as Category 4. Again, sometimes this information, when presented nonverbally, cannot be detected from tape recordings.

"Nope."   "You still didn't get it."
"You missed it."   "That's wrong."
"That's not right, Jane."

Category 5   Neutral-social.

Any statement unrelated to the goals of the therapy session fall into Category 5. These usually occur when the pathologist strays from the target objective, especially if the client looses interest in the session activities or attempts to talk about events unrelated to therapy. Pathologists frequently must respond with Category 5 statements. But if the pathologist's statement is designed to evoke a target response, it would be classed as Category 2.

"Oh yeah, I saw that program too. It was really interesting."

"Gee, I like your dress, Sue. Did your mother make it?"

"I wonder what we're having to eat today."

"Why don't you like your teacher?"

"Is red your favorite color? Is that why you're wearing a red ribbon in your hair today?"

Categories 6 through 10 are representative of statements made by the clients.

Category 6   Correct response.

Any correct response is classified as a Category 6. Sometimes it may be difficult for you to decide whether a response is correct or not, especially when a client is first learning to articulate sounds. A pathologist may reward close approximations of sounds (attempts to say the sounds even though they may not be correct). Other times, the pathologist may say "good" when clearly the response is incorrect. Thus, you may experience some difficulty in determining whether a particular response is really correct. Be careful to evaluate only speech target responses as correct. If the client is asked, "Where do you live?" and answers "On Oak Street," this answer may be correct but it has nothing to do with the objective of the session, which was improving articulation. The response would be classed as an 8, a social-oriented response.

Category 7   Incorrect response.

If the client responds incorrectly, it is rated as a 7. Occasionally, it may be difficult to determine whether a response is correct or incorrect, especially during the process of shaping articulation responses. Certain language responses are also difficult to evaluate. At other times, it is easy to determine whether or not a response is wrong.

Category 8   Inappropriate-social.

This is similar to Category 5 and is used to classify those statements made by the client that are not related to the goals of the therapy session. Occasionally, young children will talk about events that are unrelated to the goals set by the pathologist. Examples are

"My daddy has one of those."   "Can I take this picture home?"

"Can I go now?"   "Let's play a different game now."

"That man's funny. He has a big nose."

Category 9   Good self-evaluative.

Occasionally, a client states that her response was correct. When this occurs, Category 9 is used. Consider the following:

> "That was good, wasn't it?"
> "I said it right."
> "I get a point, don't I?"

Category 10   Bad self-evaluative.

The client's recognition of an incorrect response is rated in this last category. Statements like the following may occur:

> "Oh-oh—I missed it."   "That wasn't right, was it?"
> "*Thop*, I mean *soap*."   "I can't say that."

Now that you have reviewed each category, you can practice evaluating a speech therapy session. In the sesssion you are to evaluate, the pathologist is attempting to help a 5-year-old girl produce /d, t, n, k/ in co-articulated sequences, such as *need a, put it in, in a, pick a,* and *a cup.* The client tends to omit medial consonants in connected speech. The session consists chiefly of the auditory models provided by the pathologist, followed by attempts from the child to imitate these models. Production of correctly co-articulated speech using the four sounds listed above is the therapy goal for this session. Follow the script of the first minute of this session as you listen to the tape. The categories have been marked for you in Table 2–1.

Now play Assignment 2.

Table 2–1. *Script of the first minute of therapy (P = pathologist, C = child).*

Category

2	P. I need a—say that for me.
6	C. need a
3, 2	P. I need a—right.
	Make a—make a
6	C. make a
3, 2	P. good—I want a
6	C. make a
3, 2	P. I want a—good. This one's I pick a

6	C. I pick a
3, 2	P. good—I take a, take a
7	C. ake a
2	P. I took a
7	C. Ta
4, 1, 2	P. Pretty close, pretty close. OK, let's start with this one. Put it in a. Let's pick a card—pick a card. What is that?

Category

_____ 1. C: boat

_____ 2. P: A boat, O.K., let's put it right here. We'll leave these up here. Put it here. Put it in a boat. A boat.

_____ 3. C: a boat

_____ 4. P: Good. In a boat, in a boat,

_____ 5. C: in a boat

_____ 6. P: Good, in a boat

_____ 7. C: in a boat

_____ 8. P: Good, in a boat

_____ 9. C: in a boat

_____ 10. P: Good, in a boat

_____ 11. C: in a boat

_____ 12. P: Good, put it

_____ 13. C: put it

_____ 14. P: Good, put it in a boat. Put it.

_____ 15. C: in a boat

_____ 16. P: Oh, no, put it

_____ 17. C: in

_____ 18. P: Oh, you say the whole thing. Put it, put, it.

_____ 19. C: in

_____ 20. P: Let's go back to the beginning. A boat.

_____ 21. C: a boat

———— 22. P: Good, real good. Let's pick another picture. Which one do we want now? What is that?

———— 23. C: a up

———— 24. P: Cup. Tell me cup.

———— 25. C: up

———— 26. P: c–cup

———— 27. C: cup

———— 28. P: Good, a cup

———— 29. C: a up

———— 30. P: a cup

———— 31. C: a up

———— 32. P: Pretty good, in a cup

———— 33. C: in a up

———— 34. P: In a cup

———— 35. C: tup

———— 36. P: Whoa, let's go back, K, K.

———— 37. C: in a boat

———— 38. P: You want to do *boat* instead, huh? Let's try cup, K, K, K. Make that sound for me K, K, K, K, K, K, K, K. Tell me make a

———— 39. C: make a

———— 40. P: Yea, that's the same sound. Good, cup.

———— 41. C: cup

———— 42. P: Good, that's pretty close. Let's try, a cup.

———— 43. C: ta up

———— 44. P: That's pretty close. Let's see if we can find one that's easier. Let's see, how about this one. What is that?

———— 45. C: garbage can

———— 46. P: Yea, O.K. it's a garbage truck. Let's pick it up. Yea. O.K., which one did you pick, pick a card. Pick a card. That's a truck.

———— 47. C: truck

———— 48. P: Truck, O.K. Let's put the truck on the table. Good, a truck.

———— 49. C: uck

_____ 50. P: A truck

_____ 51. C: wu

_____ 52. P: That's close. That's pretty close, truck

_____ 53. C: truck

_____ 54. P: Whoops. That's good, truck

_____ 55. C: truck

_____ 56. P: A truck

_____ 57. C: uck

_____ 58. P: That's close too. In a

_____ 59. C: in a

_____ 60. P: Good, in a

_____ 61. C: in a

_____ 62. P: Good, in a

_____ 63. C: in a

_____ 64. P: Good, in a

_____ 65. C: in a

_____ 66. P: Good, in a

_____ 67. C: in a

_____ 68. P: Good, put it in a

_____ 69. C: put it in

_____ 70. P: Put it in a

_____ 71. C: in a

_____ 72. P: O.K., try again. Put it in a

_____ 73. C: in a

_____ 74. P: No, say it after me. Put it in a

_____ 75. C: put it in

_____ 76. P: Good, put it in, put it in

_____ 77. C: put ta in

_____ 78. P: Oh, that's too soft. Let's try again, put it in a

_____ 79. C: put it in a

_____ 80. P: Good, real good, Tammy. I like to hear that, you talk so pretty. Put it in.

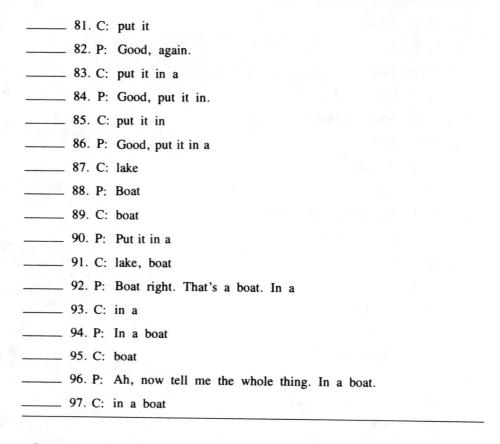

_____ 81. C: put it

_____ 82. P: Good, again.

_____ 83. C: put it in a

_____ 84. P: Good, put it in.

_____ 85. C: put it in

_____ 86. P: Good, put it in a

_____ 87. C: lake

_____ 88. P: Boat

_____ 89. C: boat

_____ 90. P: Put it in a

_____ 91. C: lake, boat

_____ 92. P: Boat right. That's a boat. In a

_____ 93. C: in a

_____ 94. P: In a boat

_____ 95. C: boat

_____ 96. P: Ah, now tell me the whole thing. In a boat.

_____ 97. C: in a boat

Just to be sure you have assigned the correct categories to the pathologist's and client's statements, check your answers with those found in the Answer Key on Table 2–5.

After the categories have been marked, the next task is to count the number of times each category occurs, that is, the number of events in each category. Refer to Table 2–2. Enter the number of events that occurred in each category for the pathologist and the client. Be sure to include those events listed during the first minute of therapy. Use the bottom line to show totals for the pathologist and client, and mark at the top of Table 2–2 the combined number of events for both participants.

Next, determine the percent each category contributed to the total. The total number of categories in this session is 156. Divide the number of events in each category by 156. Thus, the percent of Category 1 statements would be $9 \div 156 = .0576$ or 5.8% rounded off to the nearest tenth of a percent. The percent of each category should be figured and recorded in Table 2–2.

When you have finished filling the category percentages in Table 2–2, check your figures with Table 2–6 in the Answer Key.

From these data you can see that the pathologist's models (2) and good evaluative comments (3) make up just over half of the entire session. Her general descriptions (1) and negative feedback (4) are kept at a minimum, and social talk (5) is not present at

Table 2-2. *Number and percent of events in each category.*

	Pathologist			Client		
		Total Events =				
Category	No. of events	% of total	Category	No. of events	% of total
1			6		
2			7		
3			8		
4			9		
5			10		
Total events			Total events		

all. As for the client, the majority of responses are correct (6) but there is a fairly large amount of incorrect responses (7). Lack of Categories 9 and 10 might indicate the client is not monitoring her responses. This is a response class the pathologist might wish to encourage by asking the client how she would evaluate incorrect responses. Thus, these percentages provide a quick source of information to help determine what is occurring during a therapy session as well as what might be done to improve the session.

More valuable information can be obtained by observing the sequence of certain events. Boone and Prescott feel that it is wise to follow a correct response (6) with good evaluative statement (3). Therefore, many 6-3 sequences might indicate a good session. To find out how many 6-3 events occurred in the previous session, look through the category ratings and circle each 6-3 combination, like this example:

1. 2
2. 6
3. 3, 2
4. 6
5. 3, 2
6. 6
7. 3, 2

Once you have circled all the 6–3 sequences, record the total number of 6–3 events in Table 2–3.

Sometimes, either by design or by neglect, a pathologist may seldom follow a correct response (6) with verbal confirmation (3). To analyze this aspect of therapy, use a red pencil and circle all those events in which 6 is followed by an event other than 3. For example:

1. 6

2. 3,1,2

3. 7

4. 2

5. 6

6. 2

7. 6

8. 3,2

Then count the number of red circles and record that total in Table 2–3.

Table 2–3. *Analysis of correct response consequences.*

Number of 6–3 events	
Number of 6–other events	
Percent of correct responses confirmed	

You should have counted twenty-six 6–3 events and five 6–other events. To find the percent of 6–3 events, add the number of 6–3 to 6–other events. In this session, the sum is 31. Next, divide the number of 6–3 events (26) by the sum (31). Record this number in Table 2–3.*

Now that you see how to analyze events that follow a client's correct response, you should be able to analyze events that follow incorrect responses (7). Using the same procedure, draw rectangles around 7–4 events. Use a red pencil to mark 7–other events. Fill in Table 2–4 on the following page.

$$(7\text{--}4)\underline{\quad} + (7\text{--other})\underline{\quad} = (T)\underline{\quad}.$$

$$(7\text{--}4)\underline{\quad} \div (T)\underline{\quad} = \underline{\quad}\%$$

---

*83.9%.

Table 2–4. *Analysis of incorrect response consequences.*

Number of 7–4 events	
Number of 7–other events	
Percent of 7–4 events	

You should have figured eleven 7–4 events and twelve 7–other events, with a percentage of forty-eight for 7–4 events.

You also may wish to look at how many 8 events are followed by a 1 or 2 category. In this session, there were no 8 category events. If there were any, they should not have been followed by 5 category events since 8–5 sequences do not contribute toward therapy goal accomplishment. Instead, sequences like 8–1 and/or 8–2 would reflect the pathologist's efforts to return to therapy-oriented goals.

Analysis of Results for Assignment 2

Scoring a therapy session amounts to no more than busy work unless an attempt is made to evaluate the results. Based upon your computations in Tables 2–2, 2–3, and 2–4, answer the following questions:

1. According to the percent of events in Category 1, did the pathologist spend very much time explaining procedures?
2. What event occupied most of the pathologist's time?
3. Would this indicate the pathologist provided a great deal of guidance and structure in the session?
4. Compare Category 3 with Category 6. Also, look at the reward–sequence percentages you computed. Do these comparisons indicate the pathologist provided much positive feedback following the child's correct response?
5. Now compare Category 4 with Category 7, as well as the percentage of 7–4 sequences you computed. Did the pathologist provide the same amount of feedback for wrong responses?
6. Add Category 6 and Category 7. Divide the total into the Category 6 number as well as into the Category 7 number. You should have two percentages, one showing the percent of responses correct, the other the percent of responses wrong. It has been stated by several investigators that when the incorrect response rate exceeds about 20%, the task is considered to be too difficult. Would you say the task in this therapy session was too difficult for the child?
7. How would you explain the fact that there were no events in Categories 9 and 10?
8. What would the 0 entry in Category 5 indicate?
9. What would you recommend be changed in the next session?
10. Why, do you think, did the pathologist inform the child she was wrong only half the time?

Check your answers to these 10 questions with those found in the Answer Key.

Answer Key

SELECTION A

Table 2–5. *Category markings using the Boone and Prescott 10-Category System.*

1. 6	20. 1,2	39. 6	58. 4,2	77. 7
2. 1,2	21. 6	40. 3,2	59. 6	78. 4,2
3. 6	22. 3,1,2	41. 6	60. 3,2	79. 6
4. 3,2	23. 7	42. 3,2	61. 6	80. 3,2
5. 6	24. 2	43. 7	62. 3,2	81. 6
6. 3,2	25. 7	44. 4,1,2	63. 6	82. 3,2
7. 6	26. 2	45. 7	64. 3,2	83. 6
8. 3,2	27. 6	46. 1,2	65. 6	84. 3,2
9. 6	28. 3,2	47. 6	66. 3,2	85. 6
10. 3,2	29. 7	48. 1,2	67. 6	86. 3,2
11. 6	30. 2	49. 7	68. 3,2	87. 7
12. 3,2	31. 7	50. 2	69. 7	88. 2
13. 6	32. 4,2	51. 7	70. 2	89. 6
14. 3,2	33. 7	52. 4,2	71. 7	90. 2
15. 7	34. 2	53. 6	72. 2	91. 6
16. 4,2	35. 7	54. 3,2	73. 7	92. 3,2
17. 7	36. 4,1,2	55. 6	74. 4,2	93. 6
18. 4,2	37. 7	56. 2	75. 6	94. 2
19. 7	38. 1,2	57. 7	76. 3,2	95. 7
				96. 4,2
				97. 6

Table 2–6. *Number and percentage of events in each category. Total pathologist events. 101 + total child events, 55 = grand total, 156.*

	Pathologist			Client	
Category	**No. of events**	**% of total**	**Category**	**No. of events**	**% of total**
1	9	5.8	6	32	20.5
2	55	35.2	7	23	14.7
3	26	16.7	8	0	0
4	11	7.1	9	0	0
5	0	0	10	0	0
Total	101	64.8	**Total**	55	35.2

Analysis of Results from Assignment 2

1. No.
2. 2
3. Yes.
4. Yes.
5. No.

6. Yes.
7. Child is too young.
8. Pathologist was task-oriented.
9. Difficulty of the task be decreased.
10. So as not to discourage the child.

UNIT 2 STUDY QUESTIONS

1. Explain why it is important to observe speech behaviors.
2. Why are we interested in observing and describing the anatomical features of the oral mechanism?
3. List and briefly describe seven behavioral measures commonly used to describe speech responses.
4. What cautions should be taken when observing and describing behaviors?
5. List three factors that seem to be critical in predicting which children will continue to misarticulate sounds.
6. How successful have attempts been to predict which individuals will continue to stutter?
7. Why is it so difficult to develop predictive indicators for language development?
8. What observations can be made of aphasic patients that would enable us to make predictions about their progress in therapy?
9. List three environmental factors that might be responsible for the development of speech problems.
10. List seven kinds of observations we should make when conducting a behavioral diagnosis.
11. List one criticism that has been leveled at the medical model as an observational system.
12. What criticism has been leveled at behaviorists who ignore the medical model diagnostic framework?
13. Of what value is keeping data in sports and in speech therapy?
14. Why do we need to make accurate assessments of a client's behavior during speech therapy?
15. What are behavior probes?
16. List two advantages of using percentage figures in treating behavioral data. List two disadvantages.
17. Why is rate of response a better measure of behavior than percentage information?
18. Why is it better to record days than sessions?
19. Why does the line representing responses on a cumulative graph never descend?
20. List some advantages of a logarithmic graph to record data.
21. Define record floor, record ceiling, acceleration and deceleration targets, and aims as they relate to the logarithmic graph.
22. How do the concepts of response rate and response accuracy pertain to the evaluation of a speech clinician's work?
23. What three behaviors of clinicians were found to be associated with low response rate of their clients?
24. Of what use to the clinician are data obtained by using the Boone-Prescott analysis system?
25. How does Schubert's ABC system differ from the Boone-Prescott system?
26. What procedure does the W-PACC use in evaluating clinic effectiveness?
27. Explain the three criteria suggested for evaluating assessment instruments.

Unit 3

Preparing Instructional and Noninstructional Objectives

Objectives
The objectives of this unit are to enable you to: (1) identify instructional and noninstructional objectives, (2) construct instructional and noninstructional objectives, and (3) identify values and criticisms of using instructional objectives.

Suggested Assignments
You are to read chapter 5 in your text and complete assignment 3 at the end of the chapter. You will receive practice in writing a variety of objectives after listening to portions of therapy sessions and an interview with a speech/language pathologist.

Be prepared to discuss the advantages and criticisms of using behavioral objectives in class. Finally, answer the study questions that follow assignment 3.

5

Planning and Preparing Objectives in Speech Pathology

Anyone working in the field of education during the past few years has, or soon will, encounter the term *behavioral objective*. A behavioral objective is any educational objective which is stated in terms of behaviors which can be observed and measured. For example, the behavioral objective "to correctly name 24 out of 30 pictures within 15 minutes" states a behavior (naming) which can be measured (by counting the number of correct or incorrect responses) against a criterion (80% correct within 15 minutes). The individual either attains the objective or fails to attain it. Behavioral objectives identify goals and describe behaviors the learner should have as a result of instruction.

A synonym for the term behavioral objective is instructional objective. The latter term pertains more to the type of objective used in a school or other educational setting. Those who work in the public schools are more familiar with the term IEP (Individual Educational Plan) than behavioral objective. In writing an IEP for a child, one must write instructional objectives as part of the plan. It makes little difference whether we use the term behavioral objective, instructional objective, or IEP in our discussion of objectives in this chapter. All three terms specify what we intend to accomplish with a child during the educational process and when we plan to accomplish the objective. The same guidelines of writing objectives apply.

Most speech clinicians have had some experience in writing objectives as part of their lesson plans in clinical practicum courses. Recently, increased interest has been shown in formulating clear, concise, operational speech-therapy objectives.

Andrews (1971), for example, points out the need for teaching student clinicians to write objectives in measurable performance terms. Well-written objectives, he contends, allow both the clinician and the supervisor to know the precise goal of the session, as well as when the goal has been achieved. A workbook designed by ASHA (American Speech and Hearing Association, 1973) aimed at training supervisors and speech clinicians to better plan their activities through writing instructional and program objectives has emphasized the importance of writing objectives. Many public schools now require that all teachers, including speech clinicians, write performance objectives as part of their regular teaching duties. In fact, 23 states already have passed legislation that includes requirements that teachers write performance objectives. Behavioral objectives are included as a basic ingredient of many commercially developed instructional programs available to speech clinicians. Most federal grant applications which pertain to any form of instruction require that objectives be clearly indicated and tied to performance measures.

It may appear that writing objectives is a newly added feature to the educational process, but this is not the case, unless you consider a 75-year-old practice as new. Educational objectives, as they were better known, were introduced at the turn of the twentieth century, a result of the work of Thorndike and the individual testing movement. It was at this time that the scientific method began to influence trends in education, causing educators to carefully scrutinize their goals. No longer was faculty learning a sound rationale for curriculum development.

It was in 1924 that the influential educator Bobbitt (1924) proposed a curriculum in terms of identifying specific learning skills. He divided skills into units, organized the units into experiences, and provided these experiences to children. He demonstrated how educational objectives were to be formulated and identified nine areas of educational objectives. From these areas, he wrote 160 major educational objectives, ranging from "Ability to use language in all ways required for proper and efficient participation in community life," to "Ability to entertain one's friends and to respond to entertainment of one's friends." Following Bobbitt's example, Pendleton (Eisner, 1967) listed 1,581 social objectives for English, and Guiler (Eisner, 1967) identified over 300 objectives for arithmetic in grades one through six.

The movement to identify large numbers of specific objectives collapsed during the 1930s. It seemed teachers could hardly manage 50 objectives, not to mention hundreds. A new view of the child as an emerging, changing, and growing entity came into being about this time, wielding a death blow to the "machine-oriented" approach specific objectives encouraged.

After 10 to 15 years of rather aimless experimentation with various educational models, curriculum specialists looked at educational objectives once again and laid down guidelines for writing objectives. Tyler's (1951) influential book identified several general objectives and a number of objectives of lesser importance which he felt educators should strive to achieve. This was followed by Bloom's (1956) handbook, which identified objectives in the cognitive domain, and still later, another handbook was written describing behavioral objectives in the affective domain (Krathwohl et al., 1964). The appearance of Mager's (1962) concise book, *Preparing Instructional Objectives,* which outlined in simple fashion the basic requirements for writing behavioral objectives and the importance of attaching objective criterion measures, strongly influenced educators in their search for the clarifying objectives. B. F. Skinner (1953) provided the theoretical and research support for returning to the "efficiency of training" so popular in the 1920s. Tyler (1951) provided the credence and rationale to restart the movement, and taxonomists like Bloom (1956) provided bibles that permitted leading educators, chiefly Mager (1962) and Popham (1967b), to promote it (Alpren & Baron, 1974).

It was during the 1950s and 1960s that parents expressed deep concern about the quality of education in the nation's schools, especially with regard to basic mathematical and reading skills. They sought accountability measures from the schools and welcomed pronouncements about efficient instruction and objective measurement techniques. Behavioral objectives offered a way to aid the learner in achieving educational goals; through criterion reference testing, clinicians could determine precisely when goals were achieved. Within the past few years, systems for competence-based education represent the ultimate development in the specifications of behavioral objectives and measurement technique. An excellent illustration of the use of Competence Based Teacher Education (CBTE) is found in the statewide teacher-training program of special education in New York (Creamer & Gilmore, 1974). A total of 287 competences were identified for educators involved in special education. Behavioral objectives were written for each competency, from housekeeping skills for the educable mentally retarded, to specifying the pros and cons of various careers for those in special education programs.

The behavioral objective movement received additional support from federal agencies as billions of dollars were poured into school programs through grant support. Unless schools provided direct evidence of clearly stated behavioral objectives, chances of receiving monies for programs were almost nil. State and local government agencies also demanded that school officials clearly state their goals and objectives. Threats in the form of mandates and denying credentials to teacher-training institutions were powerful motivators which forced educators into specifying their objectives. Few institutions have been untouched by the movement. This power play from the federal government through the Office of Education and by state governmental agencies provided the necessary support for the curriculum reform movement of the late 1950s and early 1960s.

Those who work in the public schools are well aware of the Public Law 94-142 as outlined in the Federal Register (1977). This law requires the development of written statements about the educational needs of handicapped children and implementation of educational objectives to meet those needs. These written statements must be completed before services are provided, then implemented as soon as possible. The statements must include the following: (a) a statement about the child's level of performance abilities; (b) specification of both annual and short-term goals; (c) objective criteria and evaluative procedures for determining when the goals are achieved. Those who work in the schools and other public agencies have no choice whether or not they wish to write objectives: the task is mandatory.

Numerous papers and books have been written about the use of behavioral objectives and competency in education. The materials are designed to develop in educators the necessary skills to write behavioral objectives and to identify competencies in education (Baker & Popham, 1973; Bloom, 1956; Biggs et al., 1967; Dickson & Saxe, 1974; McAshan, 1970; Houston & Howsam, 1973; Mager, 1962,

1973; Popham, 1967b, 1969). Plowman (1968–69) for example, wrote a series of eight units on behavioral objectives, planned as teacher-growth handbooks in seven academic areas including biology, social studies, reading, science, English, mathematics, art, and music.

The effects of the behavioral objective movement have touched almost every speech clinician. Evidence of these effects are plentiful—one example is a series of articulation correction programs written by speech clinicians in Las Vegas, Nevada, as part of a federally funded project (Lundquist, 1973). It contains three general operational objectives and two behavioral objectives, plus a large number of specific objectives pertaining to each program. Gordon and Williams (Cooper, 1972) list 68 behavioral objectives to be mastered by Ohio speech clinicians who attended special workshops to develop precision articulation skills.

There can be no doubt about the widespread influence of the *behavioral objective movement.* Its influence can be seen in every aspect of the education process. According to administrators and teachers attending the 1973 summer session at the Northern Illinois University in DeKalb, it was found that 95.8% of the educators were familiar with behavioral objectives through their course work (Frey, 1974). At least 90% said they used behavioral objectives to varying degrees in their teaching. It would be interesting to know if these same percentage figures hold true for speech clinicians, especially those employed in the public schools where the movement has had its greatest impact. Certainly, it is safe to say that almost any educator who has anything to do with the instructional process will soon be asked to write behavioral objectives.

Values of Writing
Instructional Objectives

Instructional objectives serve three chief functions: (1) to provide direction in the form of concise goals in teaching and curriculum development; (2) to provide guidance in evaluation of goals; and (3) to facilitate the student's learning. Mager (1962) contends that unless objectives are clearly stated before instruction is attempted, it is difficult to select appropriate instructional materials or evaluate the results of instruction. Behavioral objectives help the teacher identify *what* the students are to be doing when instruction has ended. Not only does writing behavioral objectives assist the teacher in organizing her teaching, these objectives also aid the student in identifying what the teacher feels is important to learn.

Many educators believe that without well-stated behavioral objectives, it is impossible to determine whether or not any learning has taken place. Objectives provide us with guidelines for evaluating the effects of instruction. Plowman (1968–1969) feels the most important thing a teacher can do is modify behavior toward prescribed goals by, "defining, teaching to, and evaluating pupil progress and instruction in the light of behavioral objectives."

Of course, listing all the studies showing the advantages of using behavioral objectives does not really mean much unless there are data which support the hypothetical advantages. Unfortunately, I know no research project in speech pathology that reports concrete evidence either for, or against, the use of behavioral objectives.

This has not been the case in other areas of education. Consider the first proposed advantage of using behavioral objectives: a means for improving teaching. McNeil (1967) reported a series of three studies which provided evidence that the use of operational definitions of instructional goals, including specification of criterion measures in the supervisory process, is accompanied by more favorable assessment of teachers by supervisors. Another result of using behavioral objectives was that greater gains were achieved by the learner when behavioral objectives were used. These studies dealt with supervisors who were helping their student teachers teach punctuation skills to their pupils. These results could not be considered a valid test of the influence of behavioral objectives primarily because McNeil told the student teachers that their course grade would be determined by the performance of their pupils, rather than from the usual supervisor recommendation. Because the results of these studies are related primarily to student motivation for good grades, it is difficult to draw any valid conclusions about the benefits of using behavioral objectives.

A second study by Baker (1969) investigated whether or not using behavioral objectives had a beneficial effect on learning certain concepts in social studies. Eighteen high school teachers were randomly assigned to one of three groups. One group was given five nonbehavioral objectives like the following: to understand the difference between descriptive and causal hypothesis. The other two groups were given five different behavioral objectives each, such as: when given a hypothesis, the student can identify it as either descriptive or causal. The teachers were told to teach the material defined in the objectives. The students were then measured on five basic skills and 18 transfer skills relating to the objectives. The scores of all groups were compared statistically. No significant differences were found among any of the groups; the use of behavioral objectives had no impact upon the quality of teaching. Baker felt perhaps the teachers did not fully understand the behavioral objectives or maybe they were not rewarded for producing student change. They may have relied on inadequate instructional models, negating any positive effects behavioral objectives might have had.

There are serious design problems one must consider when conducting research to test the usefulness of behavioral objectives. If one group of teachers is given behavioral objectives and another group given nonbehavioral objectives, the effects of student performance of each group can be compared. Such a design is clearly biased against teachers who receive the nonbehavioral objective since they might have thought of observable ways to test the nonbehavioral objective other than those selected by the researcher.

With regard to the second hypothetical advantage of using behavioral objectives, that they aid in evaluating the student's performance, their use would seem to be extremely valuable. Popham and Husek (1969) issued a convincing argument for using criterion referenced tests which are related directly to behavioral objectives. They feel we learn much more about the individual and about strategies we should employ by using these types of measures. Mager (1973) provides additional support stressing the importance of using correctness of the match between objectives and performance as an evaluational technique. But when one looks for data to support these positions, there seems to be little interest in finding out whether these advantages are real or just theoretical. No data are available on this subject at present.

The third role of using behavioral objectives is that of facilitating learning on the part of the student. Specifically, does communicating behavioral objectives to the learner facilitate, or enhance, his learning? Duchastel and Merrill (1973) present an extensive review of all major studies conducted in this area. Their findings are somewhat discouraging with respect to the value of using behavioral objectives with the intent of facilitating learning. Results of the approximately 40 studies reviewed were inconsistent to say the least. Studies which found no significant difference between experimental and control groups were as numerous as those which found a difference. Three factors which may have accounted for the discrepancies among studies were analyzed. The first was the varying types of subject matter considered. It appeared irrelevant whether the subject matter was chemistry, social studies, mathematics, or English. Level of schooling was examined. Here again, it made no difference whether the students were primary, secondary, college, or adult learners. Finally, it did not seem to matter whether results were analyzed within 10 minutes after instruction or after many weeks; the results were still inconsistent.

Duchastel and Merrill (1973) concluded that presenting objectives to students may help facilitate learning and are almost never harmful; consequently, if it is convenient to provide objectives, it should be done. It is possible that having objectives available could provide some organization to subject matter. Objectives may also aid the learner in providing feedback about successful completion of the objective. One possible explanation offered for the disparaging results is in the manner in which objectives are defined and presented to the learner. Nevertheless, assumptions about the facilitative effect objectives have upon the learner seem to be questionable in view of research data.

What does this mean to the speech clinician? It has been common practice for speech clinicians initiating articulation therapy to help children understand the nature of their speech problems (Van Riper, 1963). Anderson and Newby (1973) point out the necessity of making the individual aware of his speech problem before effective speech therapy can be initiated. In a sense, this procedure amounts to the same thing as presenting a behavioral objective to the individual with the expectation that this act will in some way facilitate learning. While not attempting to investigate this problem directly, I found in an experimental study involving the use of an instructional program designed to correct lisping behavior, that explaining the behavioral objective to first-grade children may not serve any useful function (Mowrer, 1964). Children who lisped were first given a criterion test; then they received three 20-minute lessons designed to correct lisping; and finally, they were tested again. At no time was it explained to these children that they had a speech problem or that the objective of this program was to change their pronunciation of /s/. Under certain conditions, some of the children who scored zero correct /s/ productions on the pretest produced 100% correct /s/ sounds on the posttest. They were then asked if they knew why they were attending the sessions. None could give any reasons. When asked if they were aware that the purpose was to change their /s/ sound, they stated they did not know they were supposed to say a sound differently. They were also unaware of the fact that they misarticulated a sound.

The point here is that even though some experts tell us that explaining the objective of instruction is supposed to be enhance learning, the fact is that a discussion of objectives with the learner may be unnecessary. Nevertheless, there may be times when explaining the objective to the learner may indeed facilitate learning. Young children may not even comprehend our objective, whereas some older children and adults might be able to work more constructively if they have a clear idea of what is expected of them. As Duchastel and Merrill (1973) point out, probably no harm can be done in letting the learner know what is expected of him; but at this time, we cannot place much credence in the value of using behavioral objectives as a facilitator to learning.

So where does all this leave you with respect to the value of using behavioral objectives? The advantages behavioral objectives offer seem obvious, at least for tasks requiring performance activities. It seems very logical to specify exactly what we wish to accomplish by our instruction and to administer criterion tests which will enable us to determine whether or not we have been successful. Yet, the research giving credibility to this concept is lacking. Until such research data are presented, it appears we must rely upon good judgment with respect to the use of behavioral objectives. Reflecting upon the lack of research in support of behavioral objectives, McNeil (1967) said, "Personal bias and power remain the chief determiners of educational objectives."

Criticism of Using Behavioral Objectives

While proponents of behavioral objectives cite the obvious value in the teacher's knowing educational goals and how to evaluate when she reaches them, another group of educators worry that using precise objectives may hinder the full development of the student and force the teacher to be a mechanistic, inflexible technician.

One of the leading critics of behavioral objectives, E. W. Eisner (1967), lists three major reasons why use of behavioral objectives is ill-advised: (1) The instructional process is dynamic, complex, and ever changing, yielding outcomes too numerous to be specified in behavioral terms. Just to list all possible behaviors would be an enormous, time-consuming task; (2) In some subjects, especially the arts, it is not possible to specify behavioral outcomes. Furthermore, the stultifying effect of predetermined, artistic outcomes would be undesirable. Perhaps uniformity is desirable in mathematics and spelling, but where creativity is the end product, behavioral objectives would be inappropriate; and (3) Not all educational outcomes are measurable. Consider values, ethical attitudes, or mores—how can we develop empirical tests for these areas? If we view the child as an art product and the teacher as the critic, then a major task for the teacher is to help reveal the qualities of the child to himself and to others. The teacher would serve as an appraiser of the changes and improvements made by the child. Of course, it is much easier to measure skills in extracting square roots than to evaluate a child's ability to write poetry.

A different criticism of behavioral objectives was leveled by McDonald (1965). Noticing that it was common practice for objectives to be determined before instruction, thereby providing the basis for instruction, he felt we really could not know what the objectives are until after instruction is completed. No matter what we attempt to do, we only know what we want to accomplish after the fact. Writing objectives prior to instruction is a heuristic device which initiates action but becomes altered as instruction progresses.

R. L. Ebel (1967), another strong critic of behavioral objectives, feels their contribution to effective teaching is vastly overrated. He maintains if objectives are written in detail, they become far too numerous. One could spend large amounts of time just writing them. Ebel stated, "few teachers are actually as foolishly dependent on stated objectives as educational theorists have sometimes urged them to be." Broad-range objectives are necessary but of little use to the teacher in his day-to-day teaching, he contends. Ebel feels attempts to state behavioral objectives explicitly in advance of teaching is, "seldom educationally rewarding." Measurement devices are also of questionable value. All too often they amount to a subjective opinion. Frequently, we do not really know when a behavioral objective is reached. In order to encourage artistic freedom, we cannot use the exacting measurements of science.

In response to Eisner's (1967) position, Hastings (1967) agrees with arguments against use of behavioral objectives. He maintains it is "rubbish" to conclude no progress can be made until we have all the goals stated in behavioral terms; attending only to prescribed, behavioral outcomes restricts the teacher's view about the essence of the education process. The use of behavioral objectives may actually deter the teacher from his job by forcing him to attend only to performance details. An education is much more than a series of behaviors, as some would have us believe.

While quick to point out the advantages of using behavioral objectives, Hilton (1974) is also cautious about their use in all conditions. He feels all goals are not subject to behavioral specification. Art, for example, enjoyment of reading, awaking an interest, developing an appreciation of past historical events, or developing an attitude of a responsible citizen, all are difficult to pin down in terms of behavioral objectives. In addition, how does one write a behavioral objective for a child's ability to organize all the material that he has learned? Hilton feels behavioral objectives have their place in education but should not be considered a panacea for all of education's ills. Wagener (1975) adopted a similar position with respect to the limited value of behavioral objectives when he stated behavioral objectives are overworked and misused. While not denying objectives are ideally suited to some situations, like transmitting skills and certain types of knowledge, their use may be inappropriate in other instances. Wagener went on to say that a well-stated behavioral objective is no guarantee that teaching methods will be effective or that students will be more involved in their studies. The sheer number of objectives that must be written is exhaustive for the busy teacher.

Aside from some educational leaders who have taken a stand against behavioral objectives, teachers have also opposed their use in spite of the massive support given the movement by federal, state, and local agencies, as well as other pressure groups. During the 1950s and 1960s, teachers tended to resist the movement by passive or devious means. Ammons (1964) found that (1) some school systems did not have educational objectives as guides for their programs; (2) school systems did not follow recommended curriculum process to develop their instructional objectives; and (3) teachers based their programs on what they customarily had done, rather than on the system's educational objectives. What seemed to be a force to support the use of objectives was not necessarily a force in the implementation of classroom curricula.

Some teachers may fight the movement and oppose its extension to areas of accountability and certification. This opposition, according to Alpren and Baron (1974), will be the death blow to the movement, especially if teacher unions withdraw their support of accountability measures. Frey's (1974) survey of 406 educators revealed that unfavorable comments about the use of operant conditioning, behavior modification, and behavioral objectives outnumbered favorable comments 12:5. Among the unfavorable comments were, "Behavioral objectives are a waste of time—tend to dehumanize students—are of little value to the affective domain—stifle creativeness." Although the majority of teachers were familiar with, and had used, behavioral objectives, their opinions about the usefulness of objectives were indecisive. Frey believes the massive fusion of behavioral objectives with all aspects of the education process, without evidence to prove their utility, may create a backlash from teachers sufficient to destroy the movement. Rath (1968) feels the requirements for specificity recommended by behavioral objective advocates are in direct conflict with teachers who consider humanism and intellectualism paramount values in education.

Alpren and Baron (1974), while acknowledging the worth of behavioral objectives, predict an early death to the movement because of two reasons: First, the excessive use of power by federal, state, and private agencies to force teachers to write and follow behavioral objectives will cause teachers to find means of bypassing, or even boycotting, administrative mandates. Second, there will be a strong reaction against the excessive claims by some educators who contend that behavioral objectives are a cure-all or panacea to answer problems of inadequate learning. Those who are concerned about relevance in education, who emphasize affective, humanistic objectivism, and who promote higher order cognitive skills strongly oppose the behavioral objective movement. By overextending their claims, planners may fail in their attempts to convince teachers, as well as the public, that behavioral objectives have universal application. Much of what is central to education lies outside the scope of behaviorism. The umbrella of efficiency and behavioral prescription cannot encompass the goals of humanism. Alpren and Baron predict even after the fall of the behavioral objective movement, it will leave an indelible mark on the educational process, and this mark will be strongly felt in the basic skills. The impact of the movement will have an influential effect upon many future generations of teachers.

But at present, the behavioral objective movement is far from over. Academic bantering continues. For each argument the opposition proposes, the proponents counter with an equally logical answer. Popham (1967a) presents 10 reasons why some educators resist the implementation of precise instructional objectives. He then provides counter arguments for each reason cited by critics. He points out the trouble with the criticisms of precise objectives is not that they are completely without foundation (in fact, there may be elements of truth in all of the criticisms) but that many teachers will use the comments of the few critics as an excuse to keep from thinking clearly about their goals and to continue to retard educational progress. The arguments pro and con cease to be academic in light of recent legislation demanding that behavioral objectives be clearly stated. The battles that may ensue might end up in court.

As the controversy rages in education concerning the use of behavioral objectives, speech clinicians, judging from the paucity of literature about the subject, seem to be relatively unconcerned about the issue. Whether this reflects indifference to or acceptance of behavioral objectives it is difficult to determine. While only one article in our professional journals has been published promoting the use of behavioral objectives (Andrews, 1971), no one has voiced any reservations or pointed out disadvantages of their use. Since speech clinicians are primarily engaged in modifying behaviors, rather than instilling values, creativeness, or humanistic ideals, the use of behavioral objectives seem ideally suited to their instructional needs. Although their application seems appropriate to speech therapy, it remains to be seen whether research data will support this use. At present, we have no such data; neither can we "borrow" supporting data from the educational field. It just is not there. It would be unwise for speech clinicians to adopt the use of behavioral objectives simply because it is something new or recommended by a few authorities in the field. The speech clinician should carefully study the purpose of using objectives, learn how to write them, and finally, put them to use. In this way, each clinician can judge for herself the worth of the endeavor. However, some clinicians will have no choice. They must prepare and evaluate behavioral objectives now. For those who must follow this pattern and others who wish to know more about the construction of behavioral objectives, the following section should help clarify specific skills needed to write these objectives.

Writing Objectives

Constructing behavioral objectives seems to be a simple matter until one confronts all the different kinds of overt and covert behaviors humans engage in daily. Bloom (1956) outlines three major behavioral domains: (1) cognitive—behaviors dealing with recall or recognition of knowledge and the development of intellectual abilities; (2) affective—behaviors that describe attitudes and values and development of appreciations and adequate adjustment; and (3) psychomotor—behaviors that are primarily concerned with physical activities. Nagel and Richman (1972) describe five categories of objectives. They include cognitive, performance, affective, consequence, and experimental. For the most part, speech clinicians are concerned with performance- or psychomotor-type objectives; consequently, our review will be limited to this type of objective. Performance objectives identify a goal and specify some performance to indicate that the goal has been achieved. McAshan (1970) divides performance objectives into two types: (1) noninstructional objectives, which are nonlearner-oriented such as goals to improve facilities, services, or creation of products, materials, equipment; and (2) behavioral objectives, which are learner-oriented and may involve teachers, supervisors, pupils, parents, or others. Both types include a goal statement and a means of evaluating goal attainment. The steps in constructing behavioral objectives, or what we list here as instructional objectives, will be presented first.

Mager's Approach to Writing Behavioral Objectives

Garvey (1968) describes behavioral objectives as a description of what the learner will be able to do as a result of the learning experience. Mager (1962) recommended that behavioral objectives, or instructional objectives as he calls them, must contain three components. They must specify (1) what the learner is supposed to be *doing;* (2) the *conditions* under which he will be doing the act; and (3) a *criterion* to indicate how well he will be doing it. Each component will be explained in detail.

The DO statement: One of the major pitfalls in writing objectives is the use of an inappropriate verb in the do statement. The "doing" has to be something which is observable. Words like *to know, to appreciate,* and *to understand* are to be avoided in favor of verbs such as to say, to count, to write, or to point. A good check on the verb used in the do statement is to ask yourself, "Can I count it?" Consider the following examples and decide whether or not the action described is something you could count.

1. to place the tongue behind the alveolar ridge
2. to concentrate on a pleasant voice quality
3. to breathe deeply
4. to identify the picture of a stove
5. to show an interest in the activity
6. to vocalize "ah"

Placement of the tongue in a certain position is a behavior we can count and would be a legitimate do statement; but how would you know when a person is concentrating? You cannot count each time he concentrates because you have no way of knowing when he is or is not concentrating. You could only count the number of times he says, "I'm concentrating." Breathing deeply is questionable as a do statement because of its vagueness. How deep is deeply? We can count breathing all right so that part is satisfactory, but deeply is difficult to measure.

In the fourth statement, "to identify" sounds clear enough, but the question is can you count someone identifying something? You say, "Sure, I count each time she points to the stove." If this is the case, then use the word *point* in preference to *identify.* Words have very precise meanings, and we should use them appropriately. They are our basic tools for precise communication. What about number 5? That one is really poor. Here again, how do you count someone showing an interest? You can count smiling, handling objects, or watching the clinician as indicators of one's interest, so list these behaviors instead. Finally, vocalizing a sound is fine. We can count it. Recall that White and Haring (1976) describe behaviors as having a definite beginning and a definite ending. They call behavior a *movement.* Attitudes, understanding, enjoying, and knowing imply no movement, and hence, cannot qualify as valid "do" statements. That is not to say these states do not exist. They do. But the only way we have of validating whether or not someone understands is to check on their performance. For example, if I tell you to stick your tongue out between your front teeth and blow over the top of your tongue, you may say "Yes, I understand what to do." How do I find out if you know what I mean? I can ask you to *do* it, or if your tongue is paralyzed, I can ask you to *point* to a picture of someone else doing it or to *count* the number of times I do it. The key issue here is that we must be able to check on the performance and measure (count) it in some way.

Do not make the mistake of describing what *you* are going to do; always specify what you want the *learner* to do. Consider the following statement:

> To present 10 picture cards to Pat.

That tells me what *you* intend to do, but what is *Pat* supposed to do? Better to state it this way:

> To name 10 picture cards when they are presented.

Now I know what it is the learner is supposed to do; I can also count the behavior.

List A below contains vague, ill-defined, undesirable verbs, while List B is made up of verbs which are appropriate for behavioral objectives:

List A		List B	
appreciate	familiarize	diagram	label
plan	realize	count	match
acquaint	communicate	write	say
understand	verbalize	put	fold
apply	discover	pour	smile
learn	know	repeat	point
like	want	walk	place
feel	realize	reach	demand

The following is a list of *do* statements which the speech clinician might use:

Point to pictures showing children engaged in action

Say /s/

Record correct responses on a score sheet

Compute error rate per minute

Speak fluently

Produce a sustained vocalization of /æ/

Ask a question

Repeat a sound

Tell a story

Say a sentence containing subject, verb, and object

The do statement then is the "verb" component of the behavioral objective. It's the action the learner should be performing.

Stating the CONDITIONS: Could you walk two miles? Most persons could answer "yes" to this question if they were physically capable of doing so, especially if they were to receive $1,000 after completing the walk. In fact, I'll offer that amount to any reader who can accomplish the two-mile walk! But before you accept the challenge, there are a few *conditions* I would like to add to the objective. First, carry a 180-pound pack; second, up the north rim of the Grand Canyon; third, in 120-degree heat; fourth, barefoot; fifth, no drinking water; sixth, without stopping; and seventh, walking backwards. You see, the conditions stated make the two-mile hike an impossible task. Of course, I could have made the conditions much easier so that almost anyone could walk the distance. The conditions, as you see, are very important.

The following are examples of the conditions we usually impose in speech therapy:

> In the presence of the speech clinician
> Using pictures
> Given two written words
> In the home environment
> With the aid of amplified speech
> When asked a question
> Given a designated articulation test
> Using two digital counters
> After observing the child in a free time activity
> When requested by the clinician
> Given a stopwatch
> While watching a 10-minute videotape selection

Conditions specify what you will provide to the individual in order to help him do the task, or they may describe what you will deny the learner. They can also pinpoint where the behavior will be performed, when it will be performed, and in whose presence it will be performed. In other words, conditions are the "adjective" statement of the behavioral objective because they describe the situation in which the behavior is to be performed.

CRITERION for success: Finally, you will need to include a statement about how well, or how accurately, you want the learner to perform the act. If I allowed you 10 days to make that two-mile hike up the Grand Canyon, I am sure many able-bodied, and even some not so able-bodied, speech clinicians could collect the $1,000 reward. But if my criterion for success was to complete the two-mile hike in 15 minutes, obviously, no one could achieve this objective. The criterion tells me what I am to expect from the learner so I'll know when, or how well, he has achieved the objective.

Frequently, a time limit is used as the criterion. The percent correct, a minimum number of actions, a proportion of items, or a date are also commonly used measures to help determine when an objective has been reached. The criterion resembles an "adverb" statement in that it states how or when the objective is to be met. It could also be considered an adjective statement because often the criterion consists of a description of "how many behaviors."

Here is a list of criterion measures you might use:

> nine out of ten correct
> five pages
> in 5 minutes
> 80% correct
> three-fourths
> 30 items
> 90% agreement
> three statements
> every sound
> 15 two-word sentences

By putting all three components together, we can state a large number of behavioral objectives clearly and concisely so anyone would know exactly what we want the learner to *do,* the *conditions* under which he is to do it, and the *criterion* for success. The following examples illustrate objectives that include these three components.

EXAMPLE 1

Suppose you are working with a child who misarticulates /s/. He has learned to say /s/ when combined with vowels, and you are ready to teach /s/ in combination with 10 words.

Analysis:

1. Do statement = name
2. Conditions = (a) pictures containing an /s/ sound
   (b) presented by the clinician
   (c) no verbal cues
3. Accuracy = 8 out of 10 correct /s/ productions

Behavioral Objective:

To name 10 pictures each containing an /s/ sound when presented by the clinician, who will provide no verbal cues. The /s/ will be produced correctly in 8 out of 10 instances.

EXAMPLE 2

For several months, you have been working with a child on a variety of tasks. The child has a language problem. One task has been to teach him the concept of the verb "push" and to use this word after you demonstrate pushing three objects and asking, "What did I do?"

Analysis:

1. Do statement = say "push"
2. Conditions   = clinician pushes object
                = clinician follows pushing with question, "What did I do?"
3. Criterion   = say "push" immediately following each of three demonstrations

Behavioral Objective:

To say "push" immediately following each of three demonstrations by the clinician who pushes an object and asks the question, "What did I do?"

EXAMPLE 3

An adult who stutters has progressed to the point where he is able to read textual material with a fair degree of fluency. You would like to set a specific goal for him during his reading practice which will include reading at least 125 words per minute for 5 minutes from the *Reader's Digest* with no more than 2% words stuttered. You want him to do this in front of three strangers.

Analysis:

1. Do statement = read aloud
2. Conditions   = any selection in *Reader's Digest*
                = in the presence of the clinician plus three strangers
3. Criteria   = 98% of the words will be spoken fluently
                = speed of 125 or more words per minute

Behavioral Objective:

To read aloud at a speed of 125 or more words per minute for 5 minutes from any selection in *Reader's Digest* in the presence of the clinician plus three strangers. At least 98% or more words will be spoken fluently.

EXAMPLE 4

You are working with a young girl who has vocal nodules as a result of vocal abuse. You have explained the four types of vocal abuse to her and how you want her to count the number of times she abuses her voice each day during the week and bring these data to you at the end of the week.

Analysis:

1. Do statement = count and record instances of vocal abuse

                                    = present card
2. Conditions   = given a wrist counter
                                    = given a score sheet
                                    = given instructions about how to score and tally instances of vocal abuse
                                    = given instructions about how to operate the wrist counter
3. Criterion   = present one scorecard on Friday afternoon, which includes 5 days of instances of vocal abuse

Behavioral Objective:

Having explained the four types of vocal abuses and provided the child with a daily score sheet and wrist counter, plus instructions about how to operate the counter and tally scores, the child is to count and record instances of vocal abuse each day for 5 days and present the completed scorecard to the clinician on the afternoon of the fifth day.

EXAMPLE 5

An aphasic patient has had difficulty in pointing to the correct picture when you have asked her to point to one picture among two others. You wish to develop an objective for a lesson in this area which will result in 80% correct picture-pointing behavior during a 10-minute practice period. You will present pictures one at a time and ask her to point to each picture after you name it. The patient must respond within 3 seconds.

Analysis:

1. Do statement = point to picture
2. Condition   = clinician will request, "Point to the _____."
3. Criteria.   = respond within 3 seconds of the command
                    = 80% correct identification during 10-minute period

Behavioral Objective:

The patient will point to a picture named by the clinician within 3 seconds after the clinician's prompt, "Point to the _____." She will be correct 80% of the time during the 10-minute practice period.

EXAMPLE 6

This time you are working with a nonverbal child who has cerebral palsy. The child has been known to vocalize on occasion but does not do so when requested. You will feed the child her meals, a spoonful at a time, and ask her to vocalize before receiving a spoonful of food. The objective is to bring the child's vocalizations under control of the clinician's vocalization of /a/. The child must respond within 10 seconds after the clinician vocalizes and must do so 100% of the time. Food and vocalization will be paired.

Analysis:

1. Do statement = vocalize
2. Condition   = presentation of spoonful of food within 10 seconds
3. Criteria   = 10 times of 10 presentations
                = within 10 seconds after clinician's vocalization of /a/.

Behavioral Objective:

Brenda will vocalize within 10 seconds upon being presented with a spoonful of food, accompanied by the clinician's vocalization of /a/ 10 times out of 10 presentations.

McAshan's Approach to Writing Behavioral Objectives

A somewhat different approach to the construction of behavioral objectives is taken by McAshan (1970). He lists advantages of two different types of behavioral objectives: (1) minimum level objectives, and (2) desired level objectives. Both include a basic goal statement and some way to evaluate achievement of the goal. The chief difference is the degree to which the evaluation is carried out. In a minimum level objective, no criterion performance is stated. McAshan points out there are many instances when goal statements do not lend themselves to a valid success level or single criterion of performance. Frequently, these objectives are prepared for system-wide use as overall program guides or for individual projects when specific criterion standards are inappropriate. Since exacting criterion standards are unnecessary, minimum behavioral objectives are much more flexible and have a wider application than objectives requiring these standards.

First, we will consider elements which are common to each objective. McAshan uses the word *goal* for Mager's term *main intent*. It refers to the central aim of the objective—the purpose. For example, one such statement might read:

> to increase auditory reception skills of aphasic patients.

After clearly identifying the intended purpose or goal for which the objective is written, three "communication checks" are made. These include (1) the intended program variable; (2) a distinct learner; and (3) an implied behavioral domain.

The program variable is the behavior, or subject under study, that is supposed to change. In the previous example, it is auditory reception skills. The learner refers to the person(s) who will do the changing. It may be a student, a patient, staff members, or a lay citizen. In the previous example, aphasic patients would be the learners.

The implied behavioral domain falls into the cognitive, affective, or psychomotor areas. In our example, auditory reception skills would imply a change in the cognitive area, since a certain amount of recall information is required.

Here is one more example of a goal:

> to improve cooperative play among preschool children during language class.

The program variable is cooperative play, the learners are preschool children, and the behavioral domain is psychomotor, since play skills are the main target.

Having clearly identified the components of the goal statement, the next step is to add an evaluation statement to the objective. Two problems emerge: What behavioral observations can serve as valid indications that change took place, and how are standards established to judge the performance? When using minimum objectives, one is concerned with only the first problem: What indicators to use. McAshan calls this an E–1 level evaluation. Both problems must be dealt with in the desired level objective, so they must contain E–1 and E–2 type evaluations, the E–2 level being performance standards. This difference in evaluation is what differentiates the minimum level from desired level. The best way to clarify this distinction is by example. First, here is a minimal behavioral objective:

> To train speech pathology majors to understand the meaning of, and be able to use, phonetic symbols to transcribe written speech.

The program variable is to understand the meaning of (note McAshan uses the word *understand* while others would reject this term) and be able to use phonetic symbols. The learner is the speech pathology major. The implied, behavioral domain is cognitive. The E–1 evaluation is to transcribe written speech.

To convert this objective with a desired level behavioral objective, we simply add the following E–2 evaluation:

> and meet the approval of the instructor.

The E–1 evaluation specified the learner would have to transcribe spoken speech in phonetic symbols, whereas the E–2 evaluation established a standard by which this work would be judged. Note that the operational success is not specified in minimal objective levels.

Now, as I did with Mager's objectives, I will present and analyze a few objectives using McAshan's suggestions:

EXAMPLE 1

You are teaching a class in anatomy and physiology of speech. You want your students to be able to correctly identify and name all the cartilages of the larynx. You plan to administer a test to find out how much they learned.

Analysis:

Program variable	= identify and name cartilages of the larynx
Learner	= speech pathology majors
Behavioral domain	= cognitive
Evaluation 1	= take a multiple-choice test
Evaluation 2	= none

Behavioral Objective:

To train speech pathology majors to identify and name all cartilages of the larynx. All students will be expected to take a multiple-choice test covering the cartilages of the larynx.

The above example is a minimum level behavioral objective since it contains only Evaluation 1.

EXAMPLE 2

You want to increase the oral reading rate of a child who stutters and keep the disfluent rate at the present level.

Analysis:

    Program variable   = reading
    Learner   = Bob
    Behavioral domain = psychomotor
    Evaluation 1   = read for 5 minutes
    Evaluation 2   = read 100 words per minute with disfluency rate below 2%

Behavioral Objective:

To increase Bob's reading rate from 80 words per minute to 100 words per minute, while keeping disfluencies below 2%, as measured by a 5-minute reading sample.

This is an example of a desired objective.

EXAMPLE 3

You want your clinicians to be able to graph correct and incorrect response data on a linear graph as percentages.

Analysis:

    Program variable   = graphing
    Learner   = clinicians
    Behavioral domain = cognitive and psychomotor
    Evaluation 1   = graph correct and incorrect response data on a
                           linear graph as percentages
    Evaluation 2   = 90% of clinicians must score 80% or better
                           on a 10-item test

Behavioral Objective:

To develop in clinicians the ability to graph percent correct and incorrect responses from a therapy session as measured by a 10-item, teacher-made test so that 90% of the clinicians score 80% or better on the test.

EXAMPLE 4

You are working with a high school boy who is very timid and can hardly be heard in class when he speaks. Your goal is to increase the loudness of his voice when he speaks in class.

Analysis:

    Program variable   = speaking
    Learner   = Bill
    Behavioral domain = psychomotor
    Evaluation 1   = speak in class loudly enough to be heard by
                           teacher and classmates
    Evaluation 2   = none

Behavioral Objective:

To increase the loudness of Bill's voice when he speaks in class so the teacher and classmates will be able to understand what he says.

EXAMPLE 5

You wish to interact with parents so that they will become more familiar with your program and take an active interest in it.

Analysis:

Program variable	= opportunity for involvement
Learner	= parents
Behavioral domain	= affective
Evaluation 1	= participating in home visits, observation of classes and attending group meetings
Evaluation 2	= as judged successful for the successful by the supervisor's contact with parents

Behavioral Objective:

To provide an opportunity for parent involvement by arranging home visits, observations in the classroom, and group parent meetings. Your supervisor will judge from contacts made with parents how successful the program is.

McAshan illustrates most of his objectives with examples of improving academic skills in the classroom, or with program-improvement objectives. His style of writing objectives does not appear to be as relevant to our needs in speech pathology as does the procedure outlined by Mager. Yet, some people may prefer McAshan's system. Both systems are presented so the reader has a choice of writing styles. Knowledge of several systems for writing behavioral objectives can also help us understand and evaluate objectives written by others.

Snyder's Approach to Writing Behavioral Objectives

Snyder (1971) offers several suggestions to pathologists just beginning to write behavioral objectives. We all state objectives every day. Asking a librarian for a certain book, ordering a meal, and coaching someone are all instances of stating objectives. One should not view writing objectives as foreign or new. If you have trouble writing the objective, try stating the problem you are trying to solve, rather than trying to write the objective you want to accomplish. Keep your statement to five words or less. Then write a simple sentence describing what is to be achieved. Qualifying and quantifying phrases can be added later. Be sure you refer directly to a person or group of people. Also, be sure you are talking about a behavior that is to be performed, that is observable, measurable, and countable. Include a criterion to indicate the objective has been met and a time period in which it should be completed.

Below are eight questions Snyder feels are important to ask yourself when writing objectives:

1. What is to be accomplished?
2. By whom?
3. When or for how long?
4. Under what conditions?
5. With what tools or materials?
6. To what extent or degree of accuracy?
7. Judged how?
8. Any special features?

Here is an example of how these questions can be used in writing behavioral objectives in speech therapy:

EXAMPLE 1

Suppose you are a supervisor of speech clinicians in a hospital setting and you want to make sure all the clinicians know what to do if a patient has a seizure.

1. What is to be accomplished?	List the steps taken in case of patient seizure.
2. By whom?	Clinician.
3. When or for how long?	At end of 3 hours of instruction and demonstration.
4. Under what conditions?	When asked to list steps.
5. With what tools or materials?	Pencil and paper.
6. To what extent or degree of accuracy?	Clinician will list 10 steps for care of patient.
7. Judge how?	Match to the answer sheet.
8. Any special features?	Certificate given upon completion of training.

From the answers to these questions, we can now construct a behavioral objective for this project.

Behavioral Objective:

Immediately following a 3-hour training session in which 10 steps for treating a patient undergoing seizure are explained and demonstrated, the clinician will be able to list on paper all 10 steps from memory as evaluated by the 10 steps listed in the instructor's manual. A certificate certifying knowledge of these steps will be awarded to each clinician upon completion of the objective.

EXAMPLE 2

Sue, who has a multiple articulation problem, frequently omits final plosive consonants. She also has other substitutions and omissions. Your immediate job is to help Sue produce the final consonants /t/, /d/, /k/ and /g/ in single-word productions.

Analysis:

1. What is to be accomplished?	Produce /t/, /d/, /k/, and /g/ in the final position of words containing these sounds.
2. By whom?	Sue.
3. When or for how long?	After three 20-minute sessions.
4. Under what conditions?	When presented with a picture by the clinician.
5. With what tools or materials?	Deck of picture cards each containing a word with a final /t/, /d/, /k/, or /g/.
6. To what extent or degree of accuracy?	85% correct final consonant production in 25 words.
7. Judge how?	As evaluated by the speech clinician.
8. Any special conditions?	No rewards or prompts provided.

Behavioral Objective:

Following three 20-minute therapy sessions, Sue will produce final /t/, /d/, /k/, and /g/ sounds in words in response to naming picture cards presented by the speech clinician. At least 85% of the above final consonants will be produced correctly in 25 words presented. No rewards or prompts will be provided.

This may seem rather lengthy in comparison to the original intent which was "to help Sue produce final consonants /t/, /d/, /k/, and /g/ in single-word productions." But the behavioral objective tells us much more than the general intent of the instruction. It specifies how we will know when we will have accomplished the goal, and it specifies some important conditions of the objective. Snyder's question-asking system is extremely helpful in learning how to construct behavioral objectives, especially for those who are just beginning to write objectives. Clinic supervisors will find this system especially helpful in teaching student clinicians how to construct behavioral objectives. Once the eight basic questions are answered, writing the objective is simple.

Short- and Long-term Objectives

There are two variations in the types of objectives you may wish to write: long-term objectives, or *terminal objectives,* and short-term objectives called *sub-objectives* or *transitional objectives.* A terminal objective would be one you wish to have accomplished when you are ready to dismiss a case. For example, Diedrich and Gerber (1974) determined that children with /s/ or /r/ errors could be dismissed from therapy when they had reached greater than 75% correct production of the target sound on a Speech Production Task (SPT), plus a 3-minute talk test for two consecutive probes, one or two weeks apart. Assuming we have a child who has an /r/ problem, the terminal objective would look like this:

The child will produce words containing /r/ in a SPT and 3-minute talk test administered by the clinician during two consecutive probes which are given one to two weeks apart. At least 75% of the child's /r/ sounds must be judged as correct.

Of course, there are many other ways to word this objective. Here's another way:

During the clinician's administration of two consecutive SPT and 3-minute talk tests, given one to two weeks apart, the child will say the /r/ sound in words correctly 75% of the time.

There will be many sub-objectives, or transitional objectives, to reach before the terminal objective is reached. These objectives are of two types: those you work toward at the end of a session or set of sessions, and those scored during therapy. The above set of examples was of the former type. After perhaps 10 to 20 minutes of therapy, you may present a test to see if you have reached your objective. The test might be 8 out of 10 correct, or less than 2% disfluent words immediately following three demonstrations. Some objectives specify criteria which must be met throughout the entire session. For example, objectives which require a certain response rate per minute during the session or a certain percent of correct responses fall into this category. There is no "test" at the end of the session since the "test" includes all of the responses made during the session. At present, there is no evidence to support one type of sub-objective (test at the end) over another (test during therapy). Part of an articulation correction program I wrote included both types of objectives (Mowrer, 1964). In the first lesson, a child had to get at least 50% of the first 50 items correct before she could proceed to the final 50 items covered during that therapy session. There was also a criterion test consisting of 10 items given only after the child had completed the first 100 items. The two objectives would look like this:

1. The child will say /s/ correctly 50% of the time when instructed by the clinician to say /s/ in isolation, with vowels, and monosyllable words during a therapy session containing 50 items.

2. The child will say /s/ correctly in 8 out of 10 words when pictures are presented by the clinicians following completion of a 100-item training session.

Both these objectives play important roles. The first objective tells us whether or not the child can benefit from the instructional program. It has been found those children who make fewer than 25 correct responses on the first 50 items are not able to pass the first criterion test. Therefore, to continue administering the program to these children after the first 50 tries would be inadvisable because the items which follow become more and more difficult as the program progresses. The value of this first behavioral objective is that it allows us to screen out those children who will probably not succeed in the program. This type of objective could only have been written after the program had been administered to several children. In most cases, the children tell us what criterion levels should be. This is an a posteriori objective.

The second objective not only tells us which children have mastered the correct /s/ production and are ready to proceed to the next part, but also tells us which concepts or skills in the program were, or were not, mastered. Analysis of objectives may provide us with diagnostic information which can be used for future instructional planning. This second objective is an *a priori* objective. It was planned beforehand as a likely indicator of the child's success in the program. Subsequent data proved it to be a valid indicator of success, so it was retained. It is possible when using the same type of instruction to test the validity of behavioral objectives. But for the most part, clinicians will be constructing them as they progress in therapy.

Evaluating objectives: Mager (1973) outlines an approach to assist the writer of objectives to assess written objectives and to apply more effective means of measuring whether or not objectives have been achieved. He presents four steps which should be carried out in decoding an objective.

First, note what it is the learner should be doing in the objective. As I mentioned before, it must be something you can observe and count. If no performance is mentioned, then it is not an objective.

The second step is to determine whether the performance is stated as the *main intent* or as an *indicator*. The main intent of an objective is the performance, which is the purpose of the objective. Performances such as to say, to point, and to read may be the main intent of an objective, but sometimes the main intent is inferred, as in the following example:

Point to the picture named by the clinician when presented with two pictures, the names of which differ only in one phoneme.

The main intent, or purpose, of this objective is to teach the person to correctly discriminate between two sounds. The performance, in this case, is pointing. But pointing is not what we want to teach the person, is it? She already knows how to point. The main intent is to teach the person how to discriminate. We can tell whether she is discriminating correctly by what she does, that is, where she points.

Consider another example; suppose you are working with an aphasic patient and you want him to correctly identify numbers when you call them out. Your objective might say, "Draw a line under the appropriate printed numbers when they are called out by the clinician." The performance is drawing lines, but you know that is not what we want to teach. Drawing lines under appropriate numbers simply indicates he can correctly identify spoken numbers. Therefore, the main intent is identifying, or recognizing, spoken numbers, while the indicator is drawing lines.

If you recall Goal 3 in the previous section, the "do" statement was count and record instances of vocal abuse. Counting and recording are simply performance indicators, a means of discriminating between speaking conditions that result in vocal abuse and those that do not. This ability to discriminate is the main intent. A similar case is found in Goal 4. Pointing to pictures is only an indicator; the main intent is to teach the aphasic patient to match certain pictures with their related spoken words.

Mager (1973) includes two parts in step 3 of his outline: (1) if the performance is an indicator, the main intent should be identified; and (2) if on the other hand, the performance is the main intent, decide whether it is an overt or covert performance. Sometimes you may write an objective, or read someone else's objective, that contains an indicator but no main intent. For example:

> Given a set of pictures, select all the pictures containing an /s/ sound.

In this case, the indicator is to select pictures; but what is the main intent? Perhaps the main intent is to discriminate from those containing /f/ sounds or maybe just choosing those pictures which contain an /s/ sound. The objective needs to be restated as follows:

> Given a set of pictures, identify those which begin with an /s/ sound by selecting only those pictures.

The second part of this step concerns overt and covert performances. Previously, performances have had to be behaviors that are observable, countable, and manipulatable. But Mager also includes covert main objectives which can be cognitive, internal, or mental. These are events that *cannot* be observed. Examples are adding figures in your head, solving a problem silently, thinking, recognizing, and the like. No one would deny we all engage in these private mental activities, but until recently, these activities were considered to be outside the realm of behaviorism. Mager suggests that behavioral objectives can be written for these events simply by adding an overt indicator to the objective. Consider the following objective:

> To recognize what a pencil is for.

The main intent is clear enough as an objective for an aphasic patient, but there is no indicator; so one way for you to find out if he has a correct concept of what a pencil is for is to simply add the following indicator:

> To recognize what a pencil is for by writing or drawing with the pencil.

A complete objective would look something like this:

> To recognize what a pencil is for by writing or drawing with the pencil each time the clinician places the pencil before the patient and says, "Show me what you do with this."

If the main intent is an overt performance, then there is no need to include an indicator; but as you can see in the illustration above, an indicator is required.

Mager's fourth step is a test of the indicator, providing you have included an indicator. The indicator should be simple and well within the person's ability to perform. If the indicator is too difficult to perform, then you cannot test the main intent. Consider this example for a third-grade child who stutters:

> Demonstrate speech fluency by reciting the Declaration of Independence.

As you can easily see, the vocabulary level contained in the Declaration of Independence is far above that of most third-grade students and, hence, would be an inappropriate indicator with which to demonstrate speech fluency. A more appropriate indicator would be reading three pages from a second-grade reading book.

Preparing Noninstructional Objectives

In our previous discussion of McAshan's approach to writing behavioral objectives, you may have noted that he grouped instructional and noninstructional objectives together making no distinction between the two in the criteria he used for writing them. In this section, we shall consider some special procedures for writing noninstructional objectives.

A sizable portion of the speech clinician's job entails planning objectives which do not pertain to direct therapy services. Setting up testing programs, improving facilities, developing instructional and public relation materials, and developing a language improvement program may all be part of the clinician's job. Supervisors and administrators work primarily with noninstructional objectives. One of the chief advantages of writing noninstructional objectives is that it facilitates planning your activities so they can be completed. Unless we set specific goals, requirements, and deadline priorities, other more pressing activities are attended to first; and by the time we get around to the projects we intended to accomplish, we have run out of time. Also, written, noninstructional objectives provide administrators with a clear picture of your goals, time requirements, and responsibilities, as well as a knowledge of when these goals have been attained.

A procedure for writing noninstructional objectives has been presented in a manual published by the American Speech and Hearing Association (1973). The procedure consists of writing an objective which includes each of the following six basic components:

1. *When* is it going to be done?
2. *Who* is going to do it?
3. *What* is going to be done?
4. *To whom* is it going to be done?
5. What will be the *criterion* for success?
6. How will the success of the accomplishment be *evaluated?*

As you can see, the six components above are similar to those suggested in the previous section by Snyder. Here again, the most practical means of clarifying the procedure is by example.

EXAMPLE 1

Suppose you are a public school speech clinician and you want to screen the speech of all kindergarten children in the Central Elementary School next year. It is now April, and you are planning your objectives for the next school year.

First, provide answers to the following questions:

1. when?   By October 3, 19XX.
2. who?   I.
3. what?   Screen speech.
4. to whom?   Kindergarten children.

5. criterion?   All.
6. evaluation?   List of children who passed and failed submitted to
                       the principal.

Noninstructional Objective:

By October, I will have screened the speech of all kindergarten children in Central Elementary School and will submit a list of those who passed and failed this test to the principal.

By including each of the six components called for, writing the objective is a relatively simple task.

EXAMPLE 2

Now consider the following objective which was taken from a list of three operational objectives included in Lundquist's (1973) report mentioned earlier:

By September 1, 19XX, program writers will be identified and will develop a comprehensive transfer program for the /r/, /l/, /θ/, /ʃ/, /tʃ/ and the paired cognate sounds that can be utilized by professionals and/or nonprofessionals in assisting students with speech defects in one or more of these sounds.

By applying the six-component system mentioned above to this objective we can determine if all conditions have been met.

1. when?   By September 1, 19XX.
2. who?   We don't know who is going to be responsible for
                       this objective.
3. what?   (a) identify program writers.
                       (b) develop comprehensive transfer programs for
                           correction of articulation problems.
4. to whom?   Whoops! We have run into a problem.
                       There appears to be two objectives in one, as indicated by
                           the "what" component. So at this level, we are confused
                           whether to put down the writers of the program or
                           the professionals and/or nonprofessionals who will be
                           assigned students.
5. criterion?   Five transfer programs.
6. evaluation?   None.

By analyzing the objective using the six components as criteria, we have a better chance of judging whether or not an objective will be clearly understood by others who will read it. In the case above, perhaps the objective was stated adequately for those involved with the project. If we judge the end result, we have to concede the adequacy of this objective because it was completed as evidenced by Lundquist's final report. But for the purpose of clarifying how to write objectives using this system, I will rewrite this objective as two objectives, each containing all six components.

1. when?   By May 1, 19XX.
2. who?   The program director.
3. what?   Identify program writers.
4. to whom?   To the superintendent.
5. criterion   One list containing six names.
6. evaluation   Approval of the superintendent.

Noninstructional Objective:

(a) By May 1, 19XX, the program director will identify six speech clinicians as program writers and submit this list to the superintendent for her approval.

The second objective would look like this:

Noninstructional Objective:

(b) By September 1, 19XX, six speech clinicians will have written comprehensive transfer programs for the /r/, /l/, /θ/, /ʃ/, /tʃ/, and the paired cognate sounds so that they can be utilized by professionals and/or nonprofessionals. A copy of each program will be submitted to the superintendent for his approval.

As you can see, nothing has been changed from the intent of the original objective, but now there is no doubt who will do what, and when it will be accomplished. Here is another example using the six components as criteria.

EXAMPLE 3

The research branch of your school district would like you to conduct studies comparing the effectiveness of providing therapy daily versus twice a week. Your job is to write a noninstructional objective for this project.

1. when?   By January 3, 19XX.
2. who?   The speech pathologist.
3. what?   Will complete a study comparing daily and biweekly
                  therapy.
4. to whom?   Children in grades 1–3 who have articulation problems.
5. criterion?   Data of results of test scores.
6. evaluation?   Statistical analysis.

Noninstructional Objective:

By January 3, 19XX, the speech pathologist in Kingston will have completed a study comparing the effects of daily versus biweekly speech therapy sessions upon the articulation skills of children grades 1–3. The data from test scores of each child in each group will be computed and compared using a *t* test to determine if a statistical difference exists between the two groups.

EXAMPLE 4

As a supervisor, you want your clinicians to become familiar with new therapy materials. One way to do this is to assign five clinicians to use therapy program X and require that they administer program X to 30 children.

1. when?	By April 4, 19XX.
2. who?	The supervisor.
3. what?	Will assign administration of program X.
4. to whom?	Speech clinicians.
5. criterion?	Five.
6. evaluation?	Agree to administer the program to 30 children.

Noninstructional Objective:

(a) By April 4, 19XX, the supervisor will have assigned to five speech clinicians the task of administering program X to 30 children who misarticulate sounds. The clinicians will have all agreed to administer the program. In this example you can see that only part of the total objective is completed. The goal here is similar to the objective written in Lundquist's report cited previously. To complete the project we will need another objective that will look like this:

1. when?	By May 25, 19XX.
2. who?	Five speech clinicians.
3. what?	Administer program X.
4. to whom?	To 30 children.
5. criterion?	Write evaluation of program X.
6. evaluation?	Submit written evaluation of program to supervisor.

Noninstructional Objective:

(b) By May 25, 19XX, five speech clinicians will have administrated program X to 30 children who misarticulate sounds and will have submitted a written evaluation of the program to the supervisor.

Summary

Having worked through the many examples of behavioral and noninstructional objectives, you should realize the systems used here to analyze objective and goal statements can be very useful to the speech clinician, supervisor, and administrator of speech pathology programs. Even college professors could benefit from using these systems to aid in planning their course presentations. Students appreciate knowing *what* is expected of them, and they also appreciate knowing *when* they have achieved an objective. Written behavioral and noninstructional objectives are helpful tools enabling us to perform our work more efficiently. In a recent review of research pertaining to preinstructional strategies used by teachers, Hartley and Davies (1976) conclude that although research data fail to support the favorable claims made by many who support the behavioral objective movement, these objectives can be of substantial aid in helping teachers better organize their work. Organization has been termed the *hallmark* of good teaching. Any procedure that makes the organization of learning matter more obvious is certainly likely to facilitate the learning of meaningful material. On the other hand, having a bona fide objective does not mean the procedures used to obtain the objective will be effective. A good objective is only the beginning. Lacking effective procedures for use following the construction of a good objective will almost certainly result in failure to reach the criterion set in the objective. Effective procedures for obtaining behavior change are presented in chapter 7.

In conclusion, I think we, as professionals, should take a careful look at the advantages systems of writing behavioral and noninstructional objectives have to offer us. We should also be observant of the criticisms of using these types of objectives in all situations. The utility of using these systems and others which may be developed is entirely dependent on the needs of the individual. Certainly we all should know how to write objectives in some systematic manner, but we should also be cautious about the amount of time we invest in writing objectives. We could spend 2 to 3 hours a day writing objectives for the cases we will see tomorrow, but is this the most advantageous way to spend time? I feel it is important to write down what we intend to do, especially when that information is to be shared by others. But it is more important that we apply an organizational system to our daily planning as a matter of routine. This system of identifying specific behaviors, establishing certain conditions, and evaluating behaviors seems to be the important point. It becomes a modus operandi for the speech clinician in therapy. If the behavior modification movement does die out, as some predict, I would agree with Alpren and Baron (1974) who contended that it will nevertheless leave an everlasting mark on the quality of education—a mark which will have very favorable results.

BIBLIOGRAPHY

Alpren, M., & Baron, B. G. The death of the behavioral objectives movement. *Intellect,* 1974, *103,* 103–104.

American Speech and Hearing Association. *Essentials of program planning, development, management and evaluation.* W. Healy, Project Director, Washington, D. C., *Asha,* 1973.

Ammons, M. An empirical study of process and product in curriculum development. *Journal of Educational Research,* 1964, *57,* 451–457.

Anderson, V. A., & Newby, H. A. *Improving the child's speech,* 2nd. ed. New York: Oxford University Press, 1973.

Andrews, J. R. Operationally written therapy goals, in supervised clinical practicum. *Asha,* 1971, *13,* 385–387.

Baker, E. L. Effects on student achievement of behavioral and nonbehavioral objectives. *Journal of Experimental Education,* 1969, *37,* 5–8.

Baker, E. L., & Popham, W. J. *Expanding dimensions of instructional objectives.* Englewood Cliffs, N.J.: Prentice-Hall, 1973.

Biggs, L. J., Champeau, P. L., Gagné, R. M., & May, M. A. *Instructional media: A procedure for the design of multi-media instruction, a critical review of research and suggestions for future research.* Pittsburgh: American Institute for Research, 1967.

Bloom, B. S. (Ed.). *Taxonomy of educational objectives, handbook I: The cognitive domain,* New York: Tongmans, Green & Co., 1956.

Bobbitt, F. *How to make a curriculum.* Boston: Houghton Mifflin, 1924.

Cooper, T. L. (Ed.). Skills for precision therapy—Articulation. Project No. V-P-73-618 of Education of the Handicapped Act, Part B. Title VI-B. Columbus: Central Ohio Special Education Resource Center, 1972.

Creamer, J. J., & Gilmore, J. T. (Eds.). *Design for competence-based education in speech education.* Syracuse, N.Y.: Syracuse University, 1974.

Dickson, G. E., & Saxe, R. W. *Partners for educational reform and renewal.* Berkeley: McCutchan, 1974.

Diedrich, W. M., & Gerber, A. J. Analysis and measurement of articulation learning. *Asha,* 1974, *16,* 568.

Duchastel, P. D., & Merrill, P. F. The effects of behavioral objectives on learning: A review of empirical studies. *Review of Education Research,* 1973, *43,* 53–69.

Ebel, R. L. Some comments. *School Review,* 1967, *75,* 261–266.

Eisner, E. W. Educational objectives: Help or hinderance. *School Review,* 1967, *75,* 250–260.

Frey, S. Behavioral objectives: Attitudes of teachers. *Clearing House* 1974, *48,* 487–490.

Garvey, J. F. The what and why of behavioral objectives. *Instructor,* 1968, *77,* 127.

Hartley, J., & Davies, I. K. Preinstructional strategies: The role of pretests, behavioral objectives, overviews and advance organizers. *Review of Educational Research,* 1976, *46,* 239–265.

Hastings, J. T. Some comments. *School Review,* 1967, *75,* 267–271.

Hilton, E. Some cautions about objectives. *Instructor,* 1974, *84,* 16.

Houston, W. R., & Howsam, R. *Competence-based teacher education.* Chicago: Science Research Associates, 1973.

Krathwohl, D., Bloom, B. S., & Masia, B. *Taxonomy of educational objectives; handbook II: The affective domain.* New York: David McKay, 1964.

Lundquist, R. L. (Project Director). *Speech therapy transfer program.* Las Vegas: Clark County School District, 1973.

Mager, R. F. *Preparing instructional objectives.* Palo Alto, Ca.: Fearon Publishers, 1962.

Mager, R. F. *Measuring instructional intent.* Belmont, Ca.: Fearon Publishers, 1973.

McAshan, H. A. *Writing behavioral objectives.* New York: Harper & Row, 1970.

McDonald, J. B. Myths about instruction. *Educational Leadership,* 1965, *22,* 613–614.

McNeil, J. D. Concomitants of using behavioral objectives in the assessment of teaching effectiveness. *Journal of Experimental Education,* 1967, *36,* 69–74.

McNeil, J. D. Forces influencing curriculum. *Review of Educational Research,* 1969, *39,* 293–318.

Mowrer, D. E. An experimental analysis of variables controlling lisping responses of children. Unpublished doctorate dissertation. Tempe, Ariz.: Arizona State University, 1964.

Nagel, T., & Richman, P. *Competency-based instruction: A strategy to eliminate failure.* Columbus: Charles E. Merrill, 1972.

PL 94-142 regulations. *Federal Register, 42,* No. 163 August 23, 1977.

Plowman, P. *Behavioral objectives extension service.* Chicago: Science Research Associates, 1968–69.

Popham, W. J. The threat-potential of precision. Paper presented at the 19th Annual Conference on Educational Research, San Diego, Ca., November 16, 1967a.

Popham, W. J. *Selecting appropriate educational objectives.* Los Angeles, Ca.: Vincent Associates, 1967b.

Popham, W. J., & Husek, H. R. Implications of criterion-referenced measurement. *Journal of Educational Measurement,* 1969, *6,* 1–9.

Popham, W. J. et al. *Instructional objectives.* AERA Monograph, Series on curriculum evaluation, *3,* Chicago: Rand McNally, 1969.

Rath, J. D. Specificity as a threat to curriculum reform. Paper presented at American Educational Research Association, Chicago, February 1968.

Skinner, B. F. *Science and human behavior.* New York: Macmillan, 1953.

Snyder, T. Procedures for writing objectives. In F. Connor, H. Rusalem, & J. Baken (Eds.). *Competency-based programming.* New York: Teachers College, Columbia University, 1971, 52–56.

Tyler, R. *Basic principles of curriculum instruction.* Chicago: University of Chicago Press, 1951.

Van Riper, C. *Speech correction principles and methods,* 4th ed. Englewood Cliffs, N.J.: Prentice-Hall, 1963.

Wagener, E. H. Accountability: Do behavioral objectives really help? *School and Community,* 1975, *61,* 15.

White, O. R., & Haring, N. G. *Exceptional teaching.* Columbus: Charles E. Merrill, 1976.

Assignment 3

Constructing and Evaluating Objectives

Overview

Writing instructional and program objectives is an effective way of organizing your therapy or work plan in order to accomplish your goal. By following certain steps, it is easy to write your objective clearly so that others know exactly what it is you intend to accomplish. This procedure will also help clarify in your own mind what activities you will pursue.

Six exercises are presented to provide you with practice in identifying and writing instructional objectives as used in therapy settings. Two more exercises are designed to help your formulate noninstructional objectives. In these two taped selections, you will hear pathologists talk about several problems that have confronted them while working in the public schools. You will be asked to pinpoint their problems and to write program objectives to solve them.

Objective: To identify the essential components of objectives in speech pathology; to write behavioral and program objectives.

Materials: Assignment 3, Selections A–1.

Suggested Reading: Mager (1962), chapters 4–6.

Description of the Session: The selections in Assignment 3 include brief portions from a variety of speech therapy sessions. Selections A through E represent attempts to modify articulation behaviors at various stages with young children. You will be asked to identify chief components of behavioral objectives that are implied in the sessions as well as to write out complete objectives for some sessions.

Selections F and G deal more with evoking certain language concepts or spoken patterns from young children. Frequently, such objectives are more difficult to write than objectives involving simple problems of articulation.

Selections H and I present speech pathologists discussing some problems they have experienced in their programs. In these cases, you will be asked to identify the problems and write program objectives that would result in the resolution of the problems.

Procedure: Educational objectives can be divided into two major categories. Into the first category fall those objectives we wish the learner to accomplish. Usually, these objectives are called *instructional objectives,* since we observe change in the learner's behavior to determine if and when the objective has been attained. Thus behavioral objectives are usually stated in terms of what the learner is supposed to do.

The second category of objectives, *noninstructional objectives,* are not concerned with instruction. The pathologist determines these objectives. The measurement indicator used to determine if and when the objective is reached is some tangible evidence, such as a report or a list of names.

SELECTION A

Mager (1962) proposes a simple format for writing instructional objectives. He suggests such objectives should state (*a*) what the learner is to *do,* (*b*) under what *conditions* is it to be done, and (*c*) how *well* the individual is to perform. In Selection A, you will note that there is a well-defined objective. You will hear the pathologist working with a first grade boy who substitutes / f / for / θ /. He has already been taught to produce the / θ / in isolation and in a few nonsense syllables. In this portion of the therapy session, incorporating the / θ / in words was the target objective. Listen to the session and then answer the questions that follow.

Play Assignment 3, Selection A.

1. What was the child supposed to do?
2. What were the conditions under which the behavior was to be performed? (Include the nature of the task as well as the nature of the stimulus condition.)
3. There was no criterion test given during this session, so it would be difficult for you to write the expected accuracy statement. Assume the pathologist desired 90% accuracy. Write a complete behavior objective for this session.
4. The child said seven words containing / θ / and / ð / sounds. All words were correct. Did the child achieve the objective according to the accuracy statement in the objective you wrote? Check your answers on p. 189.

SELECTION B

You will now hear another portion of that same therapy session. The first objective you wrote will need to be modified slightly to account for the new task that was introduced.

Play Assignment 3, Selection B now.

Questions for Selection B

1. What conditions of the objective have changed in this selection?
2. Rewrite the original objective to include these new conditions.
3. The child produced 13 correct responses and 1 incorrect one. Did the child attain the desired accuracy for the objective? Check your answers on p. 189.

SELECTION C

In this brief session, the pathologist is working with a first-grade girl who substitutes /p/ for /f/ and /b/ for /v/. You should have no difficulty writing an objective for this selection, since your objective will be very similar to Selection B. Tasks in this session include saying /f/ and /v/ in isolation, with nonsense syllables in the initial position of words. In one case *(golf)*, the /f/ in the final position is requested but do not include this task.

Play Assignment 3, Selection C.

Now, answer the following questions; then check your answers with those in the Answer Key.

Questions for Selection C

1. Assuming a 90% criterion is desired, write the behavioral objective for this session.
2. Did the child reach the objective? (17 correct, 2 incorrect)

When writing behavioral objectives, it is best to specify the exact number of words you wish to have as criterion performance. For example, after a certain amount of therapy, you might ask the child to say five words containing /f/ in the initial position, with 80% accuracy. This would follow 3 to 5 minutes of therapy.

SELECTION D

In this next selection, the pathologist has been helping an 8-year-old child blend sounds together in phrase and sentence contexts. Previously, the child omitted many final consonants. Providing practice saying short phrases and sentences that contain these final consonants should assist the child in learning to include final consonants in word strings. The main phrases chosen by the pathologist are "I have a —," and "I wanta —." The final /v/ and /t/ are the sounds the pathologist wants the child to include in the phrase as integral units. Prior to therapy, the child omitted these sounds from the final (technically, the medial) position.

Play Assignment 3, Selection D.

Question for Selection D

1. Assume your goal is to achieve 100% accuracy. Write a behavioral goal for this brief session. Check your answer on p. 190.

SELECTION E

The pre-school child you will hear in this next selection has been receiving speech therapy for the past 4 months. The original diagnosis revealed a language problem, plus a severe articulation problem involving the omission of most consonant sounds. You will note that the pathologist will be working on both articulation and language skills simultaneously. Her chief technique is to model the response for the child. For example, she works on the concept of negation ("I don't see a ———") as well as syntax features. But for our purposes in writing simple objectives, we will limit our analysis to the articulation problem consisting of omission or substitution of /d/ in the word *don't*, the /s/ in the word *see*, and the /l/ in the words *like* and *love*.

Play Assignment 3, Selection E.

Questions for Selection E

1. Write a behavioral objective for this session. Use 80% accuracy for your criterion. Check your objective with the one in the Answer Key.

To determine whether or not the child met the objective, you would need to count each occurrence of /s/, /d/, and /l/. These data are presented for you in Table 3–1.

Table 3–1. *Number of correct and incorrect /s/, /d/, and /l/ productions in Selection E.*

Target sound	Correct	Incorrect
/s/	5	8
/d/	3	6
/l/	6	4

2. Did this child meet 80% accuracy criterion?
3. What percent of her responses were correct?

Judging from the rapid progress this child was making in this therapy session, it would be unfair to set the therapy practice criterion at 80% accuracy, especially when the modeling technique is used. It would be much better to provide a criterion test following the session that would include perhaps 10 attempts saying the carrier phrases, "I like a ——," "I see a ——," and "I don't see a ——."

You will also note that the pathologist did not attempt to correct several of the other misarticulated sounds, like /f/. These sounds were not included in her behavioral objectives. Thus, we see another advantage of using behavioral objectives; they force us to stick to the task we set out to accomplish.

Check your answers on p. 190.

SELECTION F

This selection demonstrates a portion of language therapy designed to teach a child the correct use of the words *is* and *is not* in identifying pictures. In this case, the pathologist's objective is very clear-cut; there is no doubt as to what her objective is. You will note that the pathologist talks very loudly to the child. The child in this case is mentally retarded; he does not have a hearing loss. The pathologist seems to take the viewpoint that the louder she talks, the better the child will attend and thus learn. Also, note her constant repetition of simple sentence structures. Modeling appears to play an important role as the chief stimulation technique.

The main target is to teach the child the use of negation. One way you could test to see whether or not the child had this concept would be to present him with instances in which an object or feature is present and determine whether the child says "it is" or "it is not" present. Thus, the child's use of *is* or *is not* is an indicator of the possession of the concept of negation. Pay particular attention to what responses she requires of the child.

Play Assignment 3, Selection F.

Questions for Selection F

1. What does the pathologist tell the child to do?
2. What are the conditions?
3. If we wish to complete the objective, a statement would have to be made concerning how accurately the child should respond. What do you think the pathologist should require in the way of accuracy?
4. **What consequences does the pathologist usually use following incorrect responses?** Check your answers on page 190.

SELECTION G

The pathologist in this session had some definite goals in mind but did not state them in behavioral terms. The child with whom she is working is a shy preschool youngster who has only had a few speech sessions. The pathologist wants to provide a relaxed atmosphere for the child, one in which the child feels free to respond. She will provide many correct verbal models for the child and will reward the child for his verbal attempts, but she will not place rigid demands upon the child's performance as did the pathologist in Selection F.

At first, it might seem difficult to convert the goal of establishing a relaxed atmosphere into a behavioral objective framework, but if you concentrate upon what it is the pathologist wants the child to do and can identify the conditions she establishes, it should not be difficult to state her goals in behavioral terms. Focus on the indicator. What behavior do you look for in the child that would allow you to conclude that the child is relaxed? Certainly, if the child was crying, you could assume a relaxed atmosphere was not created. It becomes important when writing some behavioral objectives to clearly distinguish between the pathologist's main intent in a session and the indicators used to determine if the main intent has been achieved.

Play Assignment 3, Selection G.

Questions for Selection G

1. The pathologist had two main objectives: creating a relaxed atmosphere and evoking certain connected speech patterns. Let's take the first objective. What's wrong with using the term *creating* in an objective?
2. The pathologist presented parts of a toy car to the child and helped him assemble it during part of the session. She thus provided a high-interest activity that would increase the probability of motor responses (act of assembling the toy car) in an interactive play situation. Now you can see how to identify observable behaviors that serve as indicators of a "relaxed atmosphere." Identify at least five behaviors that show that the child was relaxed and cooperative.
3. We could lump all of these behaviors together under the term *cooperative behaviors*. If we accept "performing cooperative behaviors" as our "do" statement, exactly what would you write as the "do" portion of the behavioral objective?
4. Now we come to the conditions statement. List at least three conditions.
5. What criterion would you select? It may seem difficult to select an accuracy figure as part of the criterion; but if you think about it, you can easily come up with one. Think of the task of assembling the entire car as 100% success. Now, assume you would be satisfied with something less than that. What would you write?
6. Now you have the first objective written in behavioral terms. You see, had the pathologist failed to provide a relaxed atmosphere, the child would not have cooperated in assembling the car. He may have stared at the floor, whimpered, or tried to escape. We would use "assembling the car" not as a legitimate goal in and of itself, but only as an indicator that the child would soon follow verbal requests from the pathologist. As you know, the younger the child, the more you may need to devise similar procedures to secure cooperation (that is, a willingness to follow direction). Once this behavior is well established, you can begin to shape the child's verbal output through differential reinforcement. Rarely do you have to follow this type of procedure with older children (grades one and above). Why?

7. Now that second objective: evoking certain connected speech patterns. Obviously, the pathologist was attempting to evoke certain speech responses from the child. What were those responses?
8. How did she attempt to evoke the desired behavior?
9. Having identified the target speech behavior as well as the conditions under which it should occur, you need only add the accuracy statement in order to write the behavioral objective. Suppose we use the following statement for accuracy: five correct sentences using correct VCV (vowel-consonant-vowel) combinations. We can add a further condition by placing a time limit on this requirement, say, a 5-minute probe of the therapy session. Write the objective for the speech behavior. Begin by writing "The child will. . . . " Check your answers on p. 191.

SELECTION H

We will now consider writing program objectives. Our first step is to identify a problem. On Assignment 3, Selection H, several pathologists discuss problems in the public schools. One pathologist had just spent a rather discouraging year. Her chief concern is that she is not achieving as much progress with her clients as she would like. First listen as she identifies her problem, then answer the questions.

Play Assignment 3, Selection H.

Questions for Selection H

1. The pathologist in Selection H voices several concerns, all related to evaluating the behaviors of the children. She notes that the progress of the children was slow; she wasn't sure when she should present new tasks; and carry-over presented a problem. What, do you think, was her chief concern or problem?
2. Identifying what this pathologist needs is the next step. What do you think this need might be?
3. Having identified the problem and the need, next we must develop the program objective. An assessment device is needed in the form of criterion-referenced tests, which can be given frequently, perhaps during every session. This strategy will necessitate that she write a series of well-developed behavioral objectives that can be tested with criterion tests. Assuming this has been done, she should describe her program objective. One practical procedure to follow in writing program objectives is to answer the following questions:
   a. *When* will she have completed the objectives?
   b. *Who* will do it?
   c. *What* will she do?
   d. *To whom* is she going to do it? (In this case, it will be her.)
   e. *How* many criterion tests will be developed?
   f. *How* will she know when she has successfully completed the objectives?

By answering each of these questions, try to write a program objective that would help this pathologist solve her problem.

4. The next program objective would be written with the aim of actually using the criterion-referenced tests during therapy. If successful, this information should help eliminate much of the pathologist's confusion and frustration about whether or not children in her classes are making progress. Other goals may consist of charting data on graphs and using other teaching strategies. What would you say is the chief value of writing program objectives? Check your answers on p. 191.

SELECTION I

In the brief interview you will hear in Selection I, a pathologist tells of her frustration resulting from a case load that is too large and too little time to meet the needs of the children she services. As you listen to her complaints, be thinking about what kind of program objective she might develop.

Play Assignment 3, Selection I now.

Questions for Selection I

1. The pathologist presented a number of problems facing her in a public school. Identify as many as you can remember.
2. Program objectives could be written to aid in the solution of all of these problems; but consider only one, parent cooperation. She suggests that the other pathologist in her district was able to obtain parent cooperation. First, she will need some kind of plan to meet the need of securing parent cooperation; this plan will be the program objective. Suppose she elects to contact parents through the PTA and, as a result of these contacts, she establishes a parent aide program. Try to write an objective that would focus upon reaching this goal. Check your answers on p. 192.

Answer Key

SELECTION A

1. The child is to say /θ/ and /ð/ in the initial position of monosyllabic words. We infer from this objective: The child is to protrude his tongue between his teeth while the airstream, voiced in one case and voiceless in the other, passes centrally between the top surface of the tongue and the lower edges of the central incisors. You can see how the *do* statement could become quite complicated if we specified the precise behaviors we wanted the child to perform. The phrase, say /θ/ and /ð/, simplifies the objective. However, there are times when we do need to specify the exact behaviors we wish to evoke.
2. There are two important conditions in the brief session. One condition pertains to the nature of the task; the other was related to the nature of the stimulus conditions. The task consisted of saying /θ/ and /ð/ in the initial position of words. The stimuli consisted of models provided by the pathologist.

   Thus the conditions statement could be written as: "in the initial position in monosyllabic words, when modeled by the pathologist."
3. The child is to say /θ/ and /ð/ in the initial position in monosyllabic words with 90% accuracy when the words are modeled by the pathologist. Of course there are several different ways of stating the same objective, each perfectly acceptable. Consider another way: The child will produce with 90% accuracy /θ/ and /ð/ in the initial position of monosyllabic words following models of these words produced by the pathologist.
4. Yes. (13 ÷ 14 = 93%)

SELECTION B

1. The pathologist has requested production of the medial and final /θ/.
2. Say /θ/ and /ð/ in the initial, medial, and final position of one- and two-syllable words with 90% accuracy when the words are modeled by the pathologist.
3. Yes.

SELECTION C

1. Say /f/ and /v/ in isolation, in the initial position of nonsense syllables and in the initial position of monosyllabic words that have been modeled by the pathologist, with 90% accuracy.
2. Yes, but just barely. Seventeen responses were correct, two were incorrect, giving a total of nineteen total responses. (17 ÷ 19 = .8947, which would be 90% rounded off)

SELECTION D

1. Without the aid of auditory models, say /aɪ hæ və ____/ and /aɪ wʌ nt ə ____/ with 100% accuracy when shown pictures presented by the pathologist.

SELECTION E

1. Say /aɪ laɪ kə ____/ and /aɪ siə ____/ and /aɪ dont siə ____/ following the pathologist's auditory models of these sentences when shown picture stimuli. Accuracy rate will be 80% correct articulation of /s/, /d/, and /l/, the target phonemes in these sentences.
2. No.
3. 44% (14 ÷ 32)

SELECTION F

1. Say, "This is a———" or "This is not a ———."
2. When shown a picture and asked, "Is this a ———?" or "What is it?"
3. 100% accuracy.
4. "No," followed by the correct model.

SELECTION G

1. It doesn't tell us what the *child* should be doing.
2. engaging in social conversation
   looking at the pathologist
   smiling
   handling the pieces of the toy car
   attempting to assemble the parts of the toy car
3. Exhibit cooperative behavior. We could be more explicit, such as "exhibit five different cooperative behaviors" or we could narrow it down to "assemble a car."
4. eight pieces of a toy car
   a smiling pathologist
   gestures and verbal encouragement from the speech pathologist for the child to assemble the car
5. Criterion would be to assemble 75% of the car pieces. The accuracy figure in this case is *75%*, while *assemble* is the behavior.
6. Their cooperative behaviors are well developed and are well established from previous experiences. The pathologist need only say, "Say this after me," "Do this," "Read this" and most children will readily cooperate.
7. Sentences in the format of "I need a ——." The pathologist's intent was to evoke coarticulated speech patterns, focusing upon the VCV combination *I nee* and *eeda*.   V C V
   V C V
8. By modeling the target response several times.
9. The child will repeat sentences, "I need a ——," using correct VCV combinations in coarticulated speech during a 5-minute probe of the session following the pathologist's correct models of the sentence format.

SELECTION H

1. She was not confident her children were making progress in speech therapy.
2. She needs an effective assessment procedure that will help her identify whether or not she is reaching her intended objectives.
3. By January, 19—, I will have devised 20 criterion-referenced tests that I can use with all my clients who have articulation problems. These tests will be written on 5 × 7 index cards.

   Of course, your objective may not resemble this objective in detail; but the general idea should be similar.
4. They help you solve problems by forcing you to systematically plan practical strategies to fulfill needs.

SELECTION I

1. The following problems were identified:
   too many schools to serve
   not enough pathologists were available to serve the needs of the children
   cannot schedule children frequently enough
   parents do not cooperate
2. By March, 19—, I will have initiated a parent aide program using 10 parents who
   will serve as aides in the speech therapy program. The parents will begin working
   with children by the end of March.

UNIT 3 STUDY QUESTIONS

1. Define a behavioral objective.
2. Why did the use of writing educational objectives diminish during the 1930s?
3. What event was responsible for the recent growth in the behavioral objective movement?
4. List three advantages for using behavioral objectives.
5. What can you conclude from the experimental data available about the value of using behavioral objectives?
6. List three reasons why it may not be wise to use behavioral objectives.
7. What might cause a decline in the widespread use of writing behavioral objectives in the public school?
8. For what kind of behavior do speech clinicians usually write objectives?
9. Briefly explain the three aspects of Mager's system of writing behavioral objectives.
10. Differentiate between short- and long-term objectives.
11. Differentiate between the main intent and the indicator of the objective.
12. List three communication checks used by McAshan to evaluate objectives.
13. List three areas in which you would write noninstructional objectives.
14. What caution should we observe when we consider writing objectives?

Unit 4

Essentials of Behavior Therapy

Objectives

This unit covers a large amount of information, including the following objectives: (1) defining important terms and concepts used in behavior therapy; (2) identifying the role played by antecedent and consequent events; (3) identifying two ways the frequency of a behavior can be increased and four ways the frequency can be decreased; (4) identifying instances of positive and negative transfer of training, and (5) identifying factors that increase and decrease retention.

Suggested Assignments

Chapters 6 and 7 are assigned readings for this unit. At the end of chapter 7 you will find a summary of ten rules to follow when using behavior therapy techniques. Knowledge of these rules is especially important when you conduct speech therapy.

Assignments 4 and 5 use the tape casette. The first one, Assignment 4, is designed to aid you in learning how to evoke consonant sounds using the shaping process. This assignment will prove particularly valuable when working with clients who have articulation problems. Assignment 5 is designed to help you analyze different ways speech/language pathologists respond to the client's responses.

Finally, a list of 27 terms are presented following these two assignments along with 24 study questions. Define the terms and answer the questions.

6

Conditioning Behaviors

Description of Behavior Therapy

Without a doubt, behavior modification has been one of the most widely used procedures in education during the past two decades. It also has been a very popular technique used by psychologists to alter behavior. Psychologists prefer the term behavior therapy over behavior modification to describe the use of contingency management, the scientific methodology of learning theory, as a chief means of modifying overt behaviors. They are referred to as *behavior therapists,* and the therapy they provide is called *behavior therapy*.

In recent years, numerous books have been written by psychologists describing behavior therapy as a treatment procedure for neurotic and psychotic patients (Yates, 1970; Kanfer & Phillips, 1970; O'Leary & Wilson, 1975; Schaefer & Martin, 1969; Rimm & Masters, 1974; Lazarus, 1972; Franks, 1969). Two journals are published which are devoted exclusively to topics concerned with behavior therapy: *The Journal of Behavior Therapy* and *Experimental Psychiatry and Behavior Therapy*.

The bulk of the material in chapters 6 and 7 will be concerned with the basic concepts of behavior therapy as applied in psychology and speech pathology. It is important for the reader to clearly understand the parameters of behavior therapy as they pertain to both fields. It is appropriate, then, to begin with a brief discussion of how the term *behavior therapy* came about and what concepts are incorporated in the use of the term.

The term *behavior therapy* was first used by Lindsley (1954) and later adopted by Lazarus in 1958, who is given credit for introducing the term (Yates, 1970). It was a term first given to the use of operant conditioning procedures developed by B. F. Skinner and his associates and applied to psychotic patients in America. In England, Shapiro and his associates used the term behavior therapy to describe these procedures when applied to neurotic individuals. The term behavior therapy is seldom used in reference to a methodology employed by speech clinicians, primarily because most communication disorders do not involve neurotic or psychotic patients. Brutten (1970) used the term to describe the modification procedures he used in his treatment of stuttering.

I also prefer to use the term behavior therapy for two reasons. First, it is the term used and accepted by authorities in psychology who are engaged in modifying deviant behaviors. To invent synonyms for the same process only leads to confusion when communicating with other professionals. Second, I think behavior therapy best describes a unique methodology which professionals use to change a client's problem behaviors. Both professionals and nonprofessionals alike apply some principles of behavior therapy in their daily interaction with others; but when there is an intensive, professional commitment to remediate a behavioral problem through systematic application of operant conditioning, then behavior therapy seems to be a more appropriate term than behavior modification. While behavior modification appears to be the term favored by those in the teaching profession, behavior therapy seems more appropriate to describe the work done by those professionals involved in rehabilitation.

Having selected the term *behavior therapy* to describe a widely used procedure for changing overt behaviors, the next task is to define what the term encompasses. A popular misconception of behavior therapy, or behavior modification, has been one of doling out M & M's following correct responses or giving redeemable tokens which could be exchanged for candy, toys, or privileges. To many who tried the new method during the 1960s, the chief concern was to increase or decrease the frequency of certain behaviors primarily through the management of consequent events. A number of simplistic "how-to-do-it" texts were published to give teachers a capsuled notion of what behavior modification was all about (as an example, see Neisworth et al., 1969). Speech clinicians were exposed to terminology and basic concepts of behavior modification via several articles appearing in journals devoted to speech and hearing pathology (McReynolds, 1970; Brookshire, 1967; Holland, 1967; Girardeau & Spradlin, 1970). Revised editions of standard textbooks in speech pathology include brief, updated sections that mentioned the use of behavior modification in speech therapy (Van Riper & Irwin, 1958; Johnson et al. 1967), and a few books include chapters describing these procedures (Wolfe & Goulding, 1973; Sloane & MacAulay, 1968). However, there has rarely been a thorough presentation of the basic concepts of behavior therapy as applied to speech pathology.

Eysenck (1964) defines behavior therapy as "the attempt to alter human behavior and emotion in a beneficial manner according to the laws of modern learning theory." In contrast, Yates (1970) defines behavior therapy as the utilization of empirical and theoretical knowledge resulting from the use of the experimental method in psychology in order (1) to explain the origin and maintenance of abnormal patterns of behavior, and (2) to treat or prevent those abnormalities by means of controlled, experimental studies of the single cases. Both authorities define behavior therapy as the application of the experimental method to eliminate the problem behavior.

Kanfer and Phillips (1970) present a description of the position taken by behavior therapists as a way of defining behavior therapy. Behavior therapists are concerned chiefly with the observable, behavioral symptoms which constitute the problem. They place little emphasis on case history except the current events which may influence present behavior. They devote little attention to subjective experiences, attitudes, insights, or feelings of the client. Once a behavior is selected as target for change, a carefully planned intervention therapy program is initiated by manipulating antecedent and consequent events. Progress is monitored continuously by counting occurrences of specified behaviors under given conditions. Frequently, electronic or manually operated equipment is used to tabulate responses and accurately measure time lapses. Response rates are graphed to determine increments or decrements in response rates. These rates are compared to relevant antecedent or consequent events manipulated by the behavior therapist. Thus, the therapist can determine precisely what effects are achieved through the treatment methods used. Outcomes of therapy are judged in relation only to the specified behavioral changes which have occurred. The problem behavior is not viewed as a superficial "symptom" or indicator of some underlying problem, but simply as a learned response which can be altered through conditioning. Therefore, treatment is aimed specifically at the problem behavior disregarding a "diagnostic label."

Behavior therapies differ in their entire conception of abnormal behavior from more traditional viewpoints about neurotic and psychotic disorders. Ullman and Krasner (1969) and Lundin (1969) present a detailed discussion concerning a behavioral approach used in abnormal psychology. Basically, behavior therapists do not follow the "medical model" in that they do not attempt to discover and to eliminate the cause of the "symptom behavior." Treatment is aimed at eliminating the problem behavior rather than resolving the inner conflict of the individual's personality presumed to be the cause of the deviant behavior.

Techniques Used
in Behavior Therapy

Behavior therapies include a wide variety of techniques designed to modify specific kinds of problems. Types of abnormal behaviors treated include fetishism, homosexuality, alcoholism, smoking, phobias, mutism, temper tantrums, self-care, and rebellion to list a few. Some of the major behavior therapy techniques used for treating these problems were identified by Yates (1970) and are presented in Figure 7–1.

Most speech clinicians are familiar with the use of the operant procedure as a technique for treating speech problems. This procedure appears to be effective for modifying many speech behaviors (Sloane & MacAulay, 1968). This chapter will focus on the use of operant procedures as they apply to contingency management

Technique	Abnormalities

I. *Classical aversive conditioning*
   1. Drugs
 	
   2. Shock
 	
   3. Paralysis
	
	 Fetishism; transvestism; homosexuality; alcoholism.
	 Writer's cramp; fetishism; transvestism; sadistic fantasies; voyeurism; alcoholism; smoking; gambling.
	 Alcoholism.

II. *Instrumental escape conditioning* (shock)	Homosexuality; alcoholism; smoking.
III. *Instrumental avoidance conditioning* (shock)	Homosexuality; alcoholism.
IV. *Massed practice*	Tics; smoking; stuttering.
V. *Aversive imagery (covert* *sensitization)*	Obsessional behavior; homosexuality; alcoholism; smoking.
VI. *Aversion—relief*	Phobias; obsessional behavior; fetishism; transvestism; smoking.
VII. *Operant procedures*	1. Childhood psychoses—elimination of undesirable behaviors (time out, etc.) strengthening of desirable behaviors—teaching speech, cognitive and social skills. 2. Adult psychoses—reinstatement of speech, control of ward behavior, etc. 3. Mental deficiency—toilet training, ward behavior, self-care, remedial education, etc. 4. Children's behavior problems—temper tantrums, operant crying, head-bumping, thumbsucking, excessive scratching, excessive verbal demands, rebellious behavior, isolate behavior, regressed crawling, hyperactivity, social interaction with peers, educational retardation (classroom orientation, reading, etc.) 5. Obsessional rituals; anorexia nervosa, neurodermatitis, tics, stuttering. 6. Delinquent and antisocial behavior.
VIII. *Special techniques*	Obsessional eyebrow plucking; functional blindness, deafness, analgesia, astereognosis, anesthesia, motor paralysis, aphonia and dysphonia, retention of urine, excessive frequency of micturition, somnambulism.
IX. *Feedback control techniques*	Stuttering.

FIGURE 6–1. Some Techniques Used By Behavior Therapists And Abnormalities To Which They Have Been Applied (Reprinted By Permission Of John Wiley & Sons, From A. J. Yates, Behavior Therapy)

for the treatment of articulation, voice, language, and stuttering problems. Both classical and instrumental conditioning models have been used as part of speech therapy training, especially in the treatment of stuttering. The first part of this discussion will begin with a presentation of classical conditioning techniques.

Classical Conditioning

Most of you are probably familiar with the *classical reward conditioning* model, best illustrated by Pavlov's famous experiment involving the elicitation of salivation from dogs following the presentation of a bell. First, Pavlov presented meat powder, the unconditioned stimuli (US), and, of course, the dog salivated, the unconditioned response (UR), in anticipation of eating the meat powder. This series of events is illustrated as shown:

$$\text{(Meat powder)} \quad \text{US} \longrightarrow \text{UR} \quad \text{(salivation)}$$

He presented the meat powder several times until the dog's salivary response (UR) was firmly established. Then, he sounded a bell just before presenting the meat powder (US), and, of course, the dog salivated (UR) after seeing the meat powder. The sequence went something like this:

$$
\begin{array}{ccc}
\text{S} & \text{US} & \text{UR} \\
\text{ding} \rightarrow & \text{meat powder} \rightarrow & \text{salivation} \\
\text{ding} \rightarrow & \text{meat powder} \rightarrow & \text{salivation} \\
\text{ding} \rightarrow & \text{meat powder} \rightarrow & \text{salivation} \\
\text{ding} \rightarrow & \text{meat powder} \rightarrow & \text{salivation}
\end{array}
$$

Then he eliminated the meat powder, and the presentation of the bell alone elicited salivation.

$$
\begin{array}{cc}
\text{CS} & \text{CR} \\
\text{ding} \rightarrow & \text{salivation} \\
\text{ding} \rightarrow & \text{salivation} \\
\text{ding} \rightarrow & \text{salivation}
\end{array}
$$

In this case, the salivation that followed the bell, the bell being the conditioned stimulus (CS), was not quite as great as it was following the meat powder, so salivation following the bell was called the conditioned response (CR). This process is usually diagrammed as follows:

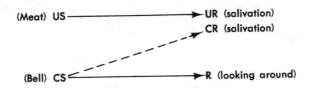

The dotted line represents the fact that the bell, through conditioning, now elicits a different response (salivation) than it did before (looking around).

Audiologists have adapted this classical conditioning experiment to assess hearing acuity in certain situations where traditional testing techniques are not adequate. But instead of presenting a reward like meat powder, they provide a slight shock to the hand (US), which is usually followed by a perspiration response (UR) measured at the fingers. Then, a moderately loud tone is presented just before shock. The shock is delivered, and the perspiration response is measured. The sequence looks like this:

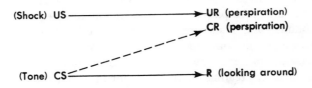

The shock is then eliminated. If the tone alone elicits perspiration, then we have been successful in conditioning the tone. The intensity of the tone is then gradually decreased until its presentation no longer elicits perspiration. This point should represent the threshold for hearing of a tone of that intensity. In this example, we have used *classical aversive conditioning* rather than reward conditioning.

Classical aversive conditioning is frequently used to treat problems of alcoholism, homosexuality, smoking, sadistic fantasies, and compulsive gambling. During the early 1930s, experiments based on the Pavlovian model were conducted which attempted to condition sight and thoughts of alcohol to electric shock in order to eliminate alcoholism. Thus, the cues associated with alcohol elicited unpleasant feelings instead of the previous pleasant sensations so that the individual responded with aversion and fear at the sight or mention of alcohol. A more recent example of the use of classical aversive conditioning is provided by a psychologist who treated a 48-year-old man who had daily suicidal ruminations. Six specific suicidal images were identified. The visual image stimulus was presented followed by electric shock, which produced an unpleasant reaction. After 350 trials, the suicidal image alone produced the unpleasant feeling so that the patient found it very unsatisfying to engage in suicidal imageries.

Brutten (1970) felt that one way in which stuttering is learned is through classical aversive conditioning. He viewed bad experiences as the unconditioned stimulus (US) which resulted in unpleasant emotional responses (UR). When words, sounds, or certain situations (CS) are paired with the (US), then the (CS) tends to elicit the (CR) by itself, disfluency being the obvious, symptomatic result.

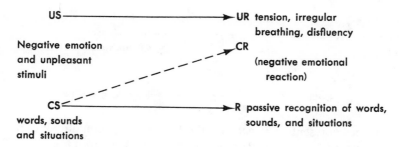

Of course, the origin of stuttering as a classically conditioned aversive response must still be considered theory since no one has yet volunteered to be classically conditioned into stuttering.

Brutten (1970) identifies two other techniques for modifying classically conditioned stuttering responses: *deconditioning* and *counter-conditioning*. Simply stated, deconditioning is a process of breaking the link between the conditioned stimulus and the unconditioned stimulus so that the conditioned stimulus no longer elicits the conditioned responses. Recall in our illustration of how certain words, sounds, or situations were said to be paired with negative emotions (US) so that eventually these words, sounds, and situations themselves produced tension and disfluent speech (CR). To break this connection, the words, sounds, and situations are to be followed by pleasant, unthreatening experiences, also associated with fluent speech. This is accomplished by creating an environment in which the conditioned stimuli (words, sounds, situations) are presented, but instead of being followed with unpleasant stimuli, pleasant consequences follow. The stutterer may be in a room by himself repeating the feared words over and over again in the absence of tension until these words become neutral stimuli as they are for fluent speakers. Situations which previously elicited tension and disfluent speech can be gradually introduced using tape recorded stimulus presentations until the stutterer can experience or talk about these situations without tension. Videotapes, as well as actual experience in the situations, can be utilized as part of the deconditioning procedures. In effect, the behavior therapist attempts to "undo" what has been classically conditioned in the past.

Counter-conditioning is the purposeful pairing of pleasant stimuli with the feared words, sounds, and situations. Rather than just breaking the old connections, new connections are conditioned. An effort is made to replace the old negative emotional response with a positive emotional response. Consequently, a feared word is first presented. If the stutterer says the word without fear, tension, or stuttering, the clinician provides praise and reward as a positive experience. The clinician carefully arranges the presentation of feared words so as not to threaten the stutterer and to insure that they will not trigger tension responses.

I used this counter-conditioning technique as part of an instructional program. The program begins by asking the stutterer to read any word from a list of monosyllabic words following the presentation of a tone which is sounded every 5 seconds. When a word is read fluently, the clinician says "Good," and another tone is sounded. This procedure is followed for 30 minutes or until the stutterer can read 360 words with 18 or less disfluencies. The counter-conditioning is accomplished by providing positive experiences in the form of the clinician's encouraging remarks following fluent utterances. Thus, previously feared words are no longer paired with unpleasant stimuli but with pleasant stimuli. The conditioning process should look like this:

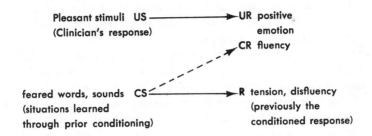

The procedure has functioned quite well in establishing fluency among stutterers, but its effects appear to be temporary unless other rehabilitative measures are taken. For the most part, speech clinicians seldom use classical conditioning techniques. They rely far more extensively on procedures utilizing instrumental conditioning.

Instrumental Conditioning

There are a number of basic differences between instrumental and classical conditioning: (1) The subject's role in classical conditioning experiments is essentially a passive one, whereas the subject plays a very active part in the learning process during instrumental conditioning (Rachman, 1963). (2) Classical conditioning has been considered the only type of learning in which automatic or involuntary responses can be modified. Instrumental conditioning, on the other hand, is viewed as the only method for modifying voluntary and skeletal muscular behaviors (Kimble, 1961). Since most of the work done by speech clinicians involves voluntary and skeletal muscular behaviors, it is easy to understand why instrumental, rather than classical, conditioning procedures occupy the clinician's chief interest. (3) A final distinction between the two types of conditioning involves reward or reinforcement. In instrumental conditioning, the act to be learned must be instrumental in securing reinforcement, whereas in classical conditioning, the subject receives the reinforcing stimulus on every training trial regardless of any response he may make.

In spite of these basic differences, several psychologists argue that the two conditioning procedures are not as different as some maintain. Inherent in both procedures is the concept of stimulus-response bond. McGeoch and Irion (1952) state that in many instances, the instrumental conditioning situation may resemble the classical conditioning situation very closely. Thus, there could be justification in classifying many classically conditioned acts as instrumental behaviors. For example, conditioned eyelid closure (an involuntary act) in response to an air puff might be classified as an instrumental act because the anticipatory closure of the lid prevents the puff of air from striking the cornea of the eye. Recent data show that an individual can gain operant control over autonomic responses such as systolic blood pressure (Shapiro et al., 1969). Katkin and Murray (1968) review experimental designs involving conditioning experiments and maintain we must modify our conclusions with respect to instrumental conditioning of autonomic responses. Autonomic responses appear to be brought under control through learning, using instrumental conditioning procedures. Since the controversy is a theoretical one and of little interest to speech clinicians, there is no need to belabor this point. I merely wish to alert you to the fact that disputes exist in reference to the establishment of the two distinct types of conditioning processes.

Instrumental conditioning is typically described as a situation in which the subject responds to a stimulus and is rewarded following the response. An experiment frequently used to illustrate *instrumental reward conditioning* involves a hungry rat inside a small cage containing a lever and a cup into which food pellets can be dispensed. The rat, in moving about the cage, may accidentally step on the lever. The lever trips the pellet dispensing mechanism, and a food pellet drops into a cup. Being hungry, the rat immediately eats the pellet and continues roaming about the cage until he again stumbles on the lever and finds another pellet, which, of course, he consumes. As you might guess, after 5 or 10 minutes of these contingencies, the rat will be pressing the lever continuously in order to secure the food pellets. When this occurs, it is said learning has taken place; the rat has been conditioned.

As you can see, the animal's behavior itself is instrumental in obtaining the reward. Since the animal "operates" on his environment, this type of conditioning is often referred to as *operant conditioning,* especially when a reward follows the response. Many believe most of our daily behaviors are conditioned in this way. We perform some operation on our environment, like squeezing a toothpaste tube, and we get rewarded for doing so. The toothpaste appears, so we continue the behavior of tube squeezing when we want toothpaste. One of the chief features of instrumental conditioning is that the consequences of the behavior serve to control the frequency of its occurrence.

The consequences may increase the frequency of the behavior, as in the case of instrumental reward conditioning cited earlier, or they may be increased through the use of *instrumental aversive conditioning*. In this latter case, let us consider a rat in a cage containing only a lever. A shock is applied to the floor of the cage, and the rat runs about the cage accidentally bumping the lever which terminates the shock. After 10 seconds, the shock is reinstated, and naturally, the rat becomes very active, probably bumping into the lever again and terminating the shock for another 10 seconds. After a number of these trials, we have a rat who keeps pressing the lever in order to avoid being shocked, having been conditioned to press the lever through instrumental aversive conditioning. This form of instrumental conditioning has also been called *avoidance training* because the subject learns to avoid the noxious stimulus (McGeoch & Irion, 1952).

When rewards are presented following a behavior and the behavior increases in frequency, the reward is called a *positive reinforcer*. When an aversive stimulus is present, or if the threat of its presentation exists so that the avoidance behavior increases in frequency, this aversive stimulus is called a *negative reinforcer*. Both types of reinforcers *increase* the frequency of the behavior. More will be said about the effects of positive and negative reinforcement later.

There is considerable evidence to indicate that vocal behaviors are learned through instrumental conditioning. Rheingold et al. (1959) recorded the frequency of vocal responses of 3-month-old infants during a six-day period. For the first two days, the vocalizations were counted but were followed with no specific consequences. During the third and fourth days, each vocalization occurring during the observation period was followed with a smile, three *tsk* sounds, and a light touch to the infant's abdomen. During these days, infant vocalizations increased. These procedures were discontinued during the fifth and sixth days, and the frequency of vocalizations returned to their original rate. It was concluded that the experimenter's smiling and other behaviors which followed the vocalizations during days three and four served as positive reinforcers that instrumentally conditioned the infant's vocal responses, i.e., caused them to increase.

Brutten (1970) you will recall pointed out he felt part of stutterer's disfluent behavior was learned through classical conditioning. He also felt many of the stutterer's behaviors were learned through instrumental conditioning as well. These two conditioning procedures formed the basis of his two-factor behavior theory and therapy. Actually, he viewed the two types of conditioning as inseparable. Classical conditioning shapes the stutterer's emotional responses, while instrumental conditioning shapes many of her overt behaviors. For example, her blocks, struggles, breath holding, and sound repetitions finally end in an utterance which allows her to escape the negative stimulation. As a result of this type of experience, according to Brutten, the stutterer will be more likely to respond in a similar way the next time she tries to escape from this circumstance. In other words, the stutterer's repetitions, hesitations, eye blinks, head nods, i.e., her stuttering behavior, is the reinforcing agent which serves to remove the strong, negative stimulation she experiences during the blockage of speech. Eventually, she learns a number of behaviors which serve to remove these unpleasant, emotional feelings and adopts a "pattern of behaviors" called *stuttering* to cope with these feelings. This type of conditioning might best be classified as *instrumental escape conditioning*.

Brutten goes on to suggest ways of conditioning fluent speech by rewarding fluent utterances and withholding reward for disfluent speech. Details of his procedures will not be discussed here. The point to be made is that both classical and instrumental conditioning models have been applied to speech disorders to explain how they originate and can best be treated. It is important that you thoroughly understand these models if you wish to use behavior therapy techniques for modifying speech behaviors.

Up to now, two types of classical conditioning have been presented (reward and aversive), and three types of instrumental conditioning (reward, aversive or avoidance, and escape) have been discussed. Kanfer and Phillips (1970) make a basic distinction between the two basic types of conditioning procedures by indicating on which side of a behavioral continuum each one operates. Basically, such a behavioral continuum consists of the following:

Stimulus—organism | response | reinforcement schedule—consequence

Classical conditioning consists of the study of the first two elements of the equation (i.e., those events which *precede* the response), while instrumental conditioning focuses on the last two elements (the events which *follow* the response). Behavior therapists who are interested in conditioning operant behaviors (instrumental conditioning) study the effects of arranging consequent, rather than antecedent, events. Indeed, the distinction between antecedent and consequent events offers a clear differentiation of classical and instrumental conditioning, and in view of the power of consequent events, it also explains the preference for instrumental conditioning. This is why the term *reinforcement* has been so widely discussed among psychologists. It is one of the most influential consequences affecting response frequency. It has been found that the most powerful techniques for controlling behavior, that is, increasing or decreasing the frequency of behavior, rest with events that occur immediately *following* the response. A massive amount of data have been reported not only in animal research, but also in the field of human learning, which relate to the effects of consequent events on overt behaviors. Procedures of manipulating consequences within the instrumental conditioning framework have been termed *operant procedures*. These procedures probably best represent what most educators call behavior modification. They are widely used in all areas of education and rehabilitation chiefly because they have been found to be so effective in changing behaviors and their effects are readily measurable. For this reason, the following section will be devoted to a detailed explanation of the management of consequent events through operant procedures.

Management of Consequent Events

Operant behaviors are behaviors whose rates can be controlled by the manipulation of the consequences which follow these behaviors. This statement may seem complicated at first, but once explained, you will see how simple it is. First of all, let us assume you have control over the consequent event, i.e., the event that immediately follows a behavior. Suppose someone wants to light a cigarette and you provide them with a lighter and tell them to push a button on the lighter. They do (operant behavior), and a flame immediately appears (consequent event). There is a strong likelihood that they will engage in the same operant behavior, button pushing, in the future when they need a light. If you control the consequences that follow button pushing, you will obviously be able to exert a strong influence over the person's button-pushing behavior. If you remove the flammable liquid so that continued button pushing results in no flame, button-pushing behavior will soon terminate. If you see to it the lighter is in good working order so that it lights every time, button pushing will continue when conditions are present requiring a flame. If you rig the lighter so it lights intermittently, you may cause the subject to push the button several times in succession. Or you may devise a lighter that delivers a strong electric shock to the person who presses the button; and that may be the last time the subject presses the button! As you can see, once you control the consequences of a behavior, you also control the frequency with which that behavior occurs. This is why behavior therapy is so popular. It allows the therapist to achieve powerful controls over the patient's behavior. But these procedures can sometimes work to the annoyance of the controller of consequences. For example, the parent who frequently provides her child with candy to pacify him when he fusses or whines will find her child whining and fussing more frequently in the future.

Much is known about the effects of manipulating consequent events. Some psychologists refer to these principles of instrumental learning as *laws* since results from thousands of studies verify that lawful relationships can be established. These laws apply equally to instrumental and classical conditioning situations. Three basic procedures found to increase or decrease behavior through management of consequent events will be discussed next. They are (1) reinforcement, (2) punishment, and (3) reinforcement and extinction combined.

Increasing the Frequency of Behaviors through Reinforcement

There can be no doubt that the most widely known procedure for increasing and sustaining a behavior is the application of *positive reinforcement* following a behavior. It is also one of the most effective means of changing behavior. There is ample evidence that humans have long known about the influence of "pleasurable stimuli" with the development of hedonistic philosophies, but not until recently have we come to understand how positive reinforcement operates and what its significance is to the development of a wide variety of behaviors.

Edward Thorndike was one of the first researchers to systematically investigate the phenomenon that a behavior followed by a "satisfying" state of affairs was more likely to occur again in the future. Clark Hull felt a reinforcing stimulus was one which reduced the drive motivating the behavior. But B. F. Skinner was by far most influential in his research-based description of positive reinforcement. He eliminated the conceptual part of Hull's definition by defining positive reinforcement as a reinforcing stimulus increasing the probability that the response it follows will occur again. In other words, by *presenting* a reinforcing stimulus following a certain response, we increase the probability that the response will occur again.

It is important to understand that a reinforcing stimulus (reinforcer) is defined solely on the basis of its actual effect on the rate of response. If the response it follows increases, the stimulus is considered a reinforcing stimulus. If there is no change in the response rate, then the stimulus, regardless of how reinforcing we think it ought to be, is not a reinforcing stimulus. It is simply a stimulus, and we must be aware that a given stimulus can change from a reinforcing stimulus to a neutral stimulus in a short time. Suppose you give a hungry child a piece of popcorn after each time she raises her hand. Upon comparing the number of times she raises her hand before presenting the popcorn and the number of times she raises her hand after receiving the popcorn during 20 trials, you would probably find that hand raising increases dramatically when the popcorn is delivered immediately following the hand-raising response. But what do you think would happen to the frequency of hand raising after 500 pieces of popcorn are delivered and consumed during one training period? As you would expect, once the child's hunger is satisfied, she will stop performing. Her desire for popcorn will be zero. Thus, whether or not popcorn will serve as a reinforcing stimulus depends entirely on the state of the child and her "desire" for the reinforcer. In other words, we cannot determine in advance what sort of event will be a reinforcing stimulus until we try it in a given situation. When an event is found that increases the frequency of response it follows, then and only then do we know that event to be a reinforcing stimulus. Reinforcers are determined empirically.

A distinction should be made between primary and secondary reinforcers. Primary reinforcers are biologically determined, unlearned stimuli such as food, sex, thirst, warmth. They are not dependent on an individual's past history of conditioning. The most universally used primary reinforcer is food. When other stimuli are paired with primary reinforcers, they too take on the properties of the primary reinforcers, and they too increase the frequency of the responses which precede them. They are called *secondary* or *conditional reinforcers*. Some of the child's early learned secondary reinforcers are the expressions on the mother's face (smiling), her vocalizations, and the sight of a milk bottle or breast. They are associated with the primary reinforcers which satisfy hunger.

Most of these secondary reinforcers are acquired through classical conditioning although secondary reinforcers are added through instrumental conditioning as well. Money, which is paired with many different primary and secondary reinforcers, is considered a *generalized reinforcer* because it can be used to reinforce so many different behaviors. A number of state hospitals and clinics have substituted tokens for money in an effort to establish a manageable secondary reinforcement program called a *token economy system*. One does not need to be concerned with whether or not a person is hungry or thirsty because tokens can be saved and used later.

Factors that Influence the Effect of Reinforcers

Four factors influence the effect of positive reinforcement upon rate of response: (1) amount of reinforcement given, (2) latency of the reinforcing stimulus, (3) number of trials, and (4) schedule during which the reinforcing stimulus is presented.

Amount of reinforcement. It can be said that in general, the greater the amount of reinforcement, the greater the strength of the response. This does not mean that more learning has occurred, only that the organism performs the task with increased vigor. Increasing the reward increases performance, whereas decreasing it decreases performance. A classic study by Guttman (1954) demonstrates this aspect of the influence of the amount of reinforcement. When he dissolved differing amounts of sugar in the same quantity of water used as a reinforcing stimulus to rats taught to press a lever in a Skinner box, he found a direct relationship between the number of bar presses per minute and the amount of sugar contained in the water.

Mentally retarded subjects who were given highly valued toys performed sorting tasks faster than those who were given low valued toys (Heber, 1959). A number of similar studies support this notion, although in some cases, it is not entirely clear whether the size of the reward, time spent in consuming it, the amount of nutrition received, or number of consummatory responses are most important where food-type reinforcers are used. Little, if any, research has been done in communication disorders to explore the effects of varying the amount of reinforcement upon number of correct responses.

Latency of the reinforcer. Latency is the amount of time that has passed between the termination of the response and the introduction of the reinforcing stimulus. Experiments using rats as subjects show that the longer the reinforcing stimulus is delayed, the less effect it has on rate of response. In other words, response strength decreases as the latency of the reinforcing stimulus increases. In some situations, performance is unaffected if the delay exceeds just a few seconds. The parent who promises the child an ice cream cone at the end of the week providing her child practices the piano everyday should not expect piano practicing to increase in frequency under those contingencies! The speech clinician can make use of the importance of reducing latency by informing her client immediately when a correct response occurs. Heaping praise on a child following a 15-minute practice session would have little effect on increasing the number of individual correct responses. For greatest effect, the praise should be immediate.

Number of trials. Response strength is a function of the number of reinforced trials presented, i.e., the more reinforced trials you provide a child, the stronger his response. Siegel and Foschee (1953) illustrated this principle in an experiment in which children were given candy following each bar press. Four different groups received either 2, 4, 8, or 16 trials and rewards. After the appropriate number of trials were completed, candy was not administered; and response strength was judged by the number of responses completed during a 3-minute period. Those who received only two reinforced trials made only a few responses during the 3-minute test period, while those who received 16 trials kept responding many times during the 3-minute period. This finding, and many others like it, verify the proverb "practice makes perfect," but it should be added that practice of the correct response followed by positive reinforcement makes perfect.

Schedules of reinforcement. Positive reinforcement can be delivered following each correct response (continuous reinforcement), or it can be delivered intermittently following a certain number of responses or following certain specified time periods. The frequency of reinforcements has a profound effect on rate of response. Morse (1966) states that these reinforcement procedures are "the most powerful techniques known for generating behavior." He felt that the reinforcement histories of individuals are the primary determinants of behavior.

Usually, continuous reinforcement is provided in order to establish a new skill. The schedule is then changed to an intermittent one, first on a variable ratio, then on a variable interval schedule, until few reinforcements are required to sustain the desired behavior. The effects of intermittent reinforcement have received a great deal of attention from behavior therapists chiefly because such schedules produce greater resistance to extinction, are more efficient in terms of cost, and reduce the possibility of satiation during training.

The two major types of intermittent schedules, ratio and interval, can each be further divided into fixed and variable intervals.

Fixed Ratio	Variable Ratio
Fixed Interval	Variable Interval

This example shows two types of ratio and interval schedules. Each has different effects on rate of response. For example, animals perform more rapidly when they receive reinforcement after every fourth correct response than they do if reinforcement follows every correct response. When reinforcement follows a fixed number of correct responses, such as every response, or every fourth, fifth, tenth, or whatever, it is called a *fixed-ratio* schedule of reinforcement. When *every* response is reinforced, it is called *continuous reinforcement* (CRF or FR-1). An FR-3 means every third response is reinforced. To develop fixed-ratio responding, it is usually necessary to begin with an FR-1 schedule and gradually proceed to larger ratios, such as FR-3, then, FR-5, FR-9, FR-12.

The rate of response data for various types of reinforcement schedules are presented in Figure 7-2.

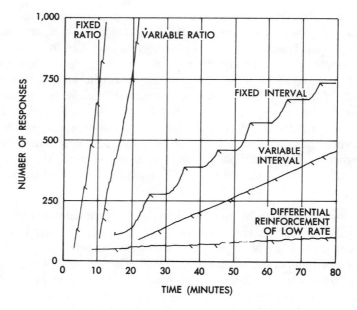

FIGURE 6-2. Effects Of Different Reinforcement Schedules Upon Pigeon Response Curves (Reprinted By Permission Of Scientific American From "Teaching Machines" By B. F. Skinner, 1961)

These data represent number of responses occurring during 10 minute time periods, the ordinate representing the number of responses and the abscissa the units of time. The responses are added cumulatively, so if five responses occur during the first minute, a dot is placed at five responses. During the second minute, three responses are produced, so a dot is placed at eight responses. If 10 responses are made during the next minute, a total of 18 responses have been made. During the fourth minute, suppose no responses occur. A dot is still placed at 18 since that represents the total number of responses accumulated during the first four minutes. In most graphing procedures, the response rate would drop to zero on the graph when no responses were produced, but this is not true on a cumulative graph. The steeper the slope of the line, the greater the number of responses produced during a time period.

As can be seen in Figure 7–2 a fixed-ratio schedule produces an extremely high rate of response.

An equally high rate of response is also produced under a *variable-ratio* schedule of reinforcement. In this schedule, reinforcement is delivered according to some varied amounts of responses, not a set amount of responses as in fixed-ratio schedules. For example, in a VR-4 schedule, reinforcement is given following an *average* of every fourth correct response. Reinforcement may be provided after two responses, then after six, three, five, two, six, and four responses, which averages out at one reinforcement to an average of every four responses (28 ÷ 7 = 4). Slot machines pay off on a variable-ratio schedule, and if you have ever visited the gambling casinos in Nevada, you will see how effective this type of schedule is in producing steady, high rates of lever-pulling responses. Door to door salespersons are also on a variable-ratio schedule of reinforcement.

Ratio schedules depend on *how much* you respond, whereas interval schedules depend on *when* you respond. Under a fixed-interval schedule of reinforcement, the number of responses is not the determinant of when a reinforcement is delivered. During a 3-minute period (FI-3), it would make no difference whether you responded 50 times or only once during the 3-minute period—you would receive only one reinforcement. As can be seen in Figure 7–2 fixed intervals generate a "scalloping" effect in that response rate is high just before reinforcement is delivered, but then drops to zero for quite some time before it gradually builds up again during expectation of another reinforcer. Suppose a supervisor visits workers once every 2 hours (FI-2) on a regular schedule. In many instances, you can expect the workers to be very busy just before the supervisor's visitation but not so busy after she leaves.

Variable-interval schedules result in even less responding over the same time unit. They function in the same way variable-ratio schedules operate, only time is the variable, not the number of responses. One of the best illustrations of an individual following a variable-interval schedule is the fisherman who patiently watches his bobber in anticipation of catching some fish (reinforcers) some time during the day. Usually, fishermen catch fish dependent upon how long they engage in the fishing behavior. They never know whether they will catch one, two, or a dozen fish, but the longer they try to catch fish, the more likely their chances of doing so. Of course, we must assume that they will be assured of catching fish sooner or later.

Several schedules can be operating alternately or concurrently to produce a complex mixture of schedules. They can be arranged to produce rapid bursts of behavior or steady responding over a long period of time. Considerable research using animals as subjects has been conducted in this area.

Unfavorable schedules of reinforcement have been suggested as responsible for many behavioral problems (Kanfer & Phillips, 1970). Some students may receive very infrequent reinforcement for studying, and eventually their study time sharply decreases. Depression has sometimes been caused from insufficient positive reinforcement from the environment. A child may develop seclusive, restrained verbal behaviors with the mother who consistently failed to respond positively to her vocal attempts at communicating with her. The same might be true of the child who is highly reinforced for producing correct speech responses in the speech therapy setting, but is rarely reinforced for producing correct responses by his mother or teacher outside that setting. The behavior therapist may elect to treat a particular problem solely through rearranging schedules of reinforcement, or she may help the person cope with new reinforcement schedules.

The effects of using various reinforcement schedules have been well validated, both in animal studies and in studies involving human subjects. The breadth and scope of these studies are far too wide to review in this chapter. The majority of studies involving human subjects have been conducted by psychologists who work with a wide variety of behavioral problems, from training subjects how to walk, to teaching language skills to nonverbal children. The massive amount of data available leaves little doubt that reinforcement scheduling can be a powerful tool for controlling and maintaining behavior rates (Morse, 1966). Kanfer and Phillips (1970) present a review of many studies demonstrating the therapeutic use of reinforcement operations.

It is surprising that the use of varying schedules of reinforcement has been mentioned so little in the literature by speech pathologists in view of how much is known about the effectiveness of these techniques. While a few reports mention the use of continuous reinforcement during studies involved in training speech skills (McLean & McLean, 1974; Appleman et al., 1975; Irwin & Griffith, 1973), reports of therapeutic procedures employing a variety of reinforcement schedules tailored specifically to maintain certain speech behaviors are almost nonexistent.

One of the few investigations of schedules of reinforcement as used in speech therapy was conducted by Horowitz (1963). She sought to determine what effect conditions of continuous versus intermittent reinforcement had on learning a new task. Using 60 mentally retarded children as subjects, each was shown a picture of a bird, cat, or dog and asked to name the picture upon hearing a buzzer sound. Thirty subjects were given continuous reinforcement following correct picture naming, and 30 were reinforced following every other correct response. Another variable introduced in the experiment was the type of reinforcement given. With respect to continuous versus intermittent reinforcement, it was found that all subjects given continuous reinforcement reached criterion performance (5 consecutive correct responses within 80 trials), while none of those subjects who received intermittent reinforcement achieved criterion performance. It would be hazardous to generalize this conclusion to all other learning situations which involve children of various intelligence levels. It may be that in learning complex vocal tasks, mentally retarded children require longer periods of continuous reinforcement before intermittent schedules can be used to maintain the desired behavior. Although evidence for use of continuous and intermittent reinforcement in speech pathology is scant, ample data have been presented in psychology to support the contention that continuous reinforcement is most effective during task acquisition.

Negative Reinforcement

Up to this point, we have discussed one type of reinforcement—positive. A positive reinforcement is usually viewed in terms of a stimulus, which is something pleasant or desirable. The behavior causes the *presentation* of the stimulus. But when the behavior causes the *removal* of a stimulus, usually an aversive stimulus like a shock, a loud noise, nagging, or some other unpleasant stimulus and as a consequence, the behavior rate increases, this process is called *negative reinforce-*

ment. Both negative and positive reinforcement cause behavior to *increase*. A simple illustration of negative reinforcement is found in a rat's lever pressing behavior. If the animal discovers that pressing behavior will terminate a shock, you will find that the rat will press the lever at a high rate. He does this in order to escape or avoid the shock. Thus, an organism's operant behavior will be found to increase when it serves to remove an aversive stimulus.

Negative reinforcement should not be confused with punishment. While both operations involve aversive stimuli (that is why they are frequently confused), they differ on (1) the effect they have upon behavior, and (2) when they are presented. The negative reinforcer (an aversive stimulus) is presented *before* the response. It becomes a negative reinforcer when it is removed and thus increases the frequency of a behavior. On the other hand, punishment (also an aversive stimulus) *follows* a behavior and tends to decrease the frequency of a response.

Negative reinforcement is commonly used as an effective procedure in treating bizarre behavioral disorders which may include sexual abnormalities, alcoholism, phobias, and autism. It has seldom been employed as a means of treating communication disorders. Several researchers reportedly have used negative reinforcement as a means of increasing stuttering or increasing fluent speech. Goldiamond (1965) demonstrated the effects of negative reinforcement on stuttering to determine whether or not stuttering was an operant behavior and could be increased through operant conditioning procedures. He presented ongoing noise which was terminated for 5 seconds following each occasion of stuttering. Stuttering increased during this period and decreased when it was no longer negatively reinforced. Martin et al. (1975) performed a similar experiment by terminating shock each time the subject stuttered. After 5 seconds, the shock was reintroduced and continued until stuttering occurred again. Results showed a marked increase in stuttering when the escape procedure was utilized prior to the punishment technique. I know of no recent therapeutic technique for the treatment of stuttering that relies on negative reinforcement to reduce the frequency of stuttering behavior. As you might suspect, the side effects of using strong aversive stimuli as negative reinforcers might create more problems than they solve in the case of stuttering. Certainly, negative reinforcement would not be recommended for the bulk of communication disorders because of the unpleasant effects strong aversive stimuli have upon individuals.

Methods of Decreasing the Frequency of Behavior

So far we have discussed two means of increasing the frequency of responses. One way is to present "pleasant" consequences following the response (positive reinforcement); the other way is to present an "aversive" stimulus which is removed as a consequence of the response (negative reinforcement). There are many times when a behavior therapist wants to reduce or eliminate a behavior such as bed wetting, hysteria, homosexual behavior, alcoholosm, tics, or phobic reactions. In the case of speech pathologists, we would like to reduce stuttering behavior, mutism, misarticulation, poor voice quality, and the like. Several procedures have been developed that effectively reduce the frequency of these behaviors.

Punishment: Punishment is one of the best known and widely used procedures for reducing or eliminating a response. As I mentioned earlier, punishment occurs when an aversive stimulus is presented immediately following the response. The effects are to make the response occur less frequently in the future when similar conditions are present. Both parents and teachers rely heavily on punishment to control the behavior of children, although they would prefer to call it *discipline*. Discipline usually implies the use of punishment techniques in contrast to the use of positive reinforcement. Punishing undesirable behaviors in an attempt to reduce or eliminate them usually produces immediate results. We are all familiar with how quickly a child terminates a behavior after he is slapped briskly on his rear end. Society, too, lays down detailed, prescribed punishments to follow a wide variety of crimes, from going through a stop sign to committing a bank robbery.

Many feel the side effects of the frequent use of punishment are very damaging to the punished individual. Punishment contingencies are viewed as generating high anxiety states and undesirable emotional reactions which may be far worse than the original behavior (Skinner, 1953). It is well known that many severe behavioral disorders are the direct result of excessive punishment, threats, anxiety states, and aversive stimulation. Because of the suspected undesirable side effects of punishment as a means of behavior control, its temporary effects, and its inadequacy in changing behavior, punishment, as a therapeutic tool, was seldom used by clinical psychologists until the last decade or two (Solomon, 1964). The use of aversive stimuli has been avoided in speech therapy as well. But recently, psychologists have taken a new look at the effectiveness of various paradigms which employ some kind of aversive stimuli as a means of reducing certain behaviors.

Punishment has been found to completely, partially, or temporarily suppress responses. But under certain conditions, punishment of escape or avoidance responses may increase, rather than suppress, the punished behavior. To be maximally effective, Azrin and Holz (1966) maintain that punishment must be: as intense as possible, presented on a FR-1 schedule, immediate, and given over brief time periods. They also recommend other responses should be made available which could be positively reinforced. Punishment suppresses old behaviors, whereas positive reinforcement strengthens new ones. By suppressing the old behaviors, new, more desirable behaviors can be encouraged. This combination of punishment and positive reinforcement appears to be a most effective technique for changing behavior. Even when punishment alone is compared with other methods for eliminating behavior, such as extinction and satiation, punishment appears to be more complete and irreversible and just as rapid and enduring (Azrin & Holz, 1966). A thorough understanding of punishment, in combination with other behavior shaping factors, may help us determine how bizarre behaviors are developed and maintained.

The effects of punishing stuttering behavior have been reported in many studies. In almost every case, punishment has been found to suppress it. Martin (1968) studied the effects of shock delivered immediately after each occasion of stuttering. He found in the five subjects studied that under conditions of shock, stuttering decreased to almost zero in a few sessions. When the shock was terminated, stuttering frequency returned to its original rate.

Flanagan et al. (1958) used a 105 decibel white noise following each occurrence of stuttering. During the end of the first 30-minute training session, stuttering was almost completely eliminated. Goldiamond (1958) reported using delayed auditory feedback as an aversive stimulus. It was introduced for 5 seconds following each stuttered word. Fluency almost doubled under these conditions as stuttering decreased. Martin and Siegel (1966) delivered shock contingent on different types of secondary stuttering features, such as nose wrinkling and tongue protrusion. They found that these behaviors decreased dramatically but returned to their original rate as soon as the shock was removed. Gross and Holland (1965) found that even when the listener was shocked, contingent upon the stutterer's disfluencies, the frequency of his disfluencies declined.

More recently, Martin et al. (1975) introduced a punishment shock condition preceding and following a shock escape condition. Punishment had the effect of reducing stuttering in both conditions with two of the subjects, but surprisingly, two other subjects actually increased the number of words stuttered during what were considered as punishing conditions, while a third subject changed very little under these conditions. The authors concluded that when several subjects are run over long periods of time, differing behavior patterns emerge. One cannot always predict what conditions will serve as punishment. As in the case presented by Martin et al., sometimes a stimulus may act as a punisher, sometimes a reinforcer, and sometimes neither one.

Punishment procedures have long been used in therapy with stutterers. Aikins (1929) reviewed some past procedures designed to eliminate stuttering through punishment as though stuttering were some manifestation of an evil spirit. Even today, Shames (1968) points out punishment of stuttering is more widespread than many would believe. He feels that confronting stutterers with their problem, forcing them into feared situations and into repeating stuttered words, and the like, are activities many speech clinicians use which have the effect of punishing the stutterer.

Van Riper (1958) states he employs a large variety of penalties in his therapy for stutterers. His purpose is to punish specific, instrumental behaviors in order to suppress them long enough to allow the clinician to substitute more appropriate behaviors. Punishment is also used as a threat, which serves as an alerting device. As positive rewards for newly developed responses increase, punishment is soon discontinued. Van Riper points out that severe punishment like shock, noise, or physical abuse should never be used.

The effect of punishment on stuttering, as a factor responsible for decreasing the frequency of a behavior, becomes more unclear as it is examined. For example, Cooper et al. (1970) followed each stuttered word with the statement "wrong." Stuttering decreased in frequency, as it also did when followed by the word *right* or even *tree*. It may be that any form of contingent attention, aversive or pleasant, may cause stuttering to decrease. This contingent attention may serve as an alerting device which aids the stutterer in reducing the stuttering act. It has also been found that just asking the stutterer to count each stuttered word as it occurs will result in a decrease of stuttered words.

Lovaas (1968), outlining a program to improve the speech of psychotic children, indicated certain times when punishment could be used to suppress deviant behaviors. They include a slap on the child's bottom or hand, a loud, stern "no," and similar actions. These actions were never administered for incorrect verbal behavior during early stages of imitation training. Later, punishment was used to suppress echolalic verbal behaviors. Many situations were created so the child could receive ample positive reinforcement during training. But in most language training programs for children, other than those classified as psychotic, there is little, if any, use of purposeful punishment of responses.

Therapy methods for other communication disorders rarely, if ever, recommend punishment as a means of modifying behavior. In discussing the treatment of articulation disorders, Van Riper (1947) mentions several punishing stimuli which could be administered following incorrectly articulated responses, but his suggested activities serve more as gentle reminders rather than punishers in the usual sense of the word. They consist of asking the individual to put a pencil from one ear to the next or to step into a trash can following the incorrect response. For the most part, punishment is viewed as an undesirable practice which has little place in speech therapy methods.

Time-out: A special type of punishment used more frequently than the presentation of aversive stimuli is *time-out*. This term, coined by Ferster (1957), who studied its effects rather extensively, is used to indicate a condition when positive reinforcers are removed. Removing the reinforcers has the same effect on behavior as presenting aversive stimuli, although some aversive stimuli like shock, used in a punishment paradigm, are a more effective and immediate suppressor of behavior. Time-out is viewed as a form of punishment because its application is contingent on a certain response and thus, acts as an aversive event.

A common procedure in time-out conditions is to place the individual in a room by herself, not allowing her to receive any rewards, such as attention, tokens, stars, or the like. But one difficulty arises if the child finds the time-out condition itself rewarding—she can engage in fantasies that may reduce the aversive character of the setting. Also, if time-out serves to remove the child from an aversive situation, she will find the time-out condition rewarding. If a child is crying because she finds sitting in class aversive, she may engage in crying in order to bring about a time-out condition. In order to be effective, there must be time-out from some reinforcing stimuli. The child must be in a situation where she is enjoying herself. If she emits an undesirable behavior, she is *removed* from the pleasant situation into a time-out condition.

You can easily see that if the child learns her destructive behavior, or if crying behavior leads to removal of the unpleasant classroom atmosphere, she may readily engage in the undesirable behavior when required to clean up, is teased by another child, etc., in order to bring about a time-out condition which will remove her from the aversive stimuli present in the classroom. Thus, what the teacher thinks should be a time-out condition, designed to eliminate the undesirable behavior, may actually turn out to be a positive reinforcer.

Patterson and White (1969) studied many clinical reports using time-out procedures and drew the following conclusions. Time-out has been more effective in eliminating undesirable behaviors in the classroom than has been the procedure of simply ignoring these behavior. Size of the time-out room is not important; supervision of the child should occur while she is in the time-out room. Finally, time-out procedures do not provide the child with imitative models, as do punishment procedures associated with physical types such as hitting and slapping. Many children learn more aversive behaviors when they are punished. For example, the child who is slapped across the face by a punitive parent may soon slap her younger brother across the face to control his behavior. Such aversive behaviors are not learned in the time-out room.

As in the case of moderate or severe punishment, time-out is seldom used by speech clinicians to eliminate or reduce undesirable speech behaviors. It has been used to reduce stuttering behaviors, as described by Curlee and Perkins (1969). The stutterer and clinician are seated in a room, and the stutterer is instructed to talk. The assumed reinforcers are the stutterer's talking to the clinician and the clinician's attention. As soon as the clinician detects an instance of stuttering, the light is turned off and both sit in silence for 30 seconds. The light is then turned on, and the stutterer resumes talking. But as you may have figured out, if the stuttering act itself is aversive and the time-out provides relief from the undesirable speech blockage situation, the time-out condition could serve as a reinforcer, rather than as a form of punishment.

Several other investigators have also used time-out in an attempt to reduce stuttering behavior. Haroldson et al. (1968) employed a period of silence as a time-out procedure contingent upon stuttering and found a marked decrease in the speech behavior of four stutterers. Martin et al. (1972), in a similar study, worked with two children under the age of five who stuttered, using the attention of a puppet as a reinforcer. Immediately following a disfluency, the puppet ceased attending to the child for 10 seconds. As a result, disfluencies decreased to almost zero.

Van Riper (1973) termed his cancellation therapy technique a time-out kind of consequence and found it to be an effective procedure with stutterers. The time-out procedure was a therapeutic technique used by Costello (1975) as the chief means of treating mild-to-moderate stutterers enrolled in the University of California Speech and Hearing Center. As long as the stutterer speaks fluently, the clinician nods, smiles, establishes eye contact, and shows interest in the conversation. When an instance of stuttering is noted, the clinician says "stop" and looks away from the stutterer for 10 seconds; no speech is allowed during this time. Therefore, two presumed reinforcers—the clinician's attention and the opportunity to speak—are withheld. Costello reported remarkable success in establishing fluent speech simply by employing these procedures.

Time-out procedures have been used with children who have language problems, especially autistic children or those children who have very poorly developed language. Sloane, Johnson, and Harris (1968) describe time-out in terms of specific teacher behaviors contingent on two consecutive, unacceptable responses. The teacher remained mute, eyes diverted, with head dropped on her chest for 60 seconds. A third consecutive failure prompted the teacher to leave the room for 1 to 2 minutes. If crying occurred during time-out, the time-out period was extended to 15 to 20 seconds after the termination of the unacceptable behavior.

Lovaas (1968) used time-out procedures to reduce echolalic responses of psychotic children being taught speech skills. The attendant's attention and the child's food were removed for a 5-second period. This procedure was also used to weaken temper tantrums. Risley and Wolf (1968) used time-out procedures as part of a program to establish functional speech in echolalic children. In an effort to reduce the crying behavior of one child, which averaged 16 minutes over each hour period, the experimenter looked away and withheld any food or toy items until the child was sitting quietly in his chair. Then the experimenter turned to the child and continued the session. By the twenty-fourth through twenty-sixth session, crying decreased to 20 seconds.

One cannot assume the exclusive use of time-out procedures will be sufficient to eliminate and to reduce undesirable behaviors. For example time-out procedures were used by Sulzbacher and Costello (1970) to reduce certain behaviors of an autistic child, such as using jargon, leaving the chair, and attending to a mirror instead of the speech clinician. These behaviors were identified as those which interferred most with speech and language training. When the child engaged in one of these behaviors, the clinician removed play materials and remained motionless while facing the floor until the undesired behaviors terminated. But the inappropriate behaviors persisted throughout 50 sessions. Then the clinician said, "No!" and "Sh!" immediately following the inappropriate behaviors, and the frequency of the disruptive behaviors decreased to zero in 15 sessions and remained at that level during the remaining 10 sessions.

Judging from a review of the literature in speech pathology, time-out procedures have been used to reduce or eliminate (1) disfluencies in the speech of stutterers, and (2) behaviors which interfere with the acquisition of language. Time-out has not been reportedly used for eliminating misarticulation or as a means of changing features of voice. This may be due to the fact that correct articulation is considered a motor skill that must be learned, and that voice problems often are a result of some physical anomaly. Nevertheless, it would be interesting to investigate whether or not time-out procedures could be of any use in modifying articulation and voice problems.

Response Cost: Whereas time-out involves removing *all* of the reinforcers from the environment, response cost is a condition in which only *one* reinforcing stimulus is removed. A common example in everyday life is the fine imposed for a traffic violation. Your response of proceeding through a stop sign without stopping may result in a $10 fine. In other words, the cost of your response is that a small portion of your reinforcer (bank account) is removed. Weiner (1962) demonstrated the effect of response cost upon the frequency of behavior by allowing a child to accumulate points on a counter as conditioned reinforcers. Then, he began subtracting a point following each response, and this resulted in immediate suppression of the response. Frequently complete termination of the response resulted.

One problem in using response cost is that the client must first be in possession of a number of reinforcers to begin with, and these reinforcers must be such that they can be removed in small and equal quantities. Removing small quantities of primary reinforcers like sex, water, or food is not only difficult in some cases, but would also be ineffective. A response cost procedure works best by withdrawing secondary reinforcers like an accumulation of points, tokens, or money. These secondary reinforcers are removed contingent on the occurrence of the undesirable behaviors. The effects of response cost as a punishment technique are similar to those found when electric shock is used.

An illustration of the use of response cost in a speech therapy situation is provided by Conley (1966). He used an instructional program to teach lisping children how to produce /s/ correctly. At the end of three instructional periods, the children could produce /s/ correctly in words but did not do so when conversing. Conley invited three peers to a session in which a lisping child was asked to tell stories. Group A was told they would all receive a plastic token each time the lisping child said /s/ correctly. They could redeem the tokens for small toys at the end of the session. Procedures for Group B were identical to those in Group A with the exception that the members of that group were told a token would be withdrawn from each member following each incorrect /s/ production (response cost). Conley found that lispers in Group B produced significantly more correct /s/ sounds than did those lispers in Group A. Of course, there were important variables to be considered other than response cost (negative comments from peers may help account for Conley's findings), but these variables were introduced by the response cost situation.

Research on the effectiveness of a response cost procedure as a means of decreasing incorrect speech responses is limited (McReynolds & Huston, 1971). The authors studied the effects of response cost on correct imitation of a verbal stimulus using two children 6 and 7 years of age. The task for one child was to articulate the word *cup* correctly; the second child was to articulate the word *ring* correctly. Two conditions were presented to each child in a multiple reversal design. In one condition, reinforcement, in the form of a token following each correct response, was provided (FR-1). In the second condition, three tokens were provided for each correct response, but one token was removed for each incorrect response. Data from this study lead the authors to conclude that token loss *per se* did not function as a punishment procedure as far as reducing the amount of incorrect responses, and that continuous reinforcement with no token loss was the most effective procedure for decreasing incorrect responses. A key observation from this study was when token gain exceeded token loss, incorrect responses diminished; but when token loss equaled token gain, the procedure was not effective. They recommended that response cost procedures not be used indiscriminately since a large number of variables can affect its efficiency.

Unfortunately, some speech clinicians apply response cost procedures without the slightest idea of what effects they have on behavior. For example, several years ago, while listening to some samples of tape recorded speech therapy sessions conducted by student clinicians, I discovered one session in which the clinician was using a combination of aversive stimuli in the form of negative reinforcement, punishment, and response cost as means of controlling the behavior of a 6-year-old child who misarticulated several consonant sounds. An analysis of verbal statements from both the child and the clinician revealed that the child's disruptive behaviors increased 60% during the second half of the session. The following are several statements made by the clinician during this session (Mowrer, 1969, pp. 103–107).

"Ah—I'll give you two (tokens) for that."
"No! I'll take them back."
"If you touch them (tokens) I'll have to take them away. Put them down! If you keep touching them, I'll have to take them away.

"Now, you lost another one. Now put them down—don't touch them . . . Come on, put them down."

The clinician asks the child to continue imitating his correct productions and after 19 trials he states:

"I'll have to take two away 'cause you didn't get that right and you're playing with them."

Following another group of about 20 more trials, the clinician further warns the child:

"Leave those alone! They aren't yours yet. You haven't won them. Chris, you're going to end up with none if you aren't careful. Sit here! Get your hands off those."

It is not surprising to discover that fewer than 20% of the responses made by this child during the session were correct. As Sajway (1969) points out in his study of the effects of schedules of loss, magnitude of loss, and prior history of the child in response to punishment procedures, response cost, if not properly programmed, may not only fail to reduce the unwanted behavior, but may lead to the development of behaviors aimed at eliminating the aversive stimuli. The child in the above example was heard making several comments that indicated he would have liked to escape from the situation. Typical among the comments were, "Do I have to do this?" and "Is it time to go yet?"

The effects of response cost as a procedure for decreasing incorrect speech responses are still relatively unknown, and the clinician should be extremely cautious in using these punishment procedures. Webster and Brutten (1974) point out response cost procedures may produce undesirable side effects and should be used with great caution as a technique for modifying stuttering behavior.

Extinction: When the reinforcers that serve to maintain a response are removed, the frequency with which the reinforced behaviors occur at first increases in rate, then gradually returns to their preconditioned rate. This process is called *extinction,* and in many ways, it resembles a time-out procedure since positive reinforcers are removed in both instances. Both also serve as punishers (Baer, 1962). A major difference is that time-out involves removal of *all* reinforcers for a certain time period following the occurrence of the undesired behavior, whereas during extinction, reinforcers are removed contingent on the specific behavior, but reinforcers are still available for other behaviors.

An example of experimental extinction frequently demonstrated in laboratories involves observing a rat's bar pressing behavior when food pellets cease to be delivered. While moving about the cage in search of food or escape, the rat may depress the bar an average of five times a minute. This rate would be the preconditioned response rate. When food is presented contingent upon bar pressing, response rate will increase sharply to something like 40 times a minute, demonstrating the effects of positive reinforcement. If the food dispensing mechanism is deactivated so that bar pressing does not result in food presentation, bar pressing behavior may actually *increase* in frequency for a short time, but will gradually decrease until it reaches the precondition rate of five responses per minute. When the rate reaches the pre-conditioned rate, the response is said to be extinguished. It is important to understand that extinction does not mean elimination of the response, just a return to its original rate. It should also be noted that response rate during extinction will not be a steady decline, but there may be periods of high response rates followed by low rates. The trend is toward a gradual decline.

It is interesting to point out here that Skinner (1956) stumbled on the effects of extinction purely by accident. The food dispensing mechanism he was using jammed during an experiment, and when he was checking response curves of various animals in his laboratory, he came across a cumulative response curve which showed high rates of behavior, a plateau, another burst of responses, and a gradual decline of responding until rate of behavior was practically zero. He quickly repaired the apparatus, but upon giving the data on the response curve more thought, he purposely disconnected the food magazines of other animals and collected additional information about extinction curves. Skinner stated, "some of the most interesting and surprising results have turned up first because of similar accidents."

Since a variety of reinforcement schedules can be used to establish and to maintain a behavior, the length of time required to extinguish a behavior will vary greatly. Also, the number of responses emitted during the conditioning period will affect the length of the extinction period. Thus, if a FR-1 schedule has been applied and only about 30 behaviors have been reinforced, extinction should occur rather rapidly when reinforcement is withheld. But if the schedule of reinforcement is gradually lengthened to an FR-10, and 1,000 behaviors have been emitted, the length of time required for extinction to occur, i.e., the number of unreinforced trials to occur before the behavior reaches its preconditional rate, will be quite lengthy. This is why we might see extinction occur rapidly with one child but not with another.

One term frequently associated with extinction, especially when schedules of reinforcement are being discussed, is *ratio strain*. If a child is learning a complex behavior and a continuous reinforcement schedule is being used, an abrupt shift to an intermittent schedule of VR-20 may result in the termination of the child's responding. In the case of the VR-20 schedule, reinforcement simply does not occur frequently enough to maintain the new behavior. The novice gambler would be especially susceptible to ratio strain. If at first he wins at the poker table, his eagerness to play more games increases. But if suddenly his luck turns sour and his wins occur with less frequency, he will soon drop out of the game. To put it another way, the ratio strain becomes so great that his behavior returns to its original rate, an occasional game. However, the compulsive gambler can tolerate large changes in reinforcement schedules. His behavior is extremely resistant to extinction. Due to his past history of conditioning, he knows the game will pay off sooner or later.

Some children seem to have a high resistance to extinction because of their unique conditioning history. Such children are observed to persevere at one task for hours even when no apparent reward is forthcoming. Sometimes behavior of this sort is labeled *maladaptive*. Many mentally retarded children are observed to engage in what we would judge to be persevering type behaviors. What we might be seeing are behaviors which are extremely tolerant of long periods of no reinforce-

ment. Of course, being able to stick to a task for long periods of time without reinforcement may be considered desirable in many circumstances. We call these people
diligent, hard workers, and industrious when they are working at tasks considered
worthwhile.

The fact that responding usually increases for a brief period immediately following withdrawal of reinforcement often discourages most individuals from continuing
the process. For example, suppose a child has been rewarded with the clinician's
attention, consisting of verbal reprimands, threats, and occásional jostling. This
attention has been contingent on seat-leaving behavior during a group language
session and the attention occurs intermittently. When attention for seat leaving is
withdrawn, seat-leaving behavior is likely to increase. The clinician's first reaction
is to conclude that extinction is not occurring and may continue to provide attention because the attention produces immediate results, i.e., the child returns to his
seat following the command, "Sit down!" Thus, the clinician has only managed to
alter the reinforcement schedule, making the behavior even more resistant to extinction. This process has been referred to as a *behavior trap* and is a common occurrence in every classroom.

The clinician must also be acutely aware that a child may find additional reinforcers that maintain his behavior other than those provided by the clinician. The
child who leaves his seat may find interesting things to do and to see, and although
he loses the clinician's attention, aversive as it might be, he may find toys in other
parts of the room, a door to exit from, other children to bother, and the like. If this
is the case, seat leaving will continue to increase in spite of the fact that one reinforcer, the clinician's attention, has been removed. Extinction functions when all
reinforcers which follow the particular behavior are removed. As you can see, in
creating such a situation, we may approach a time-out condition.

In direct opposition to perseverance of the behavior is the abrupt termination of
behavior after only one or two instances of removal of the reinforcer, especially
when the individual has been under a continuous reinforcement schedule. Dime- or
quarter-inserting behavior usually terminates after one trial followed by nondelivery
of a candy bar at a vending machine. The individual who continues coin-inserting
behavior time and time again would be considered odd indeed. This can sometimes
operate to the disadvantage of the behavior therapist if she has been reinforcing a
new response many times and following one unreinforced trial, the response rate
returns once again to the preconditioned level, which might have been at a zero
level.

One problem with extinction when used alone is that it permits neither control nor
prediction of what new responses should replace the undesirable ones that are being
extinguished. The clinician should make sure that reinforcers are readily available
for acceptable behaviors during the extinction period or else other undesirable
behaviors may develop in their place.

One undesirable response speech clinicians would like to reduce or eliminate is
stuttering behavior. Ryan (1964) reports an extinction procedure he used with a
12-year-old stutterer. He presented a penny to the subject each time he stuttered
during five reading periods. This resulted in an increase in the frequency of stuttering behavior, thereby demonstrating the effects of positive reinforcement. During
the next five readings, he stopped presenting pennies contingent upon stuttering, and
the mean number of words stuttered increased during the first four readings. On the

fifth reading, the frequency of stuttering began to decrease. Unfortunately, Ryan did not continue this extinction period beyond the fifth session; therefore, it was not possible to validate the effects of extinction in this case. Ryan predicted that if he had continued the extinction process, the frequency of stuttering would have gradually decreased.

Webster and Brutten (1974) recommend extinction as a possible procedure to help eliminate undesirable, nonverbal behaviors associated with stuttering. For example, if the stutterer wrinkles his nose frequently as part of his stuttering pattern, he is told to wrinkle his nose on purpose many times daily. The theory here is that nose wrinkling behavior will decrease since it will not be followed by a reinforcing event, that event being the ability to say a word. Unfortunately, the authors present no data regarding the effectiveness of this procedure, but merely present the idea as a therapeutic suggestion.

Very few studies in speech pathology report the effects of, or even specific use of, extinction as a technique for eliminating responses. As Spradlin and Girardeau (1970) point out, extinction is difficult to use with most vocal behavior since this behavior may be maintained by very weak reinforcers. As far as articulation therapy is concerned, one can hardly remove a reinforcer contingent on the utterance of a single sound in the stream of speech. It is far more effective to signal the occurrence of an incorrect response using a buzzer or a light. With the exception of control of echolalia, extinction procedures are employed to decrease overt disruptive behaviors rather than to decrease the frequency of certain speech behaviors.

Combined Use of Reinforcement and Extinction

When the goal of therapy is to establish new behavior patterns, it is best to use reinforcement in conjunction with extinction. This is especially true in speech therapy directed toward developing new articulatory behaviors. The particular technique may involve reinforcing the desired response and ignoring the incorrect response, or it may consist of providing information to the client when an incorrect response is made. This information may consist of a simple "no" or it may include pointing out why the response was not correct. For example, one might say, "your tongue stuck out," "you blinked your eyes," or "that was too fast."

The use of reinforcement and extinction or reinforcement plus information about the incorrect response are commonly used procedures when establishing new behaviors. These procedures are integral to two concepts, response differentiation and discrimination. To aid you in distinguishing between them each will be explained in the following sections.

Response Differentiation

The term *response differentiation* is commonly referred to as shaping a response through successive approximation. It is a process where the clinician selectively reinforces one behavior and eliminates reinforcement for another behavior. Where both desirable and undesirable responses are present, the clinician may reinforce the desirable behavior by attending to polite remarks uttered by the child and by ignoring "bad" language until undesired language responses decrease. The problem is quite different if the child has never acquired intelligible speech or has not acquired mastery over certain sounds. It may be necessary to select approximations of the desired behavior and to reinforce them "differentially." That is to say, the clinician's criterion for providing reinforcement will change as will her criterion for determining which responses go unreinforced. This process of changing criteria for various responses in the direction of some specified response is called *differential reinforcement*. Through this process, the individual can be taught to produce new behaviors. It requires that the clinician specify a number of graded tasks along a continuum of increasing difficulty or complexity.

Isaacs et al. (1960) describe a procedure for reinstating verbal behavior in a mute psychotic patient using a differential reinforcement procedure. Their goal was to evoke the word *gum* from the patient upon the presentation of, or desire for, a package of chewing gum. The patient was first reinforced for moving his eyes toward the gum; then he was reinforced for making small lip movements while looking at the gum. Making a slight sound while moving the lips was reinforced next, followed by a vocalized sound and finally, closer and closer approximations to the word *gum* were required before reinforcement was delivered. As you might suspect, this process could be a very slow one, and in some cases, there are risks that the clinician may terminate the shaping process if the steps are so small that progress seems unapparent. If this occurs, one could say ratio strain was too great for the clinician.

Documentation of the successful use of response differentiation procedures abounds in the literature, especially in the establishment of new behaviors of mentally retarded and psychotic patients. In a film produced by Meyerson (1971), each step in the process of teaching a nonambulatory retarded girl to walk is clearly portrayed in a series of events, from turning to and from opposite chairs to receive reinforcement, to walking unassisted about the room. Lee Meyerson and Nancy Kerr have also demonstrated this process in teaching speech to a nonverbal child.* Several other similar examples which demonstrate establishment of speech in nonverbal children using response differentiation techniques can be found in Sloane and MacAulay (1968).

Although several speech clinicians use this procedure to teach children how to articulate certain sounds, some do not rely on shaping procedures at all. Irwin and Griffith (1973), for example, feel that while shaping behavior is a potentially powerful technique, its use in articulation training is limited due to the difficulty of identifying the small steps from the error sound production to the correct sound. They rely more on the likelihood that the child will produce the target sound correctly in one of 20 key words. If not, traditional stimulation and phonetic placement procedures are used.

McDonald (1964) also feels it is not necessary to teach sounds through this shaping process. He relies on the prospect that the individual will produce the sound correctly when it is surrounded by other sounds that facilitate the movement patterns necessary to produce the sound. Once this occurs, the clinician has a place to begin therapy through co-articulation drills.

Most clinicians rely heavily on procedures designed to move the individual through a series of small, successive steps by rewarding behaviors which are closer

---

*Source: Unpublished manuscript, Arizona State University, 1969.

to the desired response and by ignoring those which are farther from the target sound. Van Riper and Irwin (1958) caution the beginning clinician about the dangers of rewarding a close approximation too vigorously. They report some children seem unable to make progress beyond a close approximation when the clinician provides too much praise. They also feel that in some situations such as teaching /s/ production to a child with a lateral lisp, shaping sounds may not be as appropriate as an all-or-nothing-at-all type of evaluation.

Winitz (1969) states that the process of shaping sounds can be extremely useful in articulation therapy. He illustrates how this procedure is used in teaching /χ/, a sound which is normally not in the repertoire of English speaking children. He begins by requesting the child to produce a "snorelike inspiration." This response is reinforced until a certain number are produced correctly. Next, the snorelike inspiration is uttered and is followed by a similar snorelike expiration. During the third stage, the inspired snore with an inspired /h/ is followed by the snorelike expiration. Finally, the child inhales in the usual manner and tries to produce the /χ/ phone on exhalation. Within each of the above stages, attempts which approach the criterion for the sound at that stage are reinforced, while those unlike the criterion sound are ignored. Therefore, a wide variety of responses are acceptable, but during each stage of training, less and less approximated sounds become acceptable until the final stage when only one sound, the /χ/ in this case, is reinforced. Winitz also mentions that once the uvular fricative /χ/ sound is in the child's repertoire, it is a relatively simple matter to teach the uvular plosive /k/.

One assignment I give students enrolled in a methods class is to teach someone to produce /ɝ/ using this technique of shaping a response. They select a friend and tell her to produce the vowel /ɑ/. They can provide any instruction regarding tongue placement but are not allowed to tell the person to produce /ɝ/, i.e., they cannot provide a model of the sound. By instructing the friend to place her tongue tip up and back, /ɝ/ like sounds are usually produced. The student reinforces sounds which approximate /ɝ/ and ignores those which sound like /ɑ/.

I have used the same procedure in shaping /ɝ/ with young children who distort /ɝ/. A graphic portrayal of this process is presented in Figure 7–3. Note that variations of the /ɝ/ sound are plotted on the ordinate from sounds which resemble /ʌ/ to those which resemble /ɝ/. Trials are plotted on the abscissa.

During the first two trials, a starting point is established. Then a tongue placement cue is provided, and immediately, the sound is changed slightly in the direction of /ɝ/. This response is reinforced although it is an unacceptable /ɝ/ sound. More cues are provided, and by trial 11, a fairly acceptable /ɝ/ is produced. Note that sounds produced during trials 12 and 13 were almost as good as those produced on trials 9 and 10, but now they are considered unacceptable. This demonstrates how the criterion for reinforcement changes as the individual gradually progresses. This process is continued throughout the shaping process until the desired target sound is produced, as indicated on trial 45.

Shaping sounds through response differentiation is not always the most efficient way to evoke sounds. Frequently, children who lisp can produce /s/ correctly when told to close their teeth and imitate the clinician's production of /s/ (Mowrer et al., 1968). I have found that it is best to ignore slight distortions of /s/ during the first 30 or 40 trials, while accepting teeth closure as the prime target. Within these first 40 trials, /s/ production soon begins to match the clinician's production even though

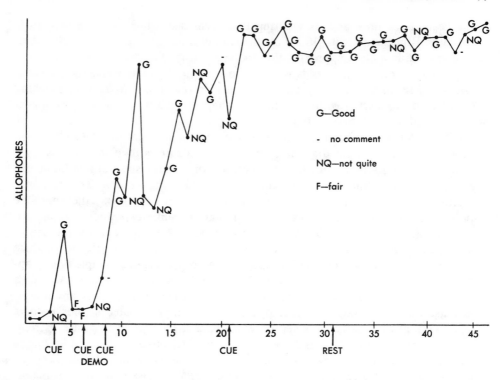

FIGURE 6–3. Graphed /ʌ/ and /ɝ/ Variants During Shaping Session 2

it still may be slightly distorted. The production of /θ/ from a child who substitutes /f/ or /s/ for /θ/ also does not usually require a shaping process.

Aside from its use in shaping articulatory responses, this process is also used extensively with those who have various voice problems. For example, Wolski and Wiley (1965) report a treatment procedure in dealing with an adolescent who was aphonic during 6 months as a result of laryngitis. First, the youth was encouraged to make soft humming sounds while chewing. Several weeks later, Wolski joined the boy while they listened to tape recordings of these sounds and let him know he approved of all sounds produced although voice quality was markedly hoarse. Wiley joined the session, and together they encouraged the boy to make more sounds until he was answering questions and conversing. He still would talk only to very few people outside the therapy setting. He was encouraged to compose short stories, which he read on the tape recorder. Their content was analyzed by the researchers. Becoming involved in discussions of various topics, the youth began to talk more freely, and episodes of whispered or inaudible speech became more and more infrequent, while the frequency of audible speech increased. Eventually, voiced speech was used exclusively with no relapses into whispered speech, and the subject was returned to the normal school environment. Treatment of similar cases is reported by Boone (1966). Smayling (1959) presented treatment procedures using this same sort of shaping process with six cases exhibiting voluntary mutism.

This process of shaping through response differentiation may not always work to our advantage. Most behavioral tantrums result from a gradual series of differential reinforcements. At first, the young infant cries in response to aversive stimuli. Crying usually brings the attention of the parent, and soon crying behavior increases because of this attention. In time, the parents ignore crying when they are convinced nothing is wrong with the child, and as a result, crying behavior normally goes through extinction. But in some cases, parents may observe that crying behavior occurs too frequently or in too many situations. They may attempt to ignore crying, hoping it will cease, but if the child cries hard enough and long enough, they may eventually "give in" and provide attention or produce what the child desires. After this occurs several times, the parents may wait longer before they finally give in, and thus, will reinforce more extreme versions of crying behavior by selectively reinforcing these extreme crying sessions. By gradually raising the point at which the child must cry before attention is provided, the parents inadvertently shape crying temper tantrums which would not normally occur. This entire process is usually complicated by other factors, such as a "good spanking" by the father, which promotes more intense crying, followed by the mother's comforting behavior. What seems like "abnormal" behaviors in children can be unwittingly shaped by well-meaning parents. Frequently, the speech clinician is confronted with such behaviors when attempting to teach speech or language skills to autistic, mentally retarded, or cerebral palsied children. Often these behaviors interfere with the therapeutic process and must be decelerated before speech therapy can be effective.

Response differentiation is an important aspect of educational training, especially in the area of motor skills. In order to teach a child to differentiate between responses, the speech clinician must first reinforce any gross or minimal behavior which approximates the desired behavior and only gradually withhold reinforcement for inappropriate behaviors while reinforcing behaviors which closer resemble the desired behavior. Suppose a child says a sound correctly only three times during 25 trials and the clinician only reinforces the child three times. This may not be sufficient reinforcement to keep the child responding. The child may simply wish to give up trying. The skilled clinician is very sensitive to the vulnerability of acquiring a new behavior and provides ample reinforcement for close approximations of the desired behavior. Thus, she prevents ratio strain. However, if one moves too slowly, too much reinforcement may be provided for intermediate behaviors, causing them to persist and to actually impede progress. The progress in shaping and acquiring new skills depends a great deal on the clinician's skill in discriminating which behaviors are to be reinforced and when reinforcement criteria should be changed, as well as when to withhold reinforcement. Unfortunately, no "hard and fast" rules exist which will assist the clinician in learning skills necessary to establish new behaviors through response differentiation.

Discrimination and Stimulus Control

The terms *differentiation* and *discrimination* are frequently confused, partly because both processes can occur simultaneously. Differentiation describes changes in a class of responses, that is to say, the individual's *responses* change. This was explained in the previous discussion of the gradual shaping of new responses. But during discrimination training, the individual learns to respond in the presence of some stimuli but not in the presence of others. Thus, *stimulus* change is most important in discrimination.

Just as in response differentiation, differential reinforcement and selective withholding of reinforcement play the important role in establishing discrimination. An individual is said to be able to discriminate among several stimuli when she consistently responds in the presence of one stimuli but not in the presence of other stimuli. When responses come under the control of specific stimuli, that is, the stimuli control whether or not the response will occur, we say the response is under stimulus control.

Recall in the previous section how parents might unwittingly shape crying tantrum behavior in their child to the point where it is considered abnormal behavior. This was accomplished through response differentiation. But suppose the child enters kindergarten and the teacher, realizing that attending to the child's tantrum behavior will only increase these behaviors, places the child in a time-out situation contingent on tantrum behavior.

As we might expect, the frequency of the tantrum behaviors increase at first and then decrease. Soon the child learns to discriminate between the two situations and exhibits tantrum behavior at home and normal behavior at school. He has learned to discriminate between how to act in one situation and how to act in another.

In discrimination training, we are interested not in rate, but the *conditions* under which a response occurs. For example, the exhibitionist is a problem not because he disrobes frequently or infrequently (rate of disrobing), but because he disrobes under inappropriate conditions, such as in public parks, bus stations, parking lots, and other public places. The problem is one of discrimination. He must learn which stimulus conditions are appropriate. The same is true of an individual's swearing behavior. We learn that swearing is appropriate on the construction site, in a business setting, or in the home, but not while conversing with acquaintances in the church lobby, or when children are present. We can say that swearing behavior is under stimulus control, i.e., we learned when to swear and when not to swear.

Discrimination training consists of conditioning a response in the presence of one stimulus and extinguishing it in the presence of another. The stimulus associated with reinforcement is abbreviated S^D (discriminative stimulus), while the stimulus which is never followed by reinforcement is abbreviated S^Δ. Construction workers are stimuli (S^D) which evoke swearing. Thus, you can easily see how positive reinforcement and extinction can be combined to alter behaviors. Much of what we know about this process has developed from laboratory experiments with animals. In fact, the procedure was used to train pigeons to guide missiles during World War II and to train dogs strapped with explosives to charge enemy tanks (Skinner, 1960).

There are many situations in which discrimination training is important in speech therapy. For example, children who talk so softly in class that they cannot be heard need to learn to speak with appropriate loudness in classroom conditions. We do not wish to increase the frequency of loud talking, nor do we need to establish a new behavior of loud talking. The child already engages in loud talking outside the classroom, but somehow the classroom has become an S^D for soft talking. Much of the work done with aphasic patients consists of discrimination training. Many can utter words, but these words are not under stimulus control. The language patterns of many retarded children are often inappropriate to the situation. A young child may approach a stranger with a lengthy conversation about how she is tormented by a classmate, but the stranger may have absolutely no notion of why the child is telling him this, nor will he be able to understand the situation. Here again, the problem is one of discrimination. The child may have good control over language skills and articulation, but because what she says is inappropriate for that particular situation, she is considered abnormal.

A great deal has been written about the subject of poor auditory discrimination, both as a cause of articulation problems, and as a necessary ingredient of a therapy program. The basic argument is some children who misarticulate sounds are unable to respond differentially to single sound changes. The child who is unable to perceive the presentation of two spoken words *soap* and *toap* as sounding different from each other is said to have a problem with auditory discrimination. The task of discrimination training is to evoke the response *different* when soap—toap are presented, and *same* when soap—soap are presented. When this is accomplished, the child's responses, "same" and "different," are under stimulus control. Winitz (1969), presents data indicating that with some children, training in learning to discriminate between two similar speech sounds may facilitate the child's ability to learn how to produce the sounds correctly. Garrett (1973), on the other hand, provides evidence to indicate that if a child is able to produce a misarticulated sound correctly in imitation of the clinician's model, i.e., he is "stimulatable," additional discrimination training does not contribute to his progress in acquisition of the correct sound.

The concept of discrimination helps us understand why some speech responses do not carry-over to speaking situations outside the training situation. Every clinician is well aware that many children articulate correctly during speech class but revert to their error sound while speaking in the classroom, on the playground, and at home. In these situations, it is said the new sound does not "carry-over" to other speaking situations. It is likely that discrimination has occurred in that the child perceives the stimuli associated with speech class as an S^D for articulating correctly, but upon returning to the classroom, the S^Ds are no longer present, so the old behavior returns. He has two behaviors: one for the clinician, and one for his teacher.

I vividly remember numerous times after administering an /s/ correction program to lisping first-grade children that they were able to articulate /s/ correctly during a criterion test, but they barely stepped outside the testing room when they said, "Can I get thome more toyth netht time?" This illustrates how discrimination can work to our disadvantage at times.

Discrimination plays an important role in early language development. Brown (1958) provides many examples of how verbal concepts are developed in young children through discrimination training. At first, the young child learns to associate the word "Daddy" with the appearance of her father. When her father enters the room or when she requests something from her father, she uses the word *Daddy*. **Through the process of generalization, which will be presented in chapter 7, the** child uses the word *Daddy* applying it to all adult male figures including the postman, an uncle, the next door neighbor, or sales clerk. But those false identifications are soon extinguished through nonreinforcement or corrective remarks on the part of the embarrassed mother, while the utterance "Daddy" in the presence of the father is reinforced. Thus, the child learns the salient features of the father stimulus and other adult males. Later, she learns to specifically identify the milkman, postman, Uncle Harry, and so on by the proper name. Discrimination has occurred.

The language clinician should take special note of this discrimination process since it is so important as a means of adding new verbal labels to the child's vocabulary. A number of language training programs make extensive use of discrimination training as an essential part of extending vocabulary.

Concluding Remarks

Behavior therapies are best noted for their use of managing contingencies as a method for controlling operant behavior. The major operations of operant conditioning and some applications of these operations in speech therapy situations have been presented in this chapter. While many of the concepts are not necessarily new ones, there has been a concerted effort during the past two or three decades to verify their usefulness in modifying behavior, both at the animal level and with human subjects. The major characteristic of this work has been the application of scientific methodology in collecting data and drawing conclusions from these findings. From the results of these investigations, we are able to both predict and control much of human behavior within educational settings. The principles employed in behavior therapy offer the speech clinician powerful tools which can be used to modify communication behaviors effectively and efficiently.

But behavior therapy is not limited solely to the management of consequent events. Maintaining behaviors once they are established is of vital importance if behavior therapy is to be successful. The next chapter will present concepts and therapy techniques designed to maintain behavior.

BIBLIOGRAPHY

Aikins, H. A. Casting out a stuttering devil. *Journal of Abnormal and Social Psychology*, 1929, *18*, 175–192.

Appelman, K., Allen, K. E., & Turner, K. D. The conditioning of language in a non-verbal child conducted in a special education classroom. *Journal of Speech and Hearing Disorders*, 1975, *40*, 3–12.

Azrin, N. H., & Holz, W. C. Punishment. In W. K. Honig (Ed.), *Operant behavior: Areas of research and application*. New York: Appleton-Century-Crofts, 1966.

Baer, D. M. Laboratory control of thumbsucking by withdrawal and re-presentation of reinforcement. *Journal of Experimental Analysis of Behavior*, 1962, *5*, 525–528.

Boone, D. Treatment of functional aphonia in a child and in an adult. *Journal of Speech and Hearing Disorders*, 1966, *31*, 69–74.

Brookshire, R. H. Speech pathology and the experimental analysis of behavior. *Journal of Speech and Hearing Disorders*, 1967, *32*, 215–227.

Brown, R. *Words and things*. Glencoe, Ill.: The Free Press, 1958.

Brutten, G. J. Two factor behavior theory and therapy. In M. Fraser (Ed.), *Conditioning in stuttering therapy*. Memphis: Speech Foundation of America, 1970.

Conley, D. *The effects of using standardized instructions to evaluate speech correction procedures*. Unpublished masters thesis, Arizona State University, 1966.

Cooper, E. B., Cady, B. B., & Robbins, C. J. The effect of the verbal stimulus words *wrong, right*, and *true* on the disfluency rates of stutterers and non-stutterers. *Journal of Speech and Hearing Research*, 1970, *13*, 239–244.

Costello, J. The establishment of fluency with time-out procedures: three case studies. *Journal of Speech and Hearing Disorders*, 1975, *40*, 216–231.

Curlee, R. F., & Perkins, W. H. Conversational rate control therapy for stuttering. *Journal of Speech and Hearing Disorders*, 1969, *34*, 245–250.

Eysenck, H. J. The nature of behavior therapy. In H. J. Eysenck (Ed.), *Experiments in behavior therapy*. London: Pergamon, 1964.

Ferster, C. B. Withdrawal of positive reinforcement as punishment. *Science*, 1957, *126*, 509.

Flanagan, B., Goldiamond, I., & Azrin, N. H. Operant stuttering: The control of stuttering behavior through response-contingent consequences. *Journal of Experimental Analysis of Behavior*, 1958, *1*, 173–178.

Franks, C. M. (Ed.), *Behavior therapy: Appraisal and status*. New York: McGraw-Hill, 1969.

Garrett, E. R. Programmed articulation therapy. In W. Wolfe & D. Goulding (Eds.), *Articulation and learning*. Springfield, Ill.: Charles C Thomas, 1973.

Girardeau, F. L., & Spradlin, J. E. (Eds.), *A functional analysis approach to speech and language*. ASHA Monographs, 1970. Washington, D.C.: American Speech and Hearing Association, 1970.

Goldiamond, I. Indicators of perception: I. Subliminal perception, subsusception, un-conscious perception, an analysis in terms of psychophysical indicator methodology. *Psychological Bulletin*, 1958, *55*, 373–411.

Goldiamond, I. Stuttering and fluency as manipulatable operant response classes. In L. Krasner & L. P. Ullman (Eds.), *Research in behavior modification*. New York: Holt, Rinehart & Winston, 1965.

Gross, M. S., & Holland, A. L. The effects of response contingent electroshock upon stuttering. *Asha*, 1965, *7*, 376.

Guttman, N. Equal reinforcing values for sucrose and glucose solutions compared with equal sweetiness values. *Journal of Comparative Physiological Psychology*, 1954, *47*, 358–361.

Haroldson, S. K., Martin, R. R., & Starr, C. D. Time-out as a punishment for stut-tering. *Journal of Speech and Hearing Research*, 1968, *11*, 560–566.

Heber, R. F. Motor task performance of high grade mentally retarded males as a function of the magnitude of incentive. *American Journal of Mental Deficiency*, 1959, *63*, 667–671.

Holland, A. Some applications of behavioral principles to clinical speech problems. *Journal of Speech and Hearing Disorders*, 1967, *32*, 11–18.

Horowitz, F. D. I. Partial and continuous reinforcement of vocal responses using candy, vocal, and smiling reinforcers among retardates. *Journal of Speech and Hearing Disorders*, Monograph Supplement, 1963, *10*, 55–69.

Irwin, J. V., & Griffith, F. A. A theoretical and operational analysis of the paired stimulus technique. In W. D. Wolfe, & D. J. Goulding (Eds.), *Articulation and learning*. Springfield, Ill.: Charles C Thomas, 1973.

Isaacs, W., Thomas, J., & Goldiamond, I. Application of operant conditioning to re-instate verbal behavior in psychotics. *Journal of Speech and Hearing Disorders*, 1960, *25*, 8–12.

Johnson, W., Brown, S., Curtis, J., Edney, C., & Keaster, J. *Speech handicapped school children*, 3rd ed. New York: Harper & Row, 1967.

Kanfer, F. H., & Phillips, J. S. *Learning foundations of behavior therapy*. New York: John Wiley & Sons, 1970.

Katkin, E. S., & Murray, E. N. Instrumental conditioning of autonomically mediated behavior: Theoretical and methodological issues. *Psychological Bulletin*, 1968, *70*, 52–68.

Kimble, G. A., *Hilgard and Marquis' conditioning and learning*, 2nd ed. New York: Appleton-Century-Crofts, 1961.

Kushner, M., & Sandler, J. Aversion therapy and the concept of punishment. *Behavior Research Therapy*, 1966, *4*, 179–186.

Lazarus, A. A. (Ed.), *Clinical behavior therapy*. New York: Brunner/Mazel, 1972.

Lindsley, O. R. *Studies in behavior therapy: Status report III*. Waltham, Mass.: Metro-politan State Hospital, 1954.

Lovaas, O. I. A program for the establishment of speech in psychotic children. In H. Sloane & B. MacAulay (Eds.), *Operant procedures in remedial speech and language training*. Boston: Houghton Mifflin, 1968.

Lundin, R. W. *Personality: A behavioral analysis*. London: MacMillan, 1969.

Martin, R. The experimental manipulation of stuttering behaviors. In H. Sloane & B. MacAulay (Eds.), *Operant procedures in remedial speech and language training*. Boston: Houghton Mifflin, 1968.

Martin, R., Kuhl, P., & Haroldson, S. An experimental treatment with two preschool stuttering children. *Journal of Speech and Hearing Research*, 1972, *15*, 743–752.

Martin, R., & Siegel, G. M. The effects of response contingent shock on stuttering. *Journal of Speech and Hearing Research*, 1966, *9*, 340–352.

Martin, R., St. Louis, K., Haroldson, S., & Hasbrouch, J. Punishment and negative reinforcement of stuttering using electric shock. *Journal of Speech and Hearing Research*, 1975, *18*, 478–490.

McDonald, E. T. *Articulation testing and treatment: A sensory-motor approach.* Pittsburgh: Stanwix House, 1964.

McGeoch, J. A., & Irion, A. L. *The psychology of human learning*, 2nd ed. New York: Longmans, Green & Co., 1952.

McLean, L. P., & McLean, J. E. A language training program for nonverbal autistic children. *Journal of Speech and Hearing Disorders*, 1974, *39*, 186–193.

McReynolds, L. Contingencies and consequences in speech therapy. *Journal of Speech and Hearing Disorders*, 1970, *35*, 12–24.

McReynolds, L. V., & Huston, K. Token loss in speech imitation training. *Journal of Speech and Hearing Disorders*, 1971, *36*, 486–495.

Meyerson, L. (Producer), *Rewards and reinforcements in learning.* Scottsdale, Ariz.: Behavior Modification Productions, 1971 (Film).

Morse, W. H. Intermittent reinforcement. In W. K. Honig (Ed.), *Operant behavior: Areas of research and application.* New York: Appleton-Century-Crofts, 1966.

Mowrer, D. E. *Modification of speech behavior: Ideas and strategies for students.* Tempe, Ariz.: Arizona State University Bookstore, 1969.

Mowrer, D. E. *Reduction of stuttering* (Tech. Rep. S-1). Tempe, Ariz.: Arizona State University Bookstore, 1971.

Mowrer, D. E., Baker, R. L., & Schutz, R. E. Operant procedures in the control of speech articulation. In H. Sloane & B. MacAulay (Eds.), *Operant procedures in remedial speech and language training.* Boston: Houghton Mifflin, 1968.

Neisworth, J. T., Deno, S. L., & Jenkins, J. R. *Student motivation and classroom management: A behavioristic approach.* Newark, Del.: Behavior Technics, 1969.

O'Leary, K. D., & Wilson, G. T. *Behavior therapy: Application and outcome.* Englewood Cliffs, N.J.: Prentice-Hall, 1975.

Patterson, G. R. & White, G. D. It's a small world: The application of "time-out for reinforcement." *Oregon Psychological Association Newsletter*, 1969, *15*, No. 2 suppl.

Rachman, S. Introduction to behavior therapy. *Behavior Research and Therapy*, 1963, *1*, 3–15.

Rheingold, H. L., Gewirtz, J. L., & Ross, H. W. Social conditioning of vocalizations in the infant. *Journal of Comparative Physiological Psychology*, 1959, *52*, 68–73.

Rimm, D. C., & Masters, J. C. *Behavior therapy: Techniques and empirical findings.* New York: Academic Press, 1974.

Risley, T., & Wolf, M. Establishing functional speech in echolalic children. In H. N. Sloane & B. MacAulay (Eds.), *Operant procedures in remedial speech and language training.* Boston: Houghton Mifflin, 1968.

Ryan, B. The construction and evaluation of a program for modifying stuttering behavior. Unpublished doctoral dissertation, Pittsburgh: University of Pittsburgh, 1964.

Sajway, T. E. *Some parameters of point loss.* Doctoral dissertation, University of Kansas, 1969.)

Schaefer, H. H., & Martin, P. L. *Behavioral therapy.* New York: McGraw-Hill, 1969.

Shames, G. Operant conditioning and stuttering. In Malcolm Fraser (Ed.), *Conditioning in stuttering therapy.* Speech Foundation of America: Memphis, Tenn., 1968.

Shapiro, D., Tursky, B., Gershon, E., & Stern, M. Effects of feedback and reinforcement on the control of human systolic blood pressure. *Science,* 1969, *163,* 588–589.

Siegel, P. S., & Foschee, J. G. The law of primary reinforcement in children. *Journal of Experimental Psychology,* 1953, *45,* 12–14.

Skinner, B. F. *Science and human behavior.* New York: Macmillan, 1953.

Skinner, B. F. A case history in scientific methods. *American Psychologist,* 1956, *11,* 221–233.

Skinner, B. F. Pigeons in a pelican. *American Psychologist,* 1960, *15,* 28–37.

Sloane, H. N., Johnson, M. K., & Harris, F. R. Remedial procedures for teaching verbal behavior to speech deficient or defective young children. In H. N. Sloane & B. MacAulay (Eds.), *Operant procedures in remedial speech and language training.* Boston: Houghton Mifflin, 1968.

Sloane, H. N., & MacAulay, B. (Eds.), *Operant procedures in remedial speech and language training.* Boston: Houghton Mifflin, 1968.

Smayling, L. M. Analysis of six cases of voluntary mutism. *Journal of Speech and Hearing Disorders,* 1959, *24,* 55–58.

Solomon, R. L. Punishment. *American Psychologist,* 1964, *19,* 239–253.

Spradlin, J. E., & Girardeau, F. L. The implications of a functional approach to speech and hearing research and therapy. *ASHA Monographs,* 1970, *14,* 70–80.

Sulzbacher, S. I., & Costello, J. M. A behavioral strategy for language training of a child with autistic behaviors. *Journal of Speech and Hearing Disorders,* 1970, *35,* 256–276.

Ullman, L. P., & Krasner, L. *A psychological approach to abnormal behavior.* Englewood Cliffs, N.J.: Prentice-Hall, 1969.

Van Riper, C. Experiments in stuttering therapy. In J. Eisenson (Ed.), *Stuttering: A symposium.* New York: Harper & Row, 1958.

Van Riper, C. *Speech correction: Principles and methods.* New York: Prentice-Hall, 1947.

Van Riper, C. *The treatment of stuttering.* Englewood Cliffs, N.J.: Prentice-Hall, 1973.

Van Riper, C., & Irwin, J. *Voice and articulation.* Englewood Cliffs, N.J.: Prentice-Hall, 1958.

Webster, L. M., & Brutten, G. J. The modification of stuttering and associated behaviors. In S. Dickson (Ed.), *Communication disorders: Remedial principles and practices.* Glenview, Ill.: Scott, Foresman, 1974.

Weiner, H. Some effects of response cost upon human operant behavior. *Journal of Experimental Analysis of Behavior,* 1962, *5,* 201–208.

Wolfe, W. D., & Goulding, D. J. *Articulation and learning.* Springfield, Ill.: Charles C Thomas, 1973.

Wolski, W., & Wiley, J. Functional aphonia in a fourteen-year-old boy: A case report. *Journal of Speech and Hearing Disorders,* 1965, *30,* 71–75.

Winitz, H. *Articulatory acquisition and behavior.* New York: Appleton-Century-Crofts, 1969.

Yates, A. J. *Behavior therapy.* New York: John Wiley & Sons, 1970.

7

Transfer
of Training
and Retention

Aside from the acquisition or elimination of behaviors and concern over rate of behaviors, the behavior therapist is equally interested in extending certain behaviors (transfer) and maintaining them for long periods of time (retention). A large portion of what we know about this topic has been derived from experiments conducted in the area of human learning prior to World War II through the work of psychologists H. Ebbinghaus, E. L. Thorndike, C. H. Judd, C. L. Hull, and many others. One danger in the present-day emphasis on behavior modification is that much of the data so carefully researched some 40 to 50 years ago are ignored simply because these studies are not representative of current trends. As a result of attempts to "modernize" therapeutic methods, many teachers overlook some sound teaching principles which have proven to be successful in the past.

This chapter reviews basic principles of learning in two well-researched areas: transfer of training and retention. A discussion of current research and practices in speech pathology will also be presented.

Transfer
of Training

Educators have known for many years that once a student learns a concept or skill, this knowledge aids him in learning new and similar concepts or skills. The fact that learning in one area facilitates learning in other areas led to the erroneous concept of "formal discipline" or faculty learning. This concept held that intensive study of Latin and mathematics resulted in the improvement of the mind and thus aided the mastery of other subjects. The more difficult the subject, the better it was supposed to be for the student. Experimental studies proved this theory to be invalid. It was also felt that the more information one possessed, the easier it would be to apply it. This concept too has since been disproven.

Soon after the turn of the twentieth century, Thorndike (1914) formulated a different concept of transfer of training which he later validated with evidence (Thorndike, 1937). Since that time, the concept of transfer of training has been thoroughly studied by psychologists so that today, we are able to explain a great deal about what factors facilitate or inhibit learning.

Positive Transfer
of Training

When learning one activity facilitates or makes the learning of another activity easier, then it is said positive transfer of training has occurred. This principle has been demonstrated many times both in the laboratory and in real-life situations. Positive transfer has also been demonstrated to occur across receptors in the same individual. For example, individuals taught to read braille letters with their right fingers are able to read letters using their left fingers immediately with almost 100% accuracy (Hulin & Katz, 1934). Learning to operate a motor scooter or mini bike facilitates learning to operate a motorcycle. Learning to play cricket facilitates learning to play baseball. Learning to memorize a list of nonsense syllables facilitates learning to memorize new lists. The number of activities which demonstrate the occurrence of positive transfer is endless. While it is important for the speech clinician to know that learning one activity may facilitate learning another activity, it is more important to be able to identify the variables involved which facilitate learning.

Thorndike's early explanation of positive transfer of training provided that when the stimuli involved in the first activity are the same or similar to those stimuli in the second activity, with the response remaining the same in both conditions, positive transfer will occur. The two stimulus situations, Thorndike said, had "identical elements." The more dissimilar the stimuli, the less transfer one could expect. As an example, we could expect to learn some foreign languages more rapidly than we learned our native language, providing the stimuli remain similar. We could expect 100% positive transfer in learning the meaning of such French words as, *champion, garage, chauffeur, lingerie, résumé, liaison, rapport, soufflé,* and *composition.* There are many French words which are similar to English words but different enough so positive transfer may not be as great as 100%. Words like *chef, sincèrement, bleu, librairie, tableau, décembre,* and *géomètrie* would be somewhat more difficult to learn than the first list above, whereas words like *mémoire, nuit, oignon, rasoir,* and *révèler* would be even more difficult. Finally, we could expect no positive transfer to occur in learning words like *santé, vivre, très, trouver, huit,* or *jambon.*

Thus, in this example, we can see that the more similar the stimuli in the two situations, i.e., English words and French words, the easier it will be to learn the second task. Conversely, the more dissimilar the stimuli, the more difficult learning the second task becomes. A series of stimuli differing from the original stimulus could be arranged on the abscissa of a graph and amount of time required to learn 10 words plotted on the ordinate (see Figure 7-1).

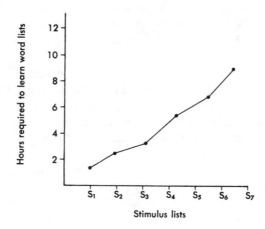

FIGURE 7-1. Number of Hours Required To Learn Stimulus Lists S₁ Through S₇, List S₁ Being Similar To English Words, List S₇ Being Dissimilar

In this case, time required to learn the English equivalent of French words is a measure of the amount of positive transfer that has occurred and according to Thorndike, this is dependent on the similarity of the two stimuli, the English words and the French words. Skinner (1953) used the term *induction* to describe transfer of training which results from "identical elements" in the stimuli. While many psychologists have referred to the condition illustrated in Figure 7-1 as a *stimulus gradient*, Skinner used the term *induction gradient*.

Another theory to explain the occurrence of positive transfer of training was put forth by Gestalt psychologists. They felt the pattern or principle is what facilitates learning, not the individual components. Harlow (1949) in his work with primates provided considerable research data to support the notion that organisms learn principles which aid them in learning new material more effectively. Suppose monkeys were presented with two stimulus objects differing in size, color, and shape. They are rewarded for picking only the larger object, regardless of color or shape. Suppose that an average of 35 trials were required before they learned to choose the largest object. Then two quite dissimilar objects are presented, again differing mainly in size, color, and shape. Fewer trials would be required for the animals to consistently pick the largest object. Thus, the principle of "largeness" is what is said to enable positive transfer to take place.

This principle has also been demonstrated in discrimination training of chickens. Chicks were taught to peck at a medium grey disk and not a lighter grey disk. If a medium grey and darker grey disk are presented, the chicks will learn to pick at the darker grey disk, not the medium grey disk as before. This further demonstrates that a principle, not so much identical elements, is what causes positive transfer.

Research data offer indications that both theories, identical elements and principle application, are plausible explanations of why positive transfer occurs.

Several variables that determine the degree to which positive transfer will occur have been investigated. One is the *amount of training* provided on the first task. A number of experiments clearly demonstrate that the greater the training on a task, the greater the amount of positive transfer that occurs on a similar task (Siipola & Israel, 1933; Melton & Irwin, 1940). This finding has lead to the conclusion that overlearning, that is, increased practice, facilitates ease with which similar material is learned.

Another important variable is the *amount of time* which lapses between original learning and presentation of the second task to be learned. Two studies, one by Bunch (1936) and one by Bunch and McCraven (1938), indicate that relatively large amounts of time delay between original learning and learning in the second condition can be tolerated without loss. Bunch found that periods of up to 90 days had little negative effect upon transfer. Whatever the subject learns during the original condition, whether it is a mode of responding or set to respond, does not seem to be adversely affected with the passage of time.

It has been found that when a person gets into a particular *set,* that is, establishes a certain postural or attentive attitude toward learning a certain task, learning a second task is facilitated (Thune, 1950). A principle or a certain method of performing called a *nonspecific factor* seems to be what is transferred to facilitate the learning of a new task. In this case, the stimuli of the two learning tasks may be quite different, but the approach to learning the task seems to be the same. A similar feature that appears to facilitate transfer of training has been labeled *mode of attack.* What is learned in one task appears to be a strategy which is used in learning other tasks—a "learning to learn." During practice in learning successive lists of verbal materials, Ward (1937) found that his subjects also learned how to follow instructions, to look for mnemonic cues, and to remain calm under failure conditions. These behaviors are often considered *tricks* of learning.

It should be pointed out that the acquisition of a principle does not automatically guarantee that this principle will be used appropriately in other situations. This fact best illustrates why the old concept of formal discipline was abandoned (Bagley, 1905). Results of school learning may transfer widely providing general knowledge is applicable to other situations; but on the other hand, there may be no transfer of training. Principles probably will not transfer if the course material taught consists of specific facts (Stroud, 1940).

Aside from transfer of general principles, similar elements in the stimulus conditions facilitate transfer. When the same response is to be made to similar stimuli, positive transfer is increased. As has been mentioned previously, the more similar the stimuli, the greater the amount of positive transfer.

Stimulus and Response Generalization

Two forms of positive transfer have been identified: (1) stimulus generalization, and (2) response generalization. *Stimulus generalization* is said to occur when a learned response to a particular stimulus tends to be evoked by stimuli which are similar to it (McGeoch & Irion, 1952). This principle has also been called *associative spread, associative generalization, law of similarity,* and *induction.*

Generalization is defined somewhat differently by Holland and Skinner (1961). If the subject is reinforced for making a certain response in the presence of a particular stimulus, he will also make that same response in the presence of similar stimuli not present during the training period even though the response is not reinforced. Practical illustrations of this principle are found in many real-life situations. We learn to put coins in pay telephones that have slots at the top of the telephone body. We are reinforced for doing so by being able to dial a number. On traveling to a foreign country, we may be confronted with different telephone body constructions which will require placing the coin in the side of the telephone body or perhaps at the bottom. The fact that we engage in coin inserting behavior (response) in the presence of all pay phones (similar stimuli) illustrates this principle of generalization. You can well understand that if we had to learn these acts all over again each time we were confronted with slightly different stimuli, we would not have time for anything other than constant relearning. Upon buying a new car, we would be forced to learn how to drive as though we had never driven a car. But fortunately, much of our learning is retained and usable in a wide variety of situations.

A further distinction is made between stimulus and response generalization. In a stimulus generalization condition, the response remains the same but the stimuli which evoke the response are slightly changed. A pigeon that has been reinforced to peck at a black surface but not a white surface will continue to peck (the same response) to shades of grey (different stimuli); but when very light shades of grey are presented, fewer and fewer pecking responses will be evoked. The amount of pecking will decrease as the grey stimulus approaches white. These data could be plotted on a graph, and the result would be a decelerating curve called a *stimulus generalization gradient*. This gradient was discussed previously.

One can find several instances of the use of stimulus generalization in articulation therapy. McLean (1970) devised an articulation training program to capitalize on the principles of stimulus generalization. He varied the stimulus conditions while attempting to keep the response the same. He selected some five mentally retarded adolescents who misarticulated sounds. Each child could produce one of the misarticulated sounds correctly in isolation. Ten words containing this sound were presented, and each child was requested to repeat the words. The four differing stimulus conditions in which the words were presented were

1. Examiner says a word to be repeated by the subject.
2. Examiner says a word at the same time as he holds a picture of the word positioned beside his mouth.
3. Examiner says a word and presents both the picture of the word plus the printed word until 20 consecutive correct productions occur, then the pictures are withdrawn.
4. Examiner says a sentence omitting one spoken word while he presents the written word to the subject. Finally, the written word is omitted and only the sentence is spoken by the examiner who withholds saying one word which is to be spoken by the subject.

The stimulus conditions could be represented by the diagram in Figure 7–2.

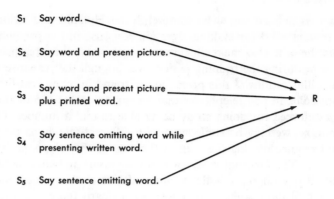

S_1 Say word.

S_2 Say word and present picture.

S_3 Say word and present picture plus printed word.

       R

S_4 Say sentence omitting word while presenting written word.

S_5 Say sentence omitting word.

FIGURE 7-2. List of Various Stimulus Conditions Which Lead To Saying Word

Data from McLean's study reveal that three out of four subjects who completed the training program showed 100% generalization to new word items when position of the sound in the new word was held constant. No generalization occurred to new words in which the position of the sound differed from training words. McLean's study clearly shows how stimulus generalization occurs as a result of articulation therapy.

Another example of stimulus generalization is found in a study of S-PACK, a lisp correction program I wrote in conjunction with two educational psychologists, Bob Baker and Dick Schutz (Mowrer, Baker, & Schutz, 1968). First-grade children who lisped were given a criterion test sampling /s/ production in 30 different conditions, from single words to connected speech. Children who lisped on all 30 items were provided instruction on correct /s/ production during three 15-minute training sessions on three consecutive days. Then they were given the 30-item criterion test again. Although 25 of the items in this test were used as training words in the instructional program, the final five items were not included in the program. We found almost 100% generalization to the five untrained words demonstrating, as McLean did, stimulus generalization.

There are several similar studies in articulation which illustrate the effects of stimulus generalization during speech therapy. Whereas most studies investigate stimulus generalization within the confines of the therapy situation, Griffiths and Craighead (1972) investigated stimulus generalization in situations outside the therapy setting. They called the former type of generalization *intrageneralization* and the latter type *extrageneralization*. This second type refers to situations in which post-tests are given in environmental settings which differ significantly from those of the therapy setting. Although one would expect stimulus generalization to occur even when subjects are tested under different environmental conditions, the authors did not find this to be the case. Intrageneralization, on the other hand, was found to occur. This may be due to the fact that only one subject was studied and that the subject was severely mentally retarded.

Similar research was conducted by Costello and Bosler (1976) in which extrageneralization was studied using three children approximately between 5 and 6 years of age. All three misarticulated /v/. Each child was given therapy in his own home by his mother and tested four times in speech clinic under four different conditions.

These tests were given after the child completed lessons 2, 4, 6, and 8. Each test consisted of 25 items which were made up of 20 words used in training plus five words which were not included in the training stimuli. The test conditions consisted of

1. Mother gave test in the speech clinic while seated across from child.
2. Examiner gave test in the speech clinic while seated across from the child.
3. Examiner gave test in large classroom outside the speech clinic area while both were seated at separate desks.
4. A second examiner (unknown to the child) gave the test in the clinic waiting room while seated in comfortable chairs.

The authors reported that some generalization occurred with all of the subjects, that is, they produced correct /v/ sounds on some of the five nontraining words. There was, on the other hand, no evidence of a stimulus gradient among the four different test conditions. It is possible the differences among the four conditions were insufficient to produce such a gradient.

Winitz (1969) maintains that children tend to group together certain features of sounds and may give the same response to two similar sounds. An investigation by Winitz and Bellerose (1963) provides support to this concept. First- and second-grade children listened to and repeated the word *shirt* during 10 trials. On the eleventh trial, he heard one of the following nonsense words: *chirt, sirt, thirt,* or *tirt,* depending on what group each was assigned to. These four words in the order given above differed more and more from the set of features found in the word *shirt,* that is, *chirt* was similar to *shirt, sirt* was less similar, *thirt* even more dissimilar, and *tirt* did not sound like *shirt* at all. As was expected, the word *shirt* was said most often when *chirt* was said, less often to *sirt,* and never to *thirt* or *tirt.* Winitz and Bellerose graphed these data revealing the existence of a typical stimulus response gradient in which each word (*chirt, sirt, thirt* and *tirt*) evoked less and less *shirt* responses.

Winitz (1969) feels that stimulus generalization may be responsible for the fact that children learn phonemes and may also account for the fact that sometimes incorrect sounds are used for correct ones. As the child learns to use sounds in word productions, he may select a sound which has similar features to the target sounds, i.e., /θ/ instead of /s/, and if rewarded, he may continue to use the similar sound in place of the correct sound. Thus, in the example above, it may be common for children to substitute *chirt* for *shirt* and perhaps *sirt* for *shirt.*

This concept that stimulus generalization may in part lead to the development of misarticulation is further supported by Crocker (1969), who presented a phonological model of articulation development in the speech of young children. He suggests that commonly substituted sounds do not occur at random but appear to follow certain rules dominated by the similarity of features contained in the correct and substituted sounds. Using this model, Crocker made several predictions about which sounds children would likely substitute for /r/, /l/, /ɚ/, /k/, /s/, /θ/, and /f/. In each case, he selected the sound which would be substituted on the basis of similarity of features and predicted the following substitutions: [w/r], vowel/[ɚ], [w or j/l] [p/f], [t/k], [θ/s], [t/s], [f/s], [tʃ/s], [f/θ]. Comparison of his predictions with studies of actual sound substitutions children make bear out the validity of his predictions. What appears to be operating here is stimulus generalization among features of sounds.

There has been some evidence to indicate that stimulus generalization occurs between sounds when they differ only on one feature. Elbert, Shelton, and Arndt (1967) found that when they provided children with instruction designed to correct the misarticulation of /s/, production of /z/, which was previously misarticulated, improved as well. These same children also misarticulated /r/, but no improvement was seen in /r/ production. Again, referring to Crocker's (1969) model, one would predict these results because /r/ develops from an entirely different set of features than those from which /s/ was derived.

Not only has the principle of stimulus generalization been demonstrated in the area of articulation, but a number of studies have shown stimulus generalization occurs under certain conditions in the speech of stutterers. Johnson and Millsapps (1937) asked stutterers to read the same passage several times in succession. Words that were stuttered were blotted out after each reading. Although the frequency of stuttered words was greatly reduced, a few of the words were still spoken disfluently. Analysis of these words revealed many of them were adjacent to the blotted out words. More importantly, these words were spoken fluently during initial readings. It would appear that a type of stimulus gradient was operating. Words in close proximity to the stuttered words also tended to evoke the disfluency.

In an effort to demonstrate the effects of response-evoking cues, Johnson, Larson, and Knott (1937) asked stutterers to read a passage to a large audience. The reading passage was surrounded by a red-colored border. When the stutterer read a different red-bordered passage to one person, more stuttering occurred than it did when a passage without a red border was used. Thus, when stimuli are similar (the red border was similar in both passages), the response, which in this case was a high rate of disfluency, generalizes to other similar reading situations.

The words on which stutterers experience difficulty do not appear to be random words. Analysis of stuttered words reveals it is possible to predict with a fair degree of accuracy which words will be disfluent. An example of stimulus generalization in stuttering is found in the fact that words associated with the stuttered words also tend to be produced disfluently. Peters and Simonson (1960) devised a study to determine the effects of pairing high probability stuttered words with low probability stuttered words. They found that significantly more stuttering occurred on low probability stuttered words when paired with high probability stuttered words than when the low probability words were paired with other low probability words. This finding lends support to the notion that stimulus generalization occurs in association learning situations.

The knowledge of rules of syntax allows the young child to make generalizations about parts of speech. This fact plays a vital part in the development of language. Berko (1958) provided a clever procedure which clearly demonstrated the effect of stimulus generalization in syntax development of children. She showed children a drawing of a birdlike creature and told them it was a "wug." Then she showed them a picture containing two of these creatures and asked them to complete the sentence, "There are two _____." Children consistently answered with the word *wugs,* thus illustrating the use of the plural marker /z/. They had generalized the rule of adding the s (in this case /z/ because of the influence of the voiced consonant /g/) to the bound morpheme to produce a plural form.

The generalization illustrated above accounts for the *s* addition to plural forms of irregular nouns such as sheeps/sheep, feets/feet, mens/men, oxes/oxen, and the like. Most of us are also familiar with the type of generalization that occurs when *ed* is added to irregular verbs to form past tense. Young children frequently make the following errors because of stimulus generalization: readed/read, runned/ran, seed/saw, laided/laid, drived/drove, and the like. As you can see, this type of stimulus generalization can act to hamper learning parts of speech which do not follow the usual rules.

Bandura (1969) points out children can construct an almost infinite number of sentences they have never heard before simply by learning a set of rules for putting words together. If children were confined simply to learning through imitation and memorizing specific utterances, then they would be unable to create new and novel sentences. For example, one child who was observed digging a hole in a sandpile wandered away briefly and returned to find his hole filled up with sand. He was heard saying, "Who undug my hole?" This is an instance of prefix generalization. In another instance, a young girl was heard saying, "Daddy, will you higher my swing?" You can see why it was perfectly logical to give the request "higher the swing" since she had previously learned "lower the swing" was correct. There are countless illustrations occurring daily which clearly depict stimulus generalization in the speech of young children. The alert speech clinician will take advantage of this principle to maximize generalization where it will aid in helping the child learn language skills.

It is important that a clear distinction be made between generalization and discrimination. They represent opposite processes. Generalization occurs because the person *does not* discriminate between two similar stimuli. Consider the individual who routinely uses profane language on his job. If his behavior generalizes, he will use curse words in the grocery store, gas station, drug store, and even in church. On the other hand, if he discriminates among these situations, generalization fails to occur and he may curse only on the job. Schedules of reinforcers and punishers play an important role in determining whether or not discrimination or generalization will occur. If discrimination is desired, then a response to one stimulus is rewarded, while a response to a similar stimulus is either unrewarded or punished. Soon the person is able to "discriminate" by responding or not responding to the appropriate stimulus. This was the case of the child who learned to discriminate between his use of the word *Daddy* for one male (his father) but not for other males. Generalization, the opposite condition, will occur when the same response is given to slightly different stimuli. For example, the child says "Bye-bye" when the father departs in the car, on his bicycle, or on foot. The stimuli are different, but the response remains the same since this response is always reinforced during occasions of departure no matter what mode of departure is taken. It could be said the child is responding to the "principle" of departing.

Thus, generalization and discrimination are very important in explaining how concepts are learned. Generalization is illustrated when members of a class of objects, such as coins, are responded to in the same general way (used for purchasing things). Discrimination is illustrated when members in each class (pennies, dimes, quarters) are identified as being different from one another. Brown (1958) presents a lengthy discussion of how children develop language concepts from both processes of generalization and discrimination. Concepts such as "chairness," "colors," "dogness," and so forth are, according to Brown, learned by making a series of generalizations and discriminations.

It becomes clear then that if it were not for stimulus generalization, we would have to teach the lisping child how to say /s/ correctly in every word containing /s/, and we would have to teach children how to say every possible sentence combination. This, of course, would be an overwhelming task. But since we can apply our knowledge to a wide variety of situations, constant relearning is unnecessary. Fortunately, stimulus generalization occurs.

The second type of generalization has been labeled *response generalization* but does not occur as frequently as stimulus generalization. When one stimulus evokes several different responses, response generalization is said to have taken place. Early investigations of this phenomenon involved studies of conditioning dogs using shock as the unconditioned stimulus. It was noted that the tone which had been paired with shock elicited not only the paw-lifting response, but a number of other responses as well including struggling with the whole body, barking, head turning, and the like. The conditioned response was quite different from the unconditioned response, which was paw lifting. It was only with additional trials that the response became more specific, that is, less generalized.

People also show evidence of response generalization. Underwood (1948) trained adults to respond with a particular word when a corresponding stimulus was presented. During later tests of retention, the adults gave different, but similar, responses to the stimuli demonstrating response generalization. For example, the first trained response to stimulus x was the word *restful*. Later, when the same stimulus x was presented, the subject replied with the response *resting* instead of *restful*. The trained response word *filmy* might later be pronounced *misty* or even *flimsy*, or perhaps *filmed*.

It has already been noted that rats give many different responses when pressing a lever to obtain a food pellet. They may press the lever with their right paw, their left paw, they may sit on the lever, press it with their chin, or engage in any number of behaviors as long as the bar is depressed; thus, the same stimulus, the lever, may evoke a variety of lever-pressing responses.

Response generalization is frequently seen in activities which involve positive bilateral transfer. Given training in some activity like writing with the right hand, an individual can easily learn to write with his left hand, or even with his foot and toes.

The concept of response generalization has rarely been mentioned in the area of speech pathology primarily because of its limited application to the treatment of speech disorders. Sommers and Kane (1974) describe learning, new sounds of words which have not been specifically taught as a process of response generalization. For example, if you teach a lisping child to say *soup, soap,* and *sun* correctly, it would be likely she would say other words beginning with /s/ correctly although she has received no training on these words. The example given by these authors may be better described as stimulus generalization if we consider the /s/ response as the same response to different stimuli, the different stimuli being the untrained words.

Winitz (1969) also refers to response generalization as a facilitating procedure which might help children acquire certain sounds although he is not entirely clear as to how this process may operate. The use of both stimulus and response generalization as an aid to teaching sounds is referred to very briefly in his book about articulation acquisition.

Although response generalization has not been mentioned in connection with stuttering behavior, it is possible this type of generalization might account for the wide variety of behaviors stutterers exhibit in certain stimulus conditions. The stutterer may respond with several different behaviors as a reaction to a feared situation. In this case, a negative reinforcer may be responsible for the individual's seeking of various responses in an attempt to escape or avoid the aversive stimulus.

One thing is clear. There is little research in speech pathology which could illustrate the effects of response generalization or its management to bring about some desired behavioral changes. Up to this point, the fact that such a principle exists is acknowledged, but we know little of its possible practical application in a therapeutic setting.

Negative Transfer of Training

The opposite of positive transfer of training is *negative transfer*. Whereas positive transfer occurs when the learning of a second task is facilitated, negative transfer occurs if learning the second task is more difficult because of what was learned during the first task. This happens when the stimuli are similar but the response is different. If you have ever had the occasion to drive an automobile in England, you realize the difficulty of learning to shift gears with the left hand instead of the right hand and to drive on the left rather than on the right side of the road. If you have had the occasion to type using a French typewriter on which many of the keys are in different locations than American typewriters, you will experience the effects of negative transfer. In these cases, many of the responses which were correct in the presence of previous stimuli are now totally inappropriate. You probably would have been able to learn to type better and faster on a French typewriter if you had never learned to type on an American machine.

The effects of negative transfer have been well illustrated in laboratory environments with animals. Using a T-shaped discrimination maze, Hunter (1922) trained rats to turn to the right when the right side of the T alley was light and to the left when the left side was darkened. An average of 268 trials were required over two consecutive days of training to reach 95% correct turning behavior. Then Hunter reversed the light and dark alleys. Now the animals had to turn right into darkness and left to the lighted alley. Thus, a new response had to be made to an old stimulus. Animals required an average of 603 trials to learn this task to the 95% criterion level. Bunch (1939) discovered similar results in other maze learning situations.

If the originally learned response is inappropriate to the new stimulus situation, then negative transfer will occur; it will take longer to learn the second task or set of responses. This is the condition that exists when we attempt to change articulation habits. The lisping child who is asked to name a picture of a sun responds [θʌn]. Then the clinician asks him to say [sʌn], a different response to the same stimulus, a picture of the sun. Thus, the child now must choose between two alternative responses /θʌn/ and /sʌn/ when confronted with the picture of a sun. One response, /θʌn/, is a strong response since it has been practiced many times in the past, while /sʌn/ is a weak, newly learned response. It is not at all surprising then to find the child produce /s/ as [s] when in the presence of the speech clinician, but a few minutes later, produce /s/ as [θ] in the classroom. One can also easily understand why, even in the presence of the speech clinician, the child may say /sθʌn/ or /θsʌn/. It could be argued, from a theoretical point of view at least, that it would be easier to teach a child to insert /s/ in place of an omission than it would be to teach an /s/ replacement for some other sound. Unfortunately, we have no data which might support this hypothesis.

One of the few authors in speech pathology who makes any mention at all about the effects of negative transfer is Winitz (1969). In writing about the effects of negative transfer on articulation learning, Winitz does not feel that traditional negative transfer paradigms exactly parallel what occurs when one sound is replaced by another. Children seem to learn sounds as an integral part of words, as morphemic units, rather than isolated, phonemic units. When presented with the word *sit,* the child responds with the correct word *sit,* but her pronunciation differs only slightly and may sound like /θɪt/. She now must learn to say /sɪt/. In the traditional negative transfer experiments involving paired word list learning, the child might first be asked to say *down* following the presentation of the word *sit* and then during task *B* she would have to learn to say *up* to the stimulus *sit.* As you can see, the responses down and up are quite different from each other, while the words *sit* and *thit* are the same words but differ only on two features.

Winitz and Bellerose (1965) devised a procedure for studying the negative effects prior learning has on acquisition of new articulatory responses. It was found that children often said [ʃfəb] when they were asked to repeat [srə́b]. It was assumed they did this because of many prior utterances of /ʃr/ combinations, but little, if any, /sr/ combinations. Thus, we might expect that learning to say syllables containing /sr/ blends might be very difficult to master, especially in cases where stimuli were present which tended to evoke the /ʃr/ blend, such as a picture of a shrub, a person shrieking, or a shirt shrinking. To test this hypothesis, three group conditions were constructed using first- and second-grade students as subjects. Children in group I were shown a picture of a shrub, and then they were asked to repeat what they heard, which was /srə́b/. Those in group II were asked simply to repeat what they heard, which was /srə́b/. Finally, children in group III were shown a picture of an unfamiliar object, which they were told was a /srə́b/.

Each correct utterance was followed by the movement of a mechanical toy car, which the authors felt would serve as a reinforcer.

Given the three conditions above, we would expect maximum negative transfer to occur with group I, less in group II, and least with group III. This is essentially what happened. While there was no significant difference between groups I and II, the number of correct responses between each of these groups differed significantly from the number of correct responses produced by children in group III. Thus, the authors concluded there is less negative transfer when a sound is taught in an unfamiliar linguistic context (learning the name of an unfamiliar object) than when taught in a more familiar linguistic context.

A second feature Winitz and Bellerose (1965) studied was the effect age had on learning the new /sr/ blend response. Under each of the three conditions above, second graders produced more correct responses (/srɔb/) than did first graders. Thus, it appears that as age increases, children are able to learn new tasks easier in spite of the detrimental effects of negative transfer.

Mowrer and Scoville (1978) made a similar finding when children were shown pictures of familiar objects and were asked to say them incorrectly. For example, a child was shown a picture of a bus and was then asked to repeat /bʌθ/. A direct relationship was found between the age of the child and his ability to respond correctly to the spoken model, even when the spoken model differed from the pictured object. The older the child, the more likely he will repeat the model spoken by the adult. On the other hand, when shown a picture of an unfamiliar object and when asked to repeat /rʌθ/, all children did so correctly demonstrating when they had no preconceived notion of how the word should sound, they followed the model presented by the examiner.

These findings lend support to the use of unfamiliar objects as stimuli in teaching new sounds in syllabic content to children who misarticulate sounds. This procedure has been advocated by many practitioners as useful in teaching or strengthening sounds children misarticulate. Van Riper (1947) recommended that nonsense syllables be practiced thoroughly before familiar words are attempted. He also suggested pictures of unfamiliar objects could be drawn and given names such as *kahto, cheerat, supee,* and *rogam.* Nonsense objects could be formed from modeling clay and given names which include the new sound. He predicted that following practice in using the new sound under these conditions, "remarkable progress will soon occur."

Although Van Riper and others who recommended the use of nonsense materials in teaching new sounds offered no experimental data to support these procedures, the data presented by Winitz and Bellerose, in addition to some of the research I have conducted, offer not only support for using these procedures, but also provide an explanation of why learning new sounds in response to old stimuli is difficult for most children.

Further evidence showing the interfering effects of negative transfer on the correct repetition of sentences is revealed in some studies by Miller and his associates (Miller & Isard, 1963; Marks & Miller, 1964). A series of three sentence types were presented to adults who were then asked to repeat them. The first sentences followed normal syntactic and semantic rules such as, "Gadgets simplify work around the house," and "Accidents kill motorists on the highways." The subjects repeated 89% of these sentences correctly. The second set of sentences were semantically incorrect but maintained correct parts of speech in their proper order. Examples were, "Gadgets kill passengers from the eyes," and "Accidents carry honey between the house." Eighty percent of these sentences were spoken correctly. Finally, the third set consisted of ungrammatical strings of words such as, "Around accidents country honey the shoot," and "On trains hive elephants the simply." Only 56% of these sentences were repeated correctly. Similar results were found when subjects were asked to memorize these types of sentences.

The clinician who works with language problems can expect similar difficulties when attempting to change children's sentence structures or sentence patterns of adults who have already learned a deviant sentence structure. It is difficult to teach the child who has said, "Me do it," to say, "I want to do it." In effect, we are expecting her to produce a new response to an old stimulus. Clearly, the adverse effects of negative transfer can be seen in the learning of new verbal responses which differ from previously learned verbal responses to the same stimuli. The best way to counteract this interference is to alter the stimuli so it will not evoke the old response. This is why nonsense material is recommended as stimulus material during initial learning experiences. Based on this information, the language clinician should use stimulus materials which are unlike the child's daily experiences. For example, the clinician might teach *ing* endings on nonsense syllables. Verbs with *ing* endings could then be taught by first presenting action pictures of stick figures engaged in activities such as kicking, running, jumping, and the like. Once correct responses are emitted in the presence of those pictures, lifelike drawings of children performing these activities are presented, followed by photographs of real children, movies of actions, and finally, the actual events themselves. If stimuli are presented in this manner, the chances of negative transfer occurring should be less likely than if attempts are made to evoke new responses under the stimulus conditions which caused the undesired response.

Although transfer of training has been discussed as an isolated event in learning, you must realize that a large number of other factors are in operation during complex human learning. For example, if learning to type is the behavior being examined, you must consider that the person under study already knows the alphabet, can read and spell, has used his fingers for a multitude of other motor acts, can understand and follow directions, and wants to learn how to type. As you can see, it would be difficult to single out only one element of transfer of training for study. The individual brings so much information, so many attitudes, and such a wide variety of skills with him that it becomes impossible to identify one single cause of learning. Add to these variables the peculiar nature of the task to be learned, the age of the individual, and his past learning experiences, the task of analyzing what occurs while learning a particular skill becomes overwhelming.

There can be no doubt our every activity is influenced by positive and negative transfer conditions. Even when an individual comprehends the fundamental nature of a problem situation (insight), transfer seems to be a major contributing factor. Perception at any level is probably never free of the influence of transfer of training. The speech clinician should be keenly aware of transfer factors as she plans her instructional procedures. Through careful planning, she can achieve maximum transfer of training and minimize the detrimental effects of negative transfer. A number of practical suggestions about taking advantage of transfer of training will be presented in chapter 8.

Retention

Retention is the term describing the persistence of behaviors which have been learned. When the behavior fails to persist, it is said the behavior or response has been forgotten. Thus, retention and forgetting are different aspects of the same process or just different terms used to describe the same data. Speech clinicians are familiar with the occasional child who, dismissed from therapy as "corrected," is soon back on the referral list. There are other children who return to speech class after 2 or 3 days and seem to have "forgotten" everything they learned previously. This seems especially true with children who come to us from special education classes.

When children and adults fail to retain much of what we teach them during speech therapy, the clinician soon becomes discouraged. One of the first questions to ask is why people forget. In searching through the literature in speech pathology for information about factors which increase or decrease amount of retention, one wonders why there is such a void of research or even opinion about retention. There has been some discussion about extending stimulus control to a variety of situations, both within and outside the clinic setting, but other than rather global, pragmatic suggestions, little has been written about this important topic. Winitz (1969), in a six-page discussion of factors relating to retention of articulatory responses, provides one of the most detailed discussions of retention found in our literature. For the most part, information about this topic comes from research conducted in the field of psychology.

Methods of Measuring Retention

Once a behavior or response has been learned, we have to be able to measure it in some way to determine if it has been retained. Generally, four different procedures have been used as measures of retention. One common procedure is the *recall* method. The individual is asked to write, or to say, everything she can remember following the original learning. This method is frequently used for testing the effects of articulation training. Usually a posttest measures how well an individual has retained correct sound production. One example of retention testing is found in a study by Shelton et al. (1967). Children were tested one week, one month, and five months following completion of articulation training in order to evaluate their retention of the correct /r/ sound. I have also conducted follow-up tests of children who received /s/ correction therapy a week after completion of testing, two weeks later, and one year later (Mowrer, 1969). Follow-up testing for the purpose of evaluating retention is a common procedure in speech research.

Sometimes an individual is asked to *reproduce* a drawing of some graphic illustration after it has been presented. This test of retention is also a measure of recall, but it is generally not used as a test in speech therapy.

Likewise, the *savings method* is seldom used in speech therapy. Ebbinghaus, one of the first psychologists to systematically investigate memory, frequently used this measure of retention. First, a task is learned to a certain criterion, say 100% correct. The number of trials required to learn the task is recorded. Then at some later time, the task is relearned to the same criterion level, 100%. If the first learning required 80 trials and the second only 40, there has been a 50% "savings" or retention of the original material. Although this type of measurement could easily be adopted to many aspects of language or articulation learning, it is seldom mentioned in the literature.

A final measurement technique commonly used by most educators is *recognition*. After learning some material, the individual is provided with several alternatives and chooses one among them as the correct answer. The choice represents successful or unsuccessful recognition. Multiple-choice examinations best illustrate this procedure. The research done in the area of speech discrimination testing might best represent this method of testing recognition. Following sessions of sound discrimination training, the child may be asked to identify whether two spoken sounds are alike or different. He is simply asked to recognize likenesses or differences between two sounds. The major drawback here is that the child has an opportunity to guess correctly 50% of the time since there are only two stimuli to judge.

The recognition method is the most sensitive retention measure. This means that if any retention of the material is present, it will appear when this measurement technique is used. On the other hand, the recall method is considered to be the least sensitive of the four. This means that scores are typically lowest when the individual must recall material previously learned. Because each measure of retention samples different aspects of learning, it is not possible to equate data of retention when different measurement procedures are used. If one is to evaluate the degree of retention over time, care must be used in selecting the same measurement technique each time retention is sampled if the data are to be compared.

Theories Of Retention

Why we remember some things and forget other things has always puzzled psychologists. Several theories attempt to explain this phenomenon. One early theory held that retention decreases as a function of the passage of time. This theory, called the *trace decay theory,* or *theory of disuse,* views unused knowledge in a manner similar to the way you might regard an unused muscle which atrophies when unused over a long period of time.

Freud felt no knowledge was actually lost, only inhibited by subconscious thoughts. This position prompted the *repression theory*. It held that under proper conditions such as hypnosis or during a period of free association, early memories which had been suppressed could be retrieved. Penfield (1958) offered support to this theory when he applied minimal currents of electricity to the cerebral cortex and found that patients were able to recall experiences that had been forgotten for long time periods. This led to the belief that much of what we learn is "buried" by new experiences.

A *trace transformation theory* developed by Bartlett (1932) maintains that remembering is an active process in which experiences are distorted or transformed to conform with one's own self-image so as to provide an individual with stability and consistency.

The most widely held theory among psychologists today is the *interference theory*. This theory explains forgetting as a process of interference from other learning, be it in the past or in the present. This seems especially true of verbal learning. In effect, any information you learn may interfere with, and be interfered by, anything else you learn. When something you learned in the past interferes with your ability to retain information, it is called *proactive inhibition*. This is almost analogous to negative transfer of training, only this latter term is used when learning new material is interfered with, whereas proactive inhibition is the term used to describe a situation in which retention of previously learned material is hindered. What a person has already learned in the past makes it difficult for him to retain newly learned material.

Winitz (1969) suggests proactive inhibition is responsible for poor retention of a newly learned sound. Theoretically, we would expect that all the years of practice a child has had in using the incorrect sound will interfere with her ability in remembering the newly learned sound. Not only will retention be affected, but learning the new sound will be more difficult because of the negative transfer effects of prior practice with the incorrect sound. It is surprising that speech clinicians experience any success in modifying articulation when so many factors play against learning and retention of the new behavior.

A second factor that Winitz (1969) contends is important but much less influential than proactive inhibition is *retroactive inhibition*. In this case, activities which occur after new learning has taken place interfere with retention of that newly learned behavior. As an example, Winitz suggests that having instructed the child how to articulate /r/ correctly in a speech therapy session, the child may leave the clinic setting and because the new /r/ sound is not reinforced in different environments, /r/ will tend to extinguish. The old response, /w/ for /r/, will be practiced instead. Further practice of /w/ for /r/ will cause retention loss, or forgetting of, the correct /r/ response. This will show up when the child is tested for retention of /r/ a few days later. This practice, using /w/ for /r/, is called an *interpolated activity*—the activity which follows the newly learned material. It is felt to be responsible for loss of retention.

There are several studies in psychology demonstrating that retention is greater if one simply rests or even sleeps following a newly learned response than if engaged in other activities following the learning experience. This accounts for the fact that you can easily remember events in the morning that you learned the night before. It also explains why as evening approaches, we tend to forget the things we learned during the morning since there were so many intervening events during the daytime hours.

Several variables affect retroactive and proactive inhibition. The more activities the person engages in between learning a task and the test of retention on that task, the less the retention. Also, if a great deal of time is spent learning the interpolated activities, retention of the originally learned activities will be slight. Another factor is the degree to which the interpolated activities are similar to the original learning. If the interpolated activities are identical to original learning tasks, then, of course, there will be no inhibition. This would be an instance of positive transfer. If the interpolated activities are very dissimilar, again, inhibition will not be strong. But in between these two extremes lie stimulus conditions which vary as to their detrimental effects upon retention. As you might suspect, determination of which interpolated activities may affect retention is extremely complex, especially when you consider that individual differences such as age, degree of motivation, past performance, and the like also affect retention.

Aside from the effects of proactive and retroactive inhibition, there are several other factors which have been shown to influence the degree to which information will be retained. As *meaningfulness* of the material increases, rate of forgetting is slower over a period of time. Thus, nonsense words are forgotten more quickly than meaningful words, and factual prose is remembered longer than either of the other two. For this reason, it would seem wise for speech clinicians to use meaningful material in their therapy sessions, rather than material that has little meaning to the child. Glancing through several texts which present therapy material for voice and articulation drill work, it is apparent that authors often show little concern about using meaningful material. A great deal of meaningless poetry is frequently presented as recommended drill material. It would make better sense to use the child's own reading book, stories she writes herself, or verbatim portions of her everyday speech instead of meaningless poems, jingles, or tongue twisters.

The *degree of learning* also affects amount of retention. One common measure of the degree of learning is the number of practice trials provided. Other measures are time a skill is practiced, the number of errors made, or the degree of skill attained. There are ample data which show that the more learning which takes place, regardless of how it is measured, the better the retention. Conversely, when small amounts of practice are provided, forgetting occurs rapidly. Several years ago, I recorded samples of two therapy sessions from each of five school speech clinicians (Mowrer, 1969). Analysis of the verbal dialogues between each speech clinician and children in their class revealed the average clinician out talked the children in their classes 10 to 1. The children's average rate of responding was 2.79 responses per minute with a range from .58 per minute (about one target response per every 2 minutes) to 6.05 per minute. Diedrich and Bangert (1976) report children they studied enrolled in public school speech therapy produced 4.6 responses per minute, but it was not specified whether this represented the total response rate or just the target sound rate. When response rate per minute was calculated for S-PACK (Mowrer et al., 1971), an effective program to correct lisping behaviors, it was found that the average rate was slightly over seven target responses per minute, almost three times more than the average rate of response evoked by the school clinicians I sampled in 1969. Of course, there are many other variables to be considered other than rate of response. The difficulty of the task, type of supportive cues presented, and mastery of the particular task are a few of the important variables that can strongly influence degree of learning as well as rate of response.

Another influential factor is the way practice is *distributed*. Available data from experiments of retention in psychology show that forgetting occurs more rapidly when tasks are learned during massed practice than when the same amount of practice time is divided up into shorter periods, that is to say, when they are distributed. Here again, we find that in many school programs, children are seen twice weekly for 20-minute periods. According to a survey of 705 public school speech clinicians (Bingham et al., 1961), it was found that of those who met with small groups of children, 33% of the clinicians provided therapy once a week, 53% offered therapy twice a week, and only 14% provided services three, four, or five times a week. Similar figures were reported for clinicians who provided individual therapy. Clearly, these speech clinicians appear to favor massed practice of one to two class periods per week to a distributed practice schedule consisting of four to five brief sessions per week. I have rarely heard of a clinician providing brief therapy sessions to the same child several times each day except during summer camp or special intensive programs. Yet, research strongly supports this notion of providing distributed practice as a means of maximizing retention.

What has been called the *affective tone* of the material to be learned seems to affect retention. This variable is related to the type of material discussed previously. Affective tone refers to the pleasantness, unpleasantness, or indifference of the material. Although psychology experiments that have been conducted to determine the effect of this variable have been somewhat subjective, there is a tendency for pleasant events to be remembered better and longer than unpleasant events or events which might be viewed with indifference. But the intensity of the affective tone is apparently more important than the quality. Strong unpleasant experiences may be retained as well as many pleasant experiences. Most of us can attest to this fact, especially in learning about touching very hot objects. You do not need many trials to retain a vivid memory of this experience. Speech clinicians should score high in the affective tone area since most provide interesting and enjoyable activities for children. A wide variety of speech games and "fun-oriented" activities are frequently used to motivate children during speech practice (Mowrer, 1970). Whether speech games and activities could be considered "intense" in affective tone is debatable when compared to the enriched classroom environments found in schools today; but at least most speech learning situations would not fall into the unpleasant category.

The *stimulus conditions* present during the period between original learning and the measurement of retention can play an important role in determining whether or not there will be a decrease in retention. For example, if the stimuli necessary to evoke the newly learned responses are not present during the interim or if new stimuli which evoke competing responses are present during this time, there will be a decrease in retention. Dulsky (1935) illustrated this principle when he asked subjects to learn a list of paired syllables. These syllables were presented on a colored background. Retention was tested using a word list on a different colored background. He found retention was much less when backgrounds were switched. Abernathy.(1940) found students tested in classrooms other than those in which they learned the material scored less on retention measures than they did when the tests were taken in the classrooms where they originally learned the material.

It could be argued that the newly learned response is simply under stimulus control when the presence of original learning stimuli has a positive effect on retention. But unless the speech clinician is aware of the powerful influence stimulus conditions have upon retention, he may neglect to use these conditions to his advantage. Also, clinicians may not be getting an accurate picture of a child's speech abilities when tested by the person who provided therapy in the same room where therapy was provided. I have noticed that some researchers guard against this condition by having a stranger to the child present during assessment of the child's speech in an environment other than the one used during therapy itself.

Speech clinicians can also take advantage of this phenomenon by making sure that many of the stimuli which were present during original learning are also present in the child's classroom. I devised a "speech pencil" to be given to children as a reward for articulating a certain sound correctly. Printed on this pencil was a variety of words containing the target sound which the clinician was attempting to teach. Hopefully, the child would be reminded of the sound he was learning, as well as the speech therapy session, each time he used his pencil in class. This represents just one attempt to maintain a facsimile of the stimulus conditions which were present during original learning.

Aside from placing stimuli in the classroom environment that may help remind the child of learning that took place in the therapy room, the clinician could increase retention by providing some of the therapy within the classroom setting or on the playground. Classroom peers could be taught to monitor the speech of the child in classroom or recess environments at certain times during the day. In this way, retention can be increased through maintaining some of the stimulus conditions under which the child learned the original target behaviors.

Finally, it has been found that providing the individual with a *preparatory set* before retention is tested will result in higher retention scores. This refers to activities the learner engages in just before retention is assessed. Suppose you wish to determine the amount of correct /s/ production in a sample of a child's conversational speech. The child should produce more correct /s/ responses if first you tell her to remember how to say her /s/'s correctly and to do her best in saying them correctly while speaking; it would be even more helpful to provide her with a brief practice period saying a few words containing /s/. This is called the *warming-up effect* and has been found to greatly increase retention scores. As you might suspect, this type of activity could strongly affect the validity of retention scores reported by researchers who attempt to assess certain therapy techniques. Those little "chats" given by the examiner while on the way to the testing room or immediately prior to the test could affect retention scores greatly.

A great deal has been written about the influence of preparation set upon the fluency rates of stutterers. It has been noted that many stutterers tense muscles surrounding the oral region just before saying a "feared" word. They appear to fix the articulators in a rigid posture rather than to make a smooth transition to the next sound. It is almost as though they think of the initial sound as an isolated event, rather than as an integral part of a word. Van Riper (1937) attempted to teach new preparatory set behaviors which would help the stutterer progress through feared words with much more ease than his former behaviors allowed. Thus, by establishing a different preparatory set just before speaking, the stutterer would be able to "remember" what to do and hence, speak fluently. This technique proved highly successful with some cases but did not seem to be effective with others; consequently, Van Riper developed other coping techniques, one of which he termed *pull-outs* and later, another technique he called *cancellation*. Although preparatory set as used in the context of a treatment of stuttering is not identical to the usual application of the term employed in most studies of retention, the effect of preparatory set on the behavior which follows it is quite similar.

I can recall how a clinician used a preparatory set of instruction to control the attention behavior of an autistic child during language therapy. The child frequently exhibited a wide variety of behaviors during the therapy which were distracting both to him and to the clinician. These included bizarre hand motions, making faces in the mirror, looking at the ceiling, and the like. Subsequently, the child was rewarded for sitting quietly, folding his hands, and looking at the clinician for 10 seconds following the command, "Show me you're ready." This period of "readiness" was extended to 1 minute in length. Thereafter, any time the child was engaging in distractable behaviors, the clinician simply said, "Show me you're ready," and the undesired behaviors would cease. From that point, the clinician would resume instruction. In the sense that the child "remembered" how he was suppose to behave, the cue "Show me you're ready" served as a preparatory set.

So far in the discussion of retention and forgetting, focus has been placed on research findings which support the position that forgetting occurs because of various interferences with learning. This does not mean to imply that these are the only factors which could account for loss of retention. There are many things which cannot be explained by principles of learning alone; for example, it could be argued that we never forget any experience we have had in the past. Skinner (1960) trained pigeons to peck at a particular spot on a target. He reinforced correct responses with birdseed until the response was conditioned. Then he placed the pigeons in cages for a period of 6 years during which no training was provided. After 6 years, the original target was presented, and the pigeons pecked the correct area with great accuracy. This has also been a common occurrence found in many psychomotor skills people learn like playing Ping-Pong, tennis, driving and the like. Long periods of time may elapse between practice periods, yet, the person can perform the task with little or no loss of skill. This is difficult to explain in terms of the interference theory.

Forgetting and Extinction

These two terms are frequently confused. During extinction, the learned response is allowed to occur, but it is not followed by reinforcement. Eventually, the response rate drops back to its preconditioned rate. During the process of forgetting, there is little opportunity to respond at all; and if the response occurs, it may or may not be followed with reinforcement. Also, extinction is usually studied immediately after learning during which time no interpolated activities are presented. Forgetting, on the other hand, is frequently studied following a much longer period from original learning, and often, interpolated activities are inserted. The persistence of a response, that is, how many responses will occur in the absence of reinforcement, is the typical measure in extinction experiments. Measures of retention are taken during one occasion at some point after learning, and then this measure is compared with the last measure taken of the original learning or some previous retention test. What the two processes do have in common is that they both result in a decrease in the rate of response. They are different chiefly in that forgetting results from a lack of opportunity to respond, whereas in extinction, many responses occur, but they are not reinforced.

Some would argue that forgetting is due to extinction plus reinforcement of incompatible responses which, of course, conflict with the original learning. Whatever the cause might be, it is fortunate that we do forget many things or our daily lives would be filled with so much trivia and conflicting thoughts that in time we would be totally unable to function. Conversely, if we forgot everything, our lives would be equally miserable. Whether we remember or forget certain things does not appear to result from chance. Although we have much to learn about variables that control retention and forgetting, we can maximize the probability that retention will be improved by following advice given to us by psychologists who have studied this phenomenon.

Factors Which Improve Retention

There are numerous things speech clinicians can do to improve retention of newly learned verbal responses. Many have already been identified; the following is a summary of these factors.

Overlearning the behavior: Countless studies indicate that retention will improve as a result of overlearning verbal material. Many teachers believe that once a skill or list of words is learned without error, learning is complete and there is no point in studying further. But this has been shown not to be the case. We reap greater benefits proportionately from small amounts of overlearning. This could be considered true up to a point. Eventually, no further benefits are derived from overlearning. Exactly what these limits are as far as learning speech skills is concerned has received little attention. Lawrence (1954) points out the optimum point of providing practice is reached when additional trials do not produce sufficient change in performance level. Providing training beyond this point merely adds to the cost of the education process without providing educational benefit. The trick is knowing when that point is reached for each individual child.

Only one investigation has specified what degree of accuracy speech clinicians should strive to reach in the area of articulation learning. Diedrich and Bangert (1975) report that clinicians could dismiss children who have /s/ or /r/ errors when they produce these sounds correctly 75% of the time as measured on a 30-item word test plus a 3-minute sample of conversational speech. Their results show less than 20% regression when tested 4 months later provided correct production rate at the time they were terminated from therapy was 75% or better. Producing the sounds at 75% accuracy could hardly be called overlearning! Perhaps overlearning is not required for adequate retention when articulation learning is involved. On the other hand, maybe overlearning should take place during each therapy session, and because of this overlearning, a 75% correct or better articulation of the target sounds is obtained. There are no empirical data to support this notion, but results of research in other areas of verbal learning would support it.

Whether or not overlearning has any effect on retention of fluent speech is not known—at least I am not aware of any research which is addressed to this issue. I believe since the stutterer does not have to learn how to speak fluently (he already speaks fluently in many situations), overlearning fluent speech may be of little assistance as far as fluency retention is concerned.

Actually, if overlearning involves more reinforced trials, especially if a variable ratio of reinforcement is used, then better retention could be explained by the fact that the response is now more resistant to extinction. It has been found that individuals whose behavior has been placed on a variable-ratio schedule develop behaviors which persist for long periods of time. In a final report by Diedrich and Bangert (1976) involving a study of some 1,400 children who misarticulated /s/ or /r/, the authors found that children in one group (rapid learners) produced less than 500 correct target responses during the first 6 weeks of therapy, which included some 3 hours of formal practice. This was sufficient to enable them to use this target sound correctly in their conversational speech. Compare this small number of responses with the estimated 876,000 incorrect /s/ or /r/ responses produced during the previous 5 years of the child's life and one could hardly say the 500 responses could represent overlearning, especially when these responses were spread out over a 6-week period!

Although recommending "overlearning" as a strategy to increase retention of the correct response seems logical, perhaps articulation learning includes some variables which may be more important than the simple provision of an overlearning condition. Frankly, I am at a loss as to explain Diedrich and Bangert's (1976) finding that such few responses can permanently alter a child's phonological system. Certainly, the listening community provides no reinforcement contingent on correct sound production. The parent or teacher may tell the child he sounds better, but this verbal reward is very infrequent and certainly not contingent on correct sound production. Perhaps with the aid of further research in the area of sound acquisition we will be able to provide better explanations of changes which occur in phonological systems.

Frequent practice: A number of studies indicate that frequent review of learned material increases retention significantly. This frequent review has the effect of limiting the detrimental effects of interpolated activities (retroactive inhibition). Figure 7-3 is a hypothetical graph showing the probable effects of daily review of material which was originally learned to 100% criterion as shown at Point A. Point B illustrates that the material is still retained at 100% accuracy 6 days later; but if no review is provided during the 6-day interval, retention may drop to only 10% (Point C). It would be nice if data were available to support this theory, but unfortunately, well-controlled empirical studies have not been conducted in speech acquisition.

As I mentioned earlier, the survey by Bingham et al. (1961) revealed that most clinicians provided therapy at intervals of once or twice weekly. Only 6% of the clinicians meet individuals and groups three, four, or five times weekly, and none

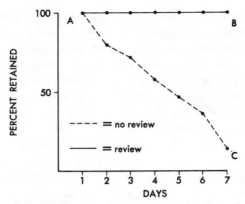

FIGURE 7-3. Hypothetical Effects Of Review And Nonreview Conditions Upon Retention

reported seeing children more than once daily. Only a few studies have investigated the effects of frequency of providing services upon progress in therapy. Even these data are questionable because there were no controls over the type of therapy given or the type of problem treated. Nevertheless, these studies will be reviewed because at present, these data represent the only work done in this area.

One early study by Backus and Dunn (1947) was an investigation of the effect of intensive group therapy versus the traditional, twice-a-week individual contact. The authors concluded that more progress was obtained in 6 weeks of daily contact than was possible during an entire school year of twice-a-week contact.

Fein et al. (1956) compared results of therapy given once a week to therapy given twice a week. The measure of progress was a subjective evaluation of each child's progress during the therapy period. Results of an opinion poll indicated that ⅔ of the clinicians felt students in the twice-a-week plan responded better to homework assignments and rapport between teachers and clinicians was better. Analysis of the final evaluations failed to reveal any significant difference between either system. Unfortunately, the lack of control over relevant variables in this study, plus the lack of data regarding actual speech improvement, render the findings meaningless. Even if differences were found, it would not be feasible to relate them to frequency of therapy alone.

Effects of intensive therapy on articulation scores of mentally retarded children were investigated by Sommers et al. (1970). One group of children received therapy four times a week. Another group was scheduled once a week, and the control group received no therapy. As you might suspect, those who received therapy four times a week (119 sessions) made larger gains on articulation pretest and posttests than either the once-a-week group (30 sessions) or the control group (0 sessions). This simply means if you provide more instruction, you should expect more progress. Had both groups received the same number of sessions over different time periods, perhaps we could have learned more about frequency of instruction.

Ausenheimer and Irwin (1971) studied the effects of providing articulation therapy twice a week (64 sessions), three times a week (96 sessions), and four times a week (128 sessions). Progress of each group of 10 children was assessed three times: at the end of 8, 16, and 32 weeks. At the end of 8 weeks, the four times a week group scored significantly higher than the other two groups. This should not be surprising in view of the fact that this group had 32 sessions while the other two had 24 and 16 respectively. Here again, this finding supports the contention that providing more therapy produces more change in articulation behavior. After 32 weeks, the twice-a-week group made the largest gains. One would expect the three times-a-week group to make larger gains. Although the children were randomly assigned to the groups, no mention was made about equating severity or type of error in each group. The authors note that several factors should be controlled in studying the effects of frequency of therapy. These include type of therapy, personality of the clinician, motivational factors, and the like. Unfortunately, this study sheds little light on the problem considered in this section, i.e., the influence of frequent instruction.

On the basis of controlled learning experiments in psychology alone, it could be recommended that clinicians could increase retention by providing frequent instruction; but bear in mind that no data are available from speech research that confirm this recommendation. It should be clearly understood that the important factor in terms of frequency of instruction is not how much instruction should be given, but the total number of instructional periods. This is similar to the massed versus distributed practice concept. One possible way of determining the effect frequency of instruction has on retention is to provide five 20-minute therapy sessions daily to one group (100 minutes total) and five sessions to another group, one session each week (100 minutes total). Retention tests could be given 1 week, 4 weeks, and 8 weeks after the final instructional period. In this way, the effects of frequency of instruction could be accurately measured.

Use of meaningful material: As has been mentioned already, experiments comparing the learning of nonsense material and meaningful words leave no doubt that meaningful material is retained much better than nonmeaningful material. It was also suggested that much of the therapy material some speech clinicians use may not aid retention of the newly learned behavior. Poetry, jingles, rhymes, and tongue twisters may be fun to say, but it is likely that these exercises may be less beneficial than we would hope. This is not to say that nonsense materials should never be used. Winitz (1969) provides evidence in support of using nonsense consonant-vowel combinations when first teaching sounds. But as soon as these combinations become stabilized in the child's repertoire, the sound should be incorporated into meaningful words. In the case of children who lisp, it has been found economical to begin with a nonsense syllable such as /ɪt'sə/, and once this can be pronounced easily, move on to meaningful phrases like /ɪt'sə bɔɪ/ /ɪt'sə kom/ /ɪt'sə mæn/ etc.

There are many ways the speech clinician can incorporate meaningful speech into her therapy lesson. One is to leave the therapy room and ask the child to take you on a "tour of the campus" as he tells you where various rooms are located. Using key words with which a child makes up his own story is another way. Reading from his school reading text would seem better than reading from some unknown text.

If we look for research to support the contention that using meaningful material in speech therapy will improve retention, we come up with much less than we were able to find under the topic of frequency of instruction. No one has attempted to explore this area as far as speech retention is concerned. Here again, we must rely solely on the findings of retention studies in psychology.

Motivation state: Retention improves if a person is highly motivated to learn the material. This was realized by Herbert Spencer as long ago as 1873 when he noted that we tend to remember pleasant events much better than unpleasant ones. Further studies verified his contention that recall for pleasant events was high. Recent studies in psychology indicate that individuals who are highly motivated recall better than those not well motivated. The motivation need not be of the pleasant variety. If a person knows she will be punished by electric shock for failure to recall an event or a behavior, she will learn and remember the act better than if no shock is associated with the response. Similarly, those who are paid a large sum of money for learning will retain the material longer than those who are paid only a small sum (Weiner, 1967).

These consequences for learning appear to increase a person's rehearsal time in between learnings, that is, how much she attends to elements in the tasks when she is not being instructed. Of course, during instruction, there is increased attention to the task also; but whether memory is facilitated or inhibited depends on the intensity of the emotion involved as well as the nature of the task, type of response, and other learning factors present.

Again, a search of the literature in speech pathology reveals that the issue of motivational state during speech acquisition has not been studied. There seem to be plenty of references to the importance of motivating children during speech therapy. These suggestions range from convincing the child he should work on his speech (Van Riper, 1947), to the use of speech games designed to make speech activities more enjoyable. Exactly to what extent these suggestions serve to enhance retention of the target response is unknown. One can say, theoretically at least, that the more the speech clinician does to increase motivation or desire to learn the materials, the better the retention should be.

It is possible that providing tokens or points contingent on correct responses may serve to increase motivation and thereby increase retention. This is especially likely if the tokens or points can be redeemed for toys or privileges which the child desires. Frequently, these rewards are shown to the child before therapy (reinforcement menu) to encourage him to work hard so he can earn one or more of them.

Concluding Remarks

In view of what we presently know about transfer of training and retention, it seems that many improvements could be made in the delivery of services to those who have communication handicaps. It is evident that a great deal more data are required before we can make positive statements regarding exactly how the speech clinician should organize and administer a speech therapy program. On the other hand, we cannot afford to wait until researchers decide to investigate these areas of learning. Some individuals have attempted to apply what we know from research findings in speech therapy and psychology. The most fruitful attempts are found in the areas of programmed instruction. This subject will be dealt with in chapters 8 and 9.

Rules to Follow Using Behavior Therapy

1. Rule of Immediacy: In order to help a child learn more efficiently, provide a reward immediately following the child's correct response. It may not be possible or even advisable to give a toy or food item, immediately, so provide a social reward, token, point, or some signal of immediate recognition.

2. Rule of Attention: Attention is a powerful social reward. Provide attention the way you would use a token, toy, or other form of recognition following a correct response. Be careful that you do not give attention to wrong or undesired behavior. This would only serve to reward the incorrect response. Attention can help children learn correct behaviors but it can also serve to reinforce undesired behavior if used inappropriately.

3. Rule of Pairing Rewards: Anything paired or associated with a reward also acquires rewarding properties. For example, if we talk to a child while feeding her, talk will become associated with food which is rewarding, and soon talk by itself will serve as a reward. Such a reward is called a secondary reinforcer.

4. Rule of Continuous Reward: At first when a behavior is being taught, reward each correct response. When the newly learned behavior is easier to produce, provide a reward every other time. Gradually decrease the frequency with which you provide a reward as learning progresses. This reduction in the schedule of reinforcement serves to maintain the behavior better than the continuous reward.

5. Rule of Selective Reward: Give a reward following the responses that are important for the child to learn. If a child is being taught to say /s/, use the reward for good /s/ productions, not for winning games or activities not related to /s/ production.

6. Rule of Small Steps: It is important to use small steps in establishing a complex behavior. At first, demand very little from the child. It may be necessary to model the desired behavior several times. By requiring small increases each day, the child can build a series of behaviors into a habit, providing rewards are presented following each bit of correct behavior.

7. Rule of Chaining: One behavior leads to another in a chain leading to a complex behavior. It is important that the reward follow the behavior that occurs at the end of the chain. Be careful that undesired behaviors are not included in the chain of desired behaviors.

8. Rule of Getting the Child's Attention: Be sure to get the child's attention (looking, listening or both) when giving directions. Looking and listening are important since children learn better when they are actively attending.

9. Rule of Imitation: Modeling desired behavior is important as a method of instruction. By rewarding the child for imitating correct models of behavior, we can improve learning.

10. Rule of Relevant Cues: It is important to use relevant cues when instructing children. For example, the cue "close your teeth when you say /s/" is important to children who lisp. Attention cues like "get ready" and "watch me" are also important. Cues provide children with a preparatory set to help them respond correctly.

BIBLIOGRAPHY

Abernathy, E. M. The effect of changed environmental conditions upon the results of college examinations. *Journal of Psychology,* 1940, *10,* 293–301.

Ausenheimer, B., & Irwin, R. B. Effect of frequencies on speech therapy on several measures of articulatory proficiency. *Language, Speech and Hearing Services in Schools,* 1971, *2,* 43–51.

Backus, O., & Dunn, H. M. Intensive group therapy in speech rehabilitation. *Journal of Speech and Hearing Disorders,* 1947, *12,* 39–60.

Bagley, W. C. *The educative process.* New York: Macmillian, 1905.

Bandura, A. Socio-learning theory of identifactory process. In D. A. Goslin (Ed.), *Handbook of socialization theory and research.* Chicago: Rand McNally, 1969.

Bartlett, F. C., *Remembering: A study in experimental and social psychology.* New York: Macmillan, 1932.

Berko, J., The child's learning of English morphology. *Word,* 1958, *14,* 150–177.

Bingham, D. S., Van Hattum, R. J., Faulk, M. E., & Taussig, E. IV. Program organization and management. *Journal of Speech and Hearing Disorders,* Monograph Supplement, 1961, *8,* 33–49.

Brown, R. *Words and things.* New York: Free Press, 1958.

Bunch, M. E. The amount of transfer in rational learning as a function of time. *Journal of Comparative Psychology,* 1936, *22,* 325–337.

Bunch, M. E. Transfer of training in the mastery of an antagonistic habit after varying intervals of time. *Journal of Comparative Psychology,* 1939, *28,* 189–200.

Bunch, M. E. & McCraven, V. G. The temporal course of transfer in the learning of memory material. *Journal of Comparative Psychology,* 1938, *25,* 481–496.

Costello, J., & Bosler, S. Generalization and articulation instruction. *Journal of Speech and Hearing Disorders,* 1976, *41,* 359–373.

Crocker, J. R. A phonological model of children's articulation competence. *Journal of Speech and Hearing Disorders,* 1969, *34,* 203–213.

Diedrich, W. M. & Bangert, C. J. Some factors which differentiate articulation learning. *Asha,* 1975, *9,* 597.

Diedrich, W. M., & Bangert, C. J. *Training speech clinicians in recording and analysis of articulatory behavior.* Washington, D.C.: U.S. Office of Education, Dept. of HEW, Grant No. OEG-0-70-1689 and OEG-0-71-1689, 1976.

Dulsky, S. G. The effect of a change of background on recall and relearning. *Journal of Experimental Psychology,* 1935, *18,* 725–740.

Elbert, M., Shelton, R. L., & Arndt, W. B. A task for evaluation of articulation change. *Journal of Speech and Hearing Research,* 1967, *10,* 281–288.

Fein, B. G., Colman, M. G., Kone, H. J., & McClintock, C. R. Effective utilization of staff time in public school speech correction. *Journal of Speech and Hearing Disorders*, 1956, *21*, 283–291.

Griffiths, H., & Craighead, W. E. Generalization in operant speech therapy for misarticulation. *Journal of Speech and Hearing Disorders*, 1972, *37*, 485–494.

Harlow, H. F. The formation of learning sets. *Psychological Review*, 1949, *56*, 51–65.

Holland, J., & Skinner, B. F. *The analysis of behavior*. New York: McGraw-Hill, 1961.

Hulin, W. S., & Katz, D. Transfer of training in reading Braille. *American Journal of Psychology*, 1934, *46*, 627–631.

Hunter, W. S. Habit interference in the white rat and in human subjects. *Journal of Comparative Psychology*, 1922, *2*, 29–59.

Johnson, W., Larson, R. P., & Knott, J. R. Studies in the psychology of stuttering: III. Certain objective cues related to the percipitation of the moment of stuttering. *Journal of Speech Disorders*, 1937, *2*, 23–25.

Johnson, W., & Millsapps, L. S. Studies in the psychology of stuttering: The role of cues representative of past stuttering in the distribution of stuttering moments during oral reading. *Journal of Speech Disorders*, 1937, *2*, 101–104.

Lawrence, D. The evaluation of training and transfer programs in terms of efficiency measures. *Psychology*, 1954, *38*, 367–383.

Marks, L. E., & Miller, G. A. The role of semantic and syntactic constraints in the memorizing of English sentences. *Journal of Verbal Learning and Verbal Behavior*, 1964, *3*, 1–5.

Melton, A. W., & Irwin, J. The influence of degree of interpolated learning on retroactive inhibition and the overt transfer of specific responses. *American Journal of Psychology*, 1940, *53*, 173–203.

McGeoch, J. A., & Irion, A. L. *The psychology of human learning*. New York: Longmans, Green & Co., 1952.

McLean, J. Extending stimulus control of phoneme articulation by operant techniques. In F. L. Girardeau & J. E. Spradlin (Eds.), *A functional analysis approach to speech and language: ASHA Monographs, 14*. Washington, D.C.: American Speech and Hearing Association, 1970.

Miller, G. A., & Isard, S. Some perceptual consequences of linguistic rules. *Journal of Verbal Learning and Verbal Behavior*, 1963, *2*, 217–228.

Mowrer, D. E. *Modification of speech behaviors: Ideas and strategies for students*. Tempe, Ariz.: Ideas, 1969.

Mowrer, D. E. An analysis of motivational techniques used by speech clinicians. *Asha*, 1970, *12*, 491–493.

Mowrer, D. E., Baker, R. L., & Schutz, R. E. Operant procedures in the control of speech articulation. In H. Sloane & B. MacAulay (Eds.), *Operant procedures in remedial speech and language training*. Boston: Houghton Mifflin, 1968.

Mowrer, D. E., Baker, R., & Schutz, R. *S-programed articulation correction kit*. Tempe, Ariz.: Ideas, 1971.

Mowrer, D. E., & Scoville, A. Response bias in children's phonological systems. *Journal of Speech and Hearing Disorders*, 1978, *43*, 473–481.

Peters, R. W., & Simonson, W. E. Generalization of stuttering behavior through associative learning. *Journal of Speech and Hearing Research*, 1960, *3*, 9–14.

Penfield, W. *The excitable cortex in conscious man*. Liverpool: Liverpool University Press, 1958.

Shelton, R. L., Elbert, M. E., & Arndt Jr., W. B. A task for evaluation of articulation change: II. Comparison of task scores during baseline and lesson series testing. *Journal of Speech and Hearing Research*, 1967, *10*, 578–585.

Siipola, E. M., & Israel, H. E. Habit-interference as dependent upon stage of training. *American Journal of Psychology*, 1933, *45*, 205–227.

Skinner, B. F. *Science and human behavior*. New York: Macmillan, 1953.

Skinner, B. F. Pigeons in a pelican. *American Psychologist*, 1960, *15*, 28–37.

Sommers, R. K., Leiss, R., Fundrella, D., Manning, W., Johnson, R., Oerther, P., Sholly, R., & Siegel, M. Factors in the effectiveness of articulation therapy with educable retarded children. *Journal of Speech and Hearing Research*, 1970, *13*, 304–316.

Sommers, R. K., & Kane, A. R. Nature and remediation of functional articulation disorders. In S. Dickson (Ed.), *Communication disorders: Remedial principles and practices*. Glenview, Ill.: Scott, Foresman, 1974.

Stroud, J. B. Experiments on learning in school situations. *Psychological Bulletin*, 1940, *37*, 777–807.

Thorndike, E. L. *The psychology of learning*. New York: Teachers College, 1914.

Thorndike, E. L. A note on assimilation and interference. *American Journal of Psychology*, 1937, *49*, 671–676.

Thune, L. E. The effect of different types of preliminary activities on subsequent learning of paired-associate material. *Journal of Experimental Psychology*, 1950, *40*, 423–438.

Underwood, B. J. Spontaneous recovery of verbal associations. *Journal of Experimental Psychology*, 1948, *38*, 429–439.

Van Riper, C. The preparatory set in stuttering. *Journal of Speech Disorders*, 1937, *2*, 149–154.

Van Riper, C. *Speech correction: Principles and methods*. New York: Prentice-Hall, 1947.

Ward, L. B. Reminiscence and rate learning. *Psychological Monograph*, 1937, *49*, 220.

Weiner, B. Motivational factors in short-term retention. Rehearsal or arousal? *Psychological Reports*, 1967, *20*, 1203–1208.

Winitz, H. *Articulatory acquisition and behavior*. New York: Appleton-Century-Crofts, 1969.

Winitz, H., & Bellerose, B. Phoneme-sound cluster learning as a function of instructional method and age. *Journal of Verbal Learning and Verbal Behavior*, 1965, *4*, 98–102.

Winitz, H., & Bellerose, B. Phoneme-sound generalization as a function of phoneme similarity and verbal unit of test and training stimuli. *Journal of Speech and Hearing Research*, 1963, *6*, 379–392.

Assignment 4

Shaping Consonant Sounds

Overview

An important task in articulation therapy is evoking consonant sounds. One effective procedure for accomplishing this task is shaping sounds through successive approximations. The strategy involves providing differential reinforcement, that is, reinforcement for sounds that approximate the desired sound and no reinforcement for sounds that do not approximate the desired sound. If this shaping process is done well, the target sound can often be evoked within a few minutes; if it is not managed successfully, it may be very difficult to evoke the correct response.

Several aspects of this process are critical, such as the cues that the pathologist provides, the immediacy and the accuracy of the feedback, and number of responses produced. Six brief therapy sessions are presented in which pathologists attempt to evoke consonants from clients. You will be asked to identify relevant events from antecedent and consequent conditions that lead to successful or unsuccessful experiences in shaping the consonant sounds.

Objective: To identify relevant cues and differential reinforcement procedures for shaping consonant sounds through successive approximation.

Materials: Tape Assignment 4, Selections A–F.

Suggested Reading: Chapter 6, pp. 223–230

Description of the Session: Selections were recorded from the first few minutes of each individual's initial therapy session. None of the individuals had received speech therapy previously. All of the children in the selections were enrolled in the first grade. Each session consists of a pathologist's attempts to evoke from an individual a target sound in isolation. In most cases, the target sound was /ɝ/.

Procedure: You will hear pathologists attempt to evoke several consonant sounds from young children and will be asked to identify the relevant cues used to evoke each sound. It is also important that you discover how verbal reinforcement is used as a consequent event. The process of successive approximation involves reinforcing a series of responses, each of which more closely approximates the target response—in this case, the correct articulation of a specific consonant sound. In each of the following selections, you will hear the pathologists attempt to evoke certain sounds. Sometimes they are successful in their attempts and at other times, they fail. Your task will be to identify critical features of each session that lead to success or failure.

SELECTION A

In this first selection, the pathologist attempts to shape the /ɝ/ sound from a first-grade child. Note which behaviors the pathologist rewards during the beginning of the session as compared to those rewarded at the end of the session.

Now play Assignment 4, Selection A.

Questions for Selection A

1. What was the goal during the first part of the session?
2. Do you feel the child would have been successful in producing /ɝ/ had the pathologist used only stimulation with the correct sound production as the chief antecedent event? Why?
3. Were "incorrect" /ɝ/ responses rewarded during this session?
4. Why would the pathologist reward incorrect responses?
5. Does the pathologist finally evoke some correct /ɝ/ sounds?
6. Many of the child's incorrect responses result in no evaluative response from the pathologist; yet closer responses usually always result in a positive statement. Why, do you think, is this done? Check your answers with those found in the Answer Key, then proceed to Selection B.

SELECTION B

The pathologist in this selection will be working with a child who has an inconsistent /f/ for /θ/ substitution. You will notice the child can produce the correct response with little difficulty; thus the shaping procedures used in Selection A were not used as extensively in this session. Also, pay attention to the type of feedback used.

Play Assignment 4, Selection B now; after listening, answer the following questions.

Questions for Selection B

1. One reason why extensive shaping procedures were not used for the /θ/ sound was because this child already had /θ/ in his repertoire. Also, /θ/ is much easier to shape than /ɝ/. What is it about /θ/ that makes it easier to shape?

2. The pathologist was very definite in providing feedback when incorrect responses were made. Why didn't he just ignore many of the incorrect responses?
3. What was the most important antecedent event used to evoke the correct /θ/ sound?
4. What was the distinctive feature of the consequent event? Check your answers with those in the Answer Key, then proceed to Selection C.

SELECTION C

In this selection, shaping procedures are again used with a first-grade boy to shape /ɝ/. In this case, the child is unable to produce a correct /ɝ/, so the sound must be shaped. Note that the same tongue position cues as those used for Selection A are used; in addition, the consequent event is heavily relied upon as a major shaping technique.

Play Assignment 4, Selection C now; then answer the following questions.

Questions for Selection C

1. What seem to be the most important antecedent event cues used to evoke /ɝ/?
2. Why, do you think, did the child respond with so many /ɝ/ attempts in such a short time?
3. There are at least four important similarities between this session (Selection C) and the first one you listened to (Selection A). Can you list them?
4. You noticed the stimulus /ɝ/ was hardly ever used as an antecedent event to evoke /ɝ/. Why, do you think, did the pathologist avoid using this sound as a stimulus?

Check your answers on p. 272: then proceed to Selection D.

SELECTION D

The ability to place accurate feedback consequent to a child's responses is very important. In this selection, the pathologist sometimes says *no* incorrectly following improved responses, yet in spite of this, the girl manages to produce several correct responses.

Play Assignment 4, Selection D, now as you listen to this pathologist attempt to shape /ɝ/.

Questions for Selection D

1. Why, do you think, was this pathologist unsuccessful in evoking /ɝ/?

2. In spite of this fault, did the child produce some acceptable /ɝ/ sounds?
3. Was the same general procedure used to shape /ɝ/ with this girl used also with the boys in Selections A and B?
   Check your answers on p. 273, then proceed to Selection E.

SELECTION E

It is very difficult to shape /ɝ/ if only the consequent event is used in the shaping process. The antecedent event, which provides important tongue position cues, does much to guide the child toward correct tongue position. In this selection, the pathologist presented the target sound once and after that purposefully gave no instructions (antecedent events) other than "try it again" and "make it different." The target sound is /ɝ/, but the child never approaches the correct sound. To shape using the consequent event only is a long, difficult task.

Now turn on Assignment 4, Selection E.

Questions for Selection E

1. The pathologist was not successful in teaching this child /ɝ/. Why not?
2. Why it is difficult to shape speech responses using only the consequent event?
3. Was the child rewarded for any of her attempts?
4. What role do you think does the knowledge that one is correct play in shaping responses? Check your answers with the Answer Key, then continue to Selection F.

SELECTION F

As an experiment to see how well a pathologist can evoke correct /ɝ/ responses from adults who already know how to say /ɝ/ (but do not know what sound the pathologist is trying to evoke), several student pathologists were asked to record their attempts with this task. In Selection F, you will hear events that transpired in one of these sessions. Note how the student pathologist tends to overcue the subject. In spite of his intellectualized description of proper tongue placement, the subject is able to produce the sound correctly near the end of the session.

Turn on Assignment 4, Selection F now as you listen to this selection.

Questions for Selection F

1. You can understand how overcueing a person with regard to tongue position might

actually interfere with a person's attempt to produce a sound. Can you list three important principles to keep in mind when using cues to shape responses?

2. Why do you suppose the pathologist talked so much?

3. If you could use any cue you wanted to for evoking the desired response, what would you say to the client?

4. **What cue, do you think, was most helpful to the individual in helping him produce /ɝ/? Check your answers on p. 273**

As you know from listening to the selections on this tape, success in shaping responses depends upon skillful use of relevant cues as well as appropriate consequences in the form of verbal feedback. Effectiveness in using effective shaping techniques also relies heavily upon experiences that involve working with a wide variety of individuals. Once these procedures are mastered, it is not difficult to evoke target sounds from children within the first 5 to 10 minutes of the initial therapy session.

Answer Key

SELECTION A

1. To correctly position the tongue.
2. Probably not. It is important to get correct tongue placement before attempting to evoke /ɝ/.
3. Yes.
4. Because they were getting closer to the /ɝ/ sound.
5. Yes.
6. So as not to discourage the child with too much negative feedback.

SELECTION B

1. The tongue position for /θ/ is clearly visible, whereas the tongue position for /ɝ/ is not visible.
2. Because this child could produce the target sound at the onset. Since the sound was in his repertoire, the pathologist could point out immediately when the response was wrong; thus the child could make necessary corrections right away.
3. The cue, "Stick your tongue out and blow" was effective in evoking /θ/.
4. The consequent events always informed the child whether he was correct or incorrect. If incorrect, information was usually provided concerning how the response should be produced correctly.

SELECTION C

1. Tongue position cues, consisting chiefly of "Lift your tongue up and back," "Keep it back there," and "Keep it back."
2. The pathologist's rapid demands and expectations for immediate responses from the child.

3. Rapid responding from child; tongue placement cues are similar; shaping, mainly through use of consequent event; much positive feedback.
4. The stimulus /ɝ/ was avoided because its use tends to evoke the error response from the child. Although the child hears /ɝ/, he's used to responding to this stimulus with the vowel /ɜ/. To him, /ɝ/ means /ɜ/; thus, the shaping procedure using the consequent event (feedback on performance) is used more extensively.

SELECTION D

1. His feedback was not always accurate and his cues were not as precise as they could have been.
2. Yes.
3. Yes.

SELECTION E

1. No relevant antecedent events were provided.
2. The child does not know what behaviors are expected of her, nor what she has to do to produce the desired behaviors.
3. No.
4. Knowledge that informs children that they are correct helps keep children responding so the pathologist can attach consequent events to their responses. Without frequent responses from children, it is impossible to shape responses.

SELECTION F

1. Keep cues simple, relevant; use them sparingly.
2. He was unsure of his ability to evoke the response by attaching differential consequent events, so he relied more heavily upon the antecedent events which require more explanation.
3. "Say /ɝ/."
4. The cue about using /g/ as a starting point for sound production.

Assignment 5

Analyzing Consequences of Behavior

Overview

There can be no doubt that the consequences we place on behavior can play an important part in determining the frequency with which a behavior will occur in the future. It is important that we carefully identify the types of feedback we provide for specific behaviors. Sometimes no feedback is provided. At other times the client is informed that the response is correct or incorrect.

Two therapy sessions have been chosen to help you identify the types of consequences pathologists provide contingent upon different types of behaviors. In the first selection, two student pathologists provide social praise contingent upon the child's attempts to produce sentences. They also desire to help the child improve his articulation skills. Unfortunately, the goals of providing an enjoyable, fun atmosphere seem to be more important than correcting articulation, as you will see when you tabulate the consequences placed upon these two behaviors.

In the second session, the pathologist very definitely provides specific consequences for specific behaviors, although often she does not provide consequences for responses. By analyzing the type and frequency of the consequences she provides, we gain some understanding of the role consequences play in therapy.

Objective: To identify behaviors that are followed by positive or negative consequences and to evaluate whether or not the consequences are appropriate to the objectives.

Materials: Tape Assignment 5, Selections A and B.

Suggested Reading: Chapter 6, pp. 207–213

SELECTION A

Description of the Session: This therapy session is somewhat unique in the fact that two rather than one undergraduate speech pathology students are conducting the

275

session with a 6-year-old boy. This child has a mild articulation problem. The two students attempt to motivate him by providing an accepting and rewarding atmosphere. Although their ultimate goal is to change speech behaviors, they seem to be more concerned that the child enjoy the session rather than obtain a great deal of practice saying sounds. As you listen to their session, remember that the students are inexperienced and nervous. They have only seen this child for a few sessions. The important point of listening to this session is to determine what type of behaviors are rewarded and what effect these consequences might have upon the frequency of the child's future response pattern.

Procedure: Table 5–1 shows the two classes of behaviors to which the two students in this session attach positive consequences. During the 3 minutes of Selection A these behaviors are identified for you. During the remaining 5 minutes, you will place marks in each behavior class that receives positive consequences.

Play Assignment 5, Selection A now, as you follow the marks made in Table 5–1.

Table 5–1. *Number of positive consequences following each class of behaviors.*

Behavior Class	Positive Consequence	Total
Making up sentences	〜〜〜 //	
Saying a word correctly	/	

Now add all the marks in the first behavior class and enter this number in the column marked 'Total' in Table 5–1. Do the same for the second behavior class. Check your answers with those in the Answer Key, Table 5–4. After having listened to the tape and compiled these data, you should be able to answer the following questions:

1. What do you feel are the chief objectives of this session from the child's standpoint?
2. What do you think was the major objective the students wanted to achieve?
3. Which behavior is followed by social praise most frequently?
4. Which behavior would you expect to increase in frequency?
5. Which behavior do you think should be followed by positive consequences if the students wish to improve articulation skills?
6. How do speech games like the one used in this session actually interfere with articulation instruction?
7. On the positive side, do you think the students established good rapport with this child? Check your answers with those found in the Answer Key. When you have finished, go on to the next exercise, Selection B.

SELECTION B

Description of the Session: The 32-year-old male client in this session has had an articulation problem all of his life because of a congenital neuromotor problem. Muscle action of the tongue, jaws, and lips are not coordinated sufficiently to produce rapid precise articulatory movements necessary for smooth co-articulation. The pathologist in this session attempts to help him learn to produce certain sound sequences in rapid succession. You will observe that the client has difficulty with this task.

Procedure: Table 5–2 lists the antecedent events used by the pathologist, the client's responses, and the pathologist's consequent events. Some of the client's behaviors are not followed by any positive or aversive consequences. This pathologist follows very closely the 3-step instructional cycle so typical of the kind of intensive drill used in behavior therapy. The pathologist's antecedent event, the client's response, and the consequent event follow one another in rapid succession.

In order to assist you in scoring occurrences of the consequent event, these consequent events have been marked for you during the first minute of therapy. During the remaining 3 minutes, you are to mark the consequent event of each response using a + (plus) mark for a correct response (good, nice, perfect, etc.), a − (minus) for an aversive consequence (No, I didn't hear it), or a zero for no consequence.

Now play Assignment 5, Selection B as you follow the information in Table 5–2.

Table 5–2. *Antecedent events and responses.*

Antecedent Event	Response	Consequent Event
what is the girl doing? back to drill work.	bouncing ball	+ ok
tell me again	bouncing ball	0
bounce	bounce	0
ing	ing ball	0
tell me again	bouncing ball	− I didn't hear the end
bounce	bouncing ball	+ that's good
again	bouncing ball	+ nice
what is he doing?	shoveling dirt	+ perfect
tell me again	shovling	− nope

Table 5–2, cont.

Antecedent Event	Response	Consequent Event
shovel	shovel ing dirt	0
again	shov	0
start again	shov-ling dirt	− no, Jack
you said shov-ling, shoveling	shov-a-ing dirt	0
tell me again	shov	0
shovel	shoveling dirt	+ perfect that time
tell me again	shoveling dirt	+ fine
again	shoveling dirt	0

and what is she doing?	bouning ball	
bounce	bouning ball	
tell me again	bouning ball	
bounce	bouncing ball	
again, bounce	bouning	
bounce	bouncing ball	
and what's he doing?	shoveling dirt	
what is she doing?	bouning ball	
bounce	boun	
bounce	bounce	
ing ball	ing ball	
bounce	bouning	
bounce	boun	
s	cing ball	
tell me again, bounce	bouncing ball	
one more time	boun	
s	cing ball	
what's he doing?	peeling ban	
bah-nan	banan	
na	na	
what's he doing?	peeling banda	

Table 5–2, cont.

Antecedent Event	Response	Consequent Event
peeling	peeling banana	
tell me again	peeling banana	
tell me again, peeling	peeling banana	
what's she doing?	bouning	
s	ing ball	
again	bouning	
s	bouncing ball	
tell me again	bouning	
start again, bounce	bouncing ball	
again	bouning	
tell me again, bounce	boun	
bounce	bounce	
tell me again	bounce	
again	bounce	
bounce	bounce	
ing	ball	
that's no fair, bounce	bounce	
ing	ing ball	
one more time	boun	
bounce	bouncing ball	
what's he doing?	peeling banana	
what's she doing?	mi-ing	
———	mixing a cake	
tell me again	mi-ing	
———	mixing cake	
let's start again, what's she doing?	bouning	
———	bouncing a ball	
tell me again	bou	
———	bounce a ball	
bouncing ball	bouning ball	

Now add all the positive consequences, including those completed for you during the first minute; add all of the aversive consequences; and add the instances of no consequences. Enter these totals in Table 5–3.

Table 5–3. *Total amount of positive, aversive, and no-consequence situations in the 4-minute therapy session.*

Consequences	Total
Positive	
Aversive	
None	

Check your answers with those found in the Answer Key, on Table 5–5. From these data, plus the information on the tape, you should be able to answer the following questions:

1. What do you think was the pathologist's chief objective in this session?
2. Do you think the client was aware of the objective?
3. Did the pathologist immediately attach consequences to the client's responses?
4. Was she consistent in her evaluations: Did right responses result in positive consequences and were wrong responses followed by negative consequences?
5. In future sessions like this one, would you expect target responses to increase and incorrect responses to decrease? Why?
6. Why, do you think, didn't this pathologist attach consequences to a third of the responses?
7. In view of the consequence totals and in view of the fact that almost two-thirds of the responses were wrong, what would you suggest the pathologist do to improve the session?
8. If articulation behaviors are considered a motor skill, is the pathologist providing the type of session conducive to developing these motor skills? How?

When you have finished answering these questions, check your answers with those found in the Answer Key. This completes the assignments for Unit 4, "Essentials of Behavior Therapy," Defining Important Terms and Study Questions follow the Answer Key.

Answer Key

SELECTION A

Table 5–4. *Number of positive consequences following each behavior class.*

Behavior Class	Total
Making up sentences	15
Saying a word correctly	4

1. Winning the game and saying sentences.
2. Saying target sounds correctly in words and in sentence context.
3. Saying sentences.
4. Saying sentences.
5. Articulating sounds in words correctly.
6. Consequences are placed on nontarget behaviors and too much time is spent on nontarget behavior activities.
7. Yes.

SELECTION B

Table 5–5. *Total amount of positive, aversive, and no-consequence situations in the 4-minute therapy session.*

Consequences	Total
Positive	24
Aversive	19
None	26

1. Her chief objective was to assist the client in correctly articulating /s/ and /l/ in the medial position of words.
2. Yes.
3. Yes.
4. Yes, with the exception that no consequences followed many responses.
5. Yes, because consequences were immediate, frequent, and accurate.
6. **Many unconsequented responses were incorrect. It would be very discouraging for the client to be told "no" so often.**
7. Change the task to make it easier for the client to achieve greater success and thus more positive consequences.
8. Yes, by providing much repetition and frequent feedback in terms of accurate consequences.

DEFINING IMPORTANT TERMS

After you have read chapters 6 and 7, write definitions for the following terms:

time-out
positive reinforcement
negative reinforcement
criterion
dependent variable
independent variable
operant behavior
extinction
incompatible behavior
punishment
successive approximation
reinforcement menu
contingency management
instructional program
emit
evoke
elicit
escape
repertoire
echoic
S^Δ
consequent event
antecedent event
behavioral objective
response chain
S^D
reinforcement schedule

UNIT 4 STUDY QUESTIONS

1. Describe the role of a behavior therapist in modifying behavior.
2. Differentiate between classical and instrumental conditioning.
3. Define an operant behavior as opposed to a reflexive behavior.
4. What do positive and negative reinforcers have in common?
5. What controls the rate of an operant behavior?
6. Stimuli that follow a response cannot be identified as reinforcers. Why not?
7. How do secondary reinforcers get established?
8. In what way is latency of reinforcement important to increasing the frequency of behavior?
9. There are many different schedules of reinforcement. What type of schedule is recommended when beginning to teach a new behavior and what type is recommended after the behavior is established?
10. Negative reinforcement is usually used to control what type of behaviors?
11. How effective are punishment procedures in reducing the frequency of a behavior?
12. How effective have time-out procedures been with stutterers?
13. How might an individual develop a persistent behavior that does not "pay off"?
14. How is differential reinforcement used in teaching new behavior?
15. Describe discrimination training and give an example to illustrate it.
16. Describe and give an example of how stimulus generalization operates with individuals who stutter.
17. Differentiate between the terms generalization and discrimination.
18. Why are nonsense syllables used in training young children to use newly learned sounds?
19. Name and describe the most common method used to measure retention of speech behaviors.
20. How is it believed that material is forgotten?
21. What factors enhance retention of material?
22. How is preparatory set used to aid in retaining a newly learned behavior?
23. Differentiate between forgetting and retention.
24. What do speech pathologists often do to affect motivational state?

Unit 5

Instructional Programming in Speech Pathology

Objectives

The objectives of this unit are to enable you to: (1) identify the basic components of programmed instruction, (2) identify basic procedures that are used in programming speech therapy materials, (3) describe at least two instructional programs written in articulation, voice, stuttering, language, and aphasia, (4) evaluate instructional programs using criterion standards, and (5) administer S-PACK as an illustration of a programmed approach to the correction of articulation disorders.

Suggested Assignment

Chapters 8 and 9 are the assigned readings for this unit. At the end of the unit is assignment 6, which is accompanied by a casette tape. This assignment should be completed after you have read both chapters. During the assignment, you will learn how to administer part of the S-PACK, an articulation correction program.

Finally, study questions are provided at the end of the unit to assist you in identifying the important concepts contained in the readings.

8

Basics of
Programming

A variety of concepts as well as a number of specific suggestions have been made concerning how teaching strategies can be improved. But unless these concepts and procedures can be unified into a plan for executing instruction, their haphazard use may have only minimal effects on increasing the effectiveness of learning. The teacher may end up with a hodgepodge collection of procedures which offer little more than a slight modernization of her methods. What is needed is an overall plan which would encompass all of the principles that have been presented in this text.

A small number of psychologists have devised means of improving instruction, developing a substantial number of instructional systems. These new instructional systems are identified by the term *programmed instruction*. Basically, this instruction consists of interaction between a student and some instructional material in which immediate feedback about the adequacy of the student's response is provided. The subject matter is arranged into a program of prearranged events or stimuli. This program may be contained in a book, on strips of paper, microfilm slides, videotape, or film loops. It may also consist of auditory material presented live or recorded on tape. Usually, there is a series of instructional items called *frames* which build cumulatively in small steps designed to help the student reach some predetermined objective.

Although instructional programs were virtually unheard of in speech pathology before 1960, an increasing amount of them have been made available to speech clinicians. Instructional programs have been written for all forms of communication disorders, from articulation to aphasia. Instructional programs have also been used extensively at all levels of education, from kindergarten to college. A variety of subjects have been taught including mathematics, reading, science, spelling, and music. A sizeable number of research studies have been conducted in an effort to evaluate the effectiveness of these new instructional systems. For example, Schramm (1964) produced an annotated bibliography of 190 research studies in the area of programmed instruction. More recently, computers have been used as the delivery system for some programmed material, leading to computer assisted instruction and computer managed instructional methods. Up to this time, no one has attempted to use the computer as a system to provide speech therapy although I am sure it is possible.

Before presenting an analysis of several programmed methods developed for use in speech pathology, the basic principles of programmed instruction will be reviewed. This should aid the reader in evaluating and possibly constructing instructional programs.

Early Development of Programmed Instruction

Although programmed instruction is usually thought of as a recent, educational innovation, its roots can be traced as far back as the early seventeenth century when Descartes wrote his "Rules for the Direction of the Intellect." According to the translation by Holdane and Ross (Descartes, 1955), Descartes suggested that difficult material should be broken down into a series of easy steps by arranging facts in an orderly fashion. Basic elements of an instructional program were also suggested by Spencer (1861) and Ebbinghaus (1885) during the nineteenth century.

It was not until 1926 that Sidney L. Pressey developed a simple device that could test, score, and also teach students, thus heralding the formal debut of programmed instruction (Pressey, 1926). His device consisted of a machine that presented a series of multiple-choice questions to the student who selected an answer by pressing one of four levers. Pressing the correct answer lever resulted in the presentation of another question, while an incorrect choice did not advance the mechanism. Thus, the student was required to select another answer until the correct lever was pressed. The student's score was based on the number of times he pressed the lever. Students in Pressey's courses studied their material in the traditional manner but took their tests on the machine. Not only did the machine serve to adequately test his students, but since they were immediately supplied with feedback about their answers (right or wrong), they also learned to discriminate between right and wrong answers, which enabled them to transfer that knowledge to other questions dealing with similar principles. Although Pressey was confident he had achieved a breakthrough in education, his ideas were met with little enthusiasm from other educators and psychologists. His failure at further attempts to improve upon his new ideas were reflected in his statement, "The writer has found from bitter experience that one person alone can accomplish relatively little, and he is regretfully dropping further work on these problems" (Pressey, 1932). Skinner (1958) felt that the general lack of knowledge among educators of that time about principles of learning accounted for the lack of support for Pressey's ideas.

It was not until 1954 that another teaching machine was introduced by Skinner (1954), but this time, it was accompanied by a teaching strategy based on principles of learning accumulated from his years of work with animals. Whereas Pressey's students simply supplemented their regular work with machine-delivered multiple-choice questions, Skinner's students were required to construct their own answers to a series of questions designed to teach *all* of the material to the student. The material was arranged as a series of increasingly complex tasks. Since the instructional material was prewritten, it was called *programmed instruction*. While both techniques developed by Pressey and Skinner featured immediate feedback, Skinner felt the entire learning process could be accomplished through programmed instruction, while Pressey considered his question-type activities as only "adjunct programs."

Shortly after Skinner's presentation of programmed instruction techniques, Norman A. Crowder (1960) introduced a modification of the Pressey-type machine, teaching concepts he called *intrinsic programming*. The student is presented a small amount of material to be studied and is then presented with a question about it. He selects an answer, and if correct, he advances to additional reading material. If he is incorrect, he is presented with supplementary material telling him why he was wrong. Thus, Crowder combined Pressey's use of study material and multiple-choice teaching tests into a self-contained, tutorial-type instructional program.

An extension of Crowder's program led to the "branch program" concept, wherein students who perform poorly on certain questions can be provided with additional information and material. Crowder refers to his program as *intrinsic* because the student's own answer determines whether a branch program should be administered or not. A program of this nature can be presented in a textbook, usually referred to as a *scrambled text*. If a student answers all of the questions correctly, he may only need to read a small portion of the text. Those who miss some questions will be required to read additional material in the text. In this way, individual differences can be met.

Extrinsic instructional programs were advocated by Skinner. This programming style depends on separate criterion tests, teacher's judgment, or criteria external to the instructional program. These criteria determine whether or not additional instructional material will be required. While Crowder preferred the use of multiple-choice questions since they make intrinsic branching easier plus the inclusion of lengthy reading material, Skinner favored short, fill-in type answers and inclusion of only occasional, brief, instructional "panels." Other than that, the differences between the two program formats could be considered as differences in style only.

From these beginnings, a sizeable number of educators have taken pen in hand to construct programmed instructional units in virtually every phase of education. During the 1960s, many educators who viewed programmed instruction as the answer to our instructional ills were disappointed, primarily because many of these new programs failed to be as effective as anticipated. This was more the result of unqualified program writers rather than the fault of the basic system involved. This fact may have been influential in lessening the impact of programmed instruction on the teaching profession. Add to this the general lack of information among many teachers with regard to basic principles of learning, it is not surprising to discover that even today, programmed instructional materials have a difficult time finding their way into the classroom. Since the advent of computers, some educators have channeled their programming efforts into computer assisted instruction, which baffles the ordinary teacher even further. One thing can be said for certain, teaching technology seems to have gone far beyond the general understanding most teachers have about how learning takes place. In my opinion, the majority of today's teachers function in ways similar to those used in the classrooms during Pressey's time. The need now appears to be that of implementing more effective instructional strategies at the level of our teacher-training institutions.

This quest will not occur without opposition. There are many educators who not only misunderstand, but also violently oppose, the programmed instruction movement. Blyth (1960) summarized this objection by stating that automation of education with teaching machines represents such a summation of horrors for some people that it blocks intelligent inquiry into the merits of teaching machines. Blyth also stated he learned more about instruction from the time he began programming than he had during his entire 27 years of teaching (Williams, 1963). Hopefully, if teachers have the opportunity to learn about basic principles of learning upon which programmed instruction is based, there may be a wider, more effective application of programmed instructional materials.

The Basis of
Programmed Instruction

Programmed instruction is an educational expression of laboratory-developed operant conditioning procedures. It represents the ultimate of control and precision in teaching. Furthermore, the entire concept of programmed instruction represents a radical departure from what might be called *traditional teaching*. This has been due chiefly to the technical maturation of operant-conditioning work generated in the 1950s, especially in the fields of experimental design and evaluation in psychology (Sidman, 1960).

In terms of the maturation of operant conditioning, there has been a steady solidification of the learning model as a conceptual scheme, chiefly, reinforcement theory. This has permitted the experimental analysis in carefully controlled laboratory situations of such variables as reinforcement, extinction, and their counterparts —stimulus discrimination, generalization, chaining, and response differentiation.

The use of new experimental designs has also strongly influenced the development of programmed instruction. There has been a decided shift away from statistical methodology as a means of controlling variance (Thoresen, 1969). Rather than using large samples as a means of controlling error, many behavioral researchers prefer to use small samples and control error by reducing the number of uncontrolled variables. Focus has been on the individual learner and intensive case studies. Emphasis has also been placed on description of processes, rather than a comparison of methods.

Research techniques in education conducted some 30 to 50 years ago grew out of traditional psychological research which emphasized tests to determine the success of a method. Literally hundreds of ability, achievement, interest, and aptitude tests were constructed and used in our schools as the chief means of "measuring," through test scores, teacher or method effectiveness. Testing was considered a means of controlled observation, but the *teaching* was left relatively uncontrolled. Today's educators are very familiar with the methodological battles that have been fought to determine which method was better—phonics or sight reading, child-centered vs. teacher-structured approaches, and so on. Even in the area of speech pathology, experimenters have sought to find the best teaching method by comparing test scores of children under each method—block vs. traditional system, operant therapy vs. traditional therapy, therapy vs. no therapy, and so on. Usually, two groups of subjects were matched for age and intelligence and tested following a particular treatment. The group obtaining the highest scores, providing the difference was statistically significant, represented the favored method.

The basic problem with the test-based strategy was that it was still not possible to identify those independent variables responsible for behavioral change. The concern for achieving better behavioral controls was an outgrowth of the work being done in operant conditioning. An interest developed in identifying those variables which controlled behavior change, and once the experimenter was in control of these variables, she could both predict behavioral outcomes and control them as well. These two factors, prediction and control, have been identified in previous chapters as the basis of a science. And this is exactly what those who undertook the scientific analysis of teaching determined to do, i.e., add the precision elements of prediction and control to education. Their vehicle was programmed instruction, an instrument that would virtually guarantee these two qualities to educators. It was a deliberate attempt to produce, or to control, a specified behavior.

The fundamental characteristics of programmed instruction consists of three basic procedures according to Skinner (1954). First, the material should be presented in small steps arranged in a logical sequence. The concept here is to build on the existing behavior of the learner, gradually introducing new material which should lead the learner toward achievement of a final goal. You may recall Skinner's use of the term *successive approximation* as descriptive of this process. Skinner's programming technique consisted of composing a number of frames in which small amounts of subject matter was presented in 20 and 30 words or less. Each frame contained one or more blanks, which the student was to complete. Overt responding on the part of the student was the second characteristic of Skinner's program. Without this active responding, Skinner felt little learning could take place. The following are examples of a few frames of the type Skinner recommends:

1. A test is considered valid if it accurately measures what it was designed to test. If it does not measure what it was supposed to measure, we say it is not a _____ test.

2. Test validity refers to how _____ a test measures the thing it is supposed to test.

Finally, Skinner's third prerequisite for an instructional program was that the student's correct response be reinforced immediately. Simple knowledge of results has been considered adequate enough, especially for adolescents and college students. Perhaps you have been exposed to programmed tests in which after writing a response, you turned the page to find the correct answer. If it matched your answer, you are supposedly rewarded and move forward to the next item. If not, you at least are presented with the correct answer, and hopefully, will profit from it. The programmer may use abundant cues to insure that the student will give the correct response. As the concept is thoroughly learned, the cues are reduced or eliminated. Thus, small steps, overt responding, and immediate reward constitute what Skinner felt were essential ingredients of an effective instructional program.

Skinner's program prerequisites have been criticized by several authorities who feel they may not be as essential to a good program as Skinner would have us believe (Barlow, 1963). It has been pointed out that presentation of large amounts of material may actually facilitate comprehension. Gilbert (1962) argues that an analytical approach to the presentation of material seems to tell the programmer more about student achievement than a synthetic, small-step approach. He feels the programmer should assume the student is very capable, and thus, large steps should be incorporated into the program. If this proves to be a false assumption, error rate will be high. Consequently, the programmer constructs smaller steps. On the other hand, if the programmer's first program consists of small steps which would result in very low error rate, it is likely that the programmer will not be able to discover that his steps may be too small. He also points out that it is advisable for the student to survey a large amount of material before attempting to learn separate parts of the material. This survey procedure is frequently suggested by educators as an excellent study technique. Finally, programs written in very small steps are apt to be considered dull and boring to everyone except the slowest student (Whaley & Malott, 1971). Also, students come to programs with varying amounts of information. Some students, therefore, require small steps, or gradual presentation of information, while others would benefit more from a program which moved rapidly from one concept to the next.

It has been suggested that it is much more important to manipulate cues than it is to concern oneself so much with the manipulation of reward schedules (Coulson, 1962). Many students who perform well in a program tend to ignore or bypass the confirmation or correction frame. My experience in delivering some highly cued instructional programs to children who lisp would substantiate the idea that an immediate, external reward, or even knowledge of results, is not always required. I found that some students acquired a correct /s/ during administration of a lisp correction program even though they were never rewarded or informed of the correctness of their response. This would indicate that the cues built into the program were adequate to evoke and to maintain the desired response.

We have known for some time that recitation definitely seems to facilitate memorization. But recent studies have questioned the validity of this statement, especially in some areas of learning. For example, Evans (1961) found that children learned to write numbers fairly well during a teaching situation designed to help them discriminate between correctly and incorrectly formed numbers although they received no practice writing the numbers. Evans et al. (1959) unexpectedly found that students who wrote down answers to frames scored more poorly on a posttest than did students who did not respond overtly. This finding was also supported by Goldbeck and Biggs (1960) and by Roe (1961). Active responding in Crowder-type programs consists of merely a button-pressing action on the part of the student, rather than construction of an answer. In this case, it is felt that "active responding" is the covert verbal behavior a student engages in when she reads instructional information contained in the frame. The button pushing or selection of a multiple-choice item simply serves to test the student's understanding of the written material. There are certainly many variables to be considered in deciding whether or not overt responses are necessary, such as the nature of the task, age of the individual, past history of the individual, and the like. There may be some instances where overt responding is required for learning to take place and some where it is not.

As you can readily see, it is difficult to establish comprehensive "rules" for constructing instructional programs. What might appear to be a rule in one learning situation may not hold true for another condition. Consequently, the naive program writer must be careful not to make the mistake of writing programs as though there were only one "correct" method of constructing them. But there are some educators today who believe that there is only one best method of teaching skills such as reading, mathematics, or writing. As most of us know, there are many effective methods of teaching these skills. Each technique has its own peculiar advantages or disadvantages. Skinner, Crowder, and Pressey each presented differing models of program construction, and each method is supported by research findings. Other models have yet to be presented. To conclude that there is one "right" or "best" model for all learning situations and for all individuals is indeed naive. A number of other educators have refined and modified some of the original conceptions of what constitutes an instructional program. For example, Fine (1962) identifies five characteristics of an instructional program:

1. constant interchange between programmer and student through program frames which require responses from the student.
2. the idea or concept presented in the program must be thoroughly mastered before advancing.
3. presents only that instructional material for which the student is ready.
4. contains needed cues, prompts, and suggestions designed to help the student respond correctly.
5. the student is reinforced for correct responses, which helps to shape and maintain newly learned behavior.

Fine likens the instructional programming technique to a tutorial situation in which ideal learning conditions exist.

Coolagan (1976) defines programmed instruction as an interaction between the student and instructional material wherein immediate feedback is provided about the adequacy of the student's response. The subject matter called the program could take many forms: a book, strip of paper, auditory material, microfilm slides, videotape, film loops, or a combination of the above. The instructional items are presented as short, informational segments called frames, each frame calling for a response from the student. A series of frames are combined to form a step or goal. A combination of steps form a large goal or level of performance. Frequently, criterion tests are used to measure the adequacy of learning which should have taken place at each step.

In an article by Costello (1977) describing the basic characteristics of programmed instruction, four major components are listed as being critical to a programmed instructional package. These components are

1. Stimulus
2. Response
3. Consequence and schedule of reinforcement
4. Criterion.

The stimulus component consists of those instructions, prompts, or cues required to evoke an expected response. During the introduction of a new task, these stimuli, sometimes called the *antecedent events,* are written so they provide a very clear indication of what the response should be. For example, the speech clinician might model the response as well as provide tongue position cues. Specific pictures designed to evoke verbal responses containing the desired sound are frequently used. Kinesthetic or tactile cues may also be provided. As the new behavior is practiced, many of the supportive cues are faded or dropped completely. For example, the clinician may say "Close your teeth and say /s/ like this: [s]" early in an articulation program, but later may simply say "Say it again." As you can see, the cue was weakened from a modeling cue, plus a placement cue, to a simple request of repetition. Usually, when a new task is presented, the stimulus instructions or cues are increased; and as the task is mastered, the cues are gradually reduced or faded. Of course, it is also assumed that new material is presented in small amounts, taking the learner through a series of increasingly difficult tasks.

Costello's second component consists of the student's response. She stresses that the programmer must clearly define what response the student should have when the program has been completed. This has often been called the *terminal behavior.* In addition to this final response, the program writer must also define a series of "sub-objectives," or behaviors which are to be learned during the program. A combination of these behaviors are referred to as successive approximations. It is important that the program writer be very familiar with constructing behavioral objectives since they clearly define the response made at each level within the program.

The amount of responses considered as errors has been an issue of much concern and considerable disagreement among program writers. Skinner (1954) favors a program in which few or no errors should occur. Students, according to Skinner, learn by making correct responses, not by making errors. The ideal program is one leading the student through a series of learning activities which allow the student to succeed at each step. Crowder, on the other hand, says, "I think it is desirable that in a routine program step (if there is such a thing) no more than 15% of the students should select a wrong answer. However, a major branch might have a question that would be failed by 90% of the students" (Coulson, 1962). This 15% figure is not far from the 10% figure set by many Skinnerian programmers. Programmers following Crowder's suggestions use error rate as a means of deciding when program branches should be used. But errors that occur as a result of poorly constructed program items are viewed by all program writers as something to be eliminated.

The consequent event following the response consists of either a reward, designed to strengthen the response, or an aversive stimulus, aimed at weakening the response. The consequent event may also consist of withholding the reward so that the response may weaken (extinction). It is at this consequent event level that a response is deliberately weakened or strengthened. You probably know from reading the previous chapters that the program writer will also attempt to manipulate the reinforcement schedule in such a way as to maximize the probability that the response will be resistant to extinction. This is done by gradually demanding more and more responses to obtain a single reward. The reward may consist of some type of extrinsic item, like a toy, candy, points, or an intrinsic reward, such as the knowledge that one is performing correctly, i.e., praise, smile, presentation of the correct answer, and the like. A token economy system may also be designed and used as part of the program package. Aversive stimuli following incorrect responses usually take the form of verbal reprimands, buzzer sounds, loss of points, and written statements such as, "You're wrong," and the like. These consequent events are frequently discussed in terms of knowledge of results and are considered by most program writers as one of the most important ingredients of an instructional program. It becomes imperative then that response parameters be defined clearly so there is no doubt about what constitutes a correct or incorrect response.

Costello's final characteristic of a program consists of the criterion level set for either advancing through the program, terminating the program, or branching into an alternative program sequence. These criteria are usually determined from test runs of the program with a small sample of subjects. For example, in one program I wrote, it was found that children who missed more than 50% of the first 50 instructional items were unable to pass any of the criterion tests contained in the remaining three program parts. Therefore, a criterion level of performance was built into the program stating that if more than 50% of the first 50 items were missed, the program was to be discontinued.

Many programs include a series of criterion tests that serve as "check points" to indicate how well the subject matter has been mastered. Such a criterion test might consist of 10 test items containing a review of the major skills covered in the program up to that point. A criterion level of performance may be set: "8 out of 10 correct items must be obtained before the subject can advance to the next section." A score below that criterion level may require that the subject repeat that section until it is mastered. Certain criterion performances in extrinsic programs route the subject through branch programs. Still other ways of dealing with criterion levels consist of keeping track of performance on each section. Suppose a program consists of 100 instructional items. The programmer may decide that the criterion level of performance for mastery of that section require that the student produce 85% of the items correctly. If the student meets this criterion, she advances to the next step or section. If not, the program items are presented again, a branch program may be presented, or the program may be terminated.

Editing
a Program

Writing the program is only a first step in developing programmed instruction. A critical stage sometimes overlooked by authors of programs consists of editing the program. This process goes beyond fact checking, proofreading, or correcting grammatical errors. Progam editing, an arduous and time-consuming task, entails thorough testing and validation of the materials contained in the program. Frequently, the program editor and program writer are the same person, but this need not be the case. In fact, it is better if someone who is somewhat naive about the subject matter acts as the editor.

When programs fail to produce the results they should, the program editor can often point out and help correct trouble spots. New program writers often get into the habit of adding more frames when students fail in certain parts of the program. But rather than increasing the number of frames, it might be better to carefully analyze the material presented *prior to* the failure site. It may be that the skills needed to succeed at the failure site were not thoroughly developed during some earlier level; perhaps the wording of the failure site items was not correct. A number of variables should be considered before attempting to write additional frames.

Another fault commonly found among inexperienced program writers is the inclusion of too many prompts. This procedure almost guarantees students will answer frames correctly, but does not succeed in teaching them anything. Consider the following example:

Phonetics is the study of speech sounds.
The study of speech sounds is called P_____.

Certainly, most students will answer this frame correctly, but chances are that learning will be minimal. Overcued programs are frequently boring and require much time to complete.

Insufficient cueing is another common fault of many new program writers. When this occurs, one can expect error rate to increase dramatically. Ambiguous cues may also be at fault. The speech clinician who uses pictures to evoke certain responses may find his pictures contain unwanted cues which evoke undesired responses.

Basescu (1963) suggests that almost anyone other than the programmer himself should test the program. The ego involvement, he points out, makes it almost impossible for most program writers to approach validation in an unbiased manner. Basescu notes that one program writer continually helped students by saying to them, "Do you remember what you learned in Unit Three?" She did not realize that it was unfair to tamper with the program sequence in this manner. I am reminded of an instance where student speech clinicians administering an instructional program gave the children many prompts while walking with them to the testing center. These prompts may have strongly influenced the children's performance during administration of the program.

The true value of the program tester is that she is willing and able to find out what is wrong with the program. Although students may be able to provide correct answers to program items, the program may not always be teaching the skills or behavior intended by the programmers. I recall the first program I wrote included the use of puppets as a means of evoking speech responses. My program editors, who happened to be two of my professors, quickly discouraged the use of puppets as irrelevant stimuli to the behavior I was trying to evoke; consequently, I switched to a more direct approach of just asking the subject to repeat items.

Size and type of population sample are also an important consideration when evaluating a program. Here, the editor places limitations on applicability of the program. Often the programmer, overjoyed by the success of his program on a small population, feels he has constructed a "universal" program applicable to all populations. I found that in developing a program for correction of the frontal lisp that it was not suitable for use with populations of lisping children who have an open bite, a severe overbite, a lateral lisp, or a /t/ substitution for /s/. It was also never tested on children who were not enrolled in regular public school classrooms. As a result, this particular program contained a sizeable number of restrictions about the population for which it could be used.

Research Results of
Programmed Instruction

The creation of instructional programs was predicted to be the answer to the educator's instructional woes during the mid-century mark. A large number of instructional programs were written, many of which found their way to both public school and college classrooms. Even encyclopedia companies offered programmed instructional kits as supplements to their books. This intense activity was soon followed by research attempts designed to evaluate the effectiveness of these programs.

One early survey of the research on programmed instruction was conducted by Schramm (1964). In reviewing approximately 190 studies, he identified 36 which compared programmed instruction to traditional instructional models. Of these studies half, or 18, showed no differences, whereas programmed instruction was favored in 17 instances. Only in one case was a traditional method considered better than programmed instruction.

In a more recent review by Lange (1972), 172 studies reported between 1960 and 1964 were analyzed. All studies compared programmed methods with traditional methods. Again half, or 49%, showed no difference, 41% showed programmed instruction to be better, and 10% found traditional methods better.

After viewing the programming movement some 20 years after its introduction, Jamison et al. (1974) concluded that programmed instruction is generally as effective as traditional instruction and may require less of the student's time to reach the same educational goal. The authors also pointed out that the current trend in research is not to compare one method with another, but to focus on techniques which improve programs, how to increase student interest, and how to adapt programmed instruction to unusual educational settings. Within the last decade, several other educational instruction systems have been developed, such as computer assisted instruction, instructional television, computer managed instruction, and even instructional radio. But all of these advances fail to add to the productivity of the present system. They do provide alternatives to traditional educational models, but they certainly have not proved that they can play an important role in American schools. Perhaps further refinement of this new educational technology will alter this conclusion.

Maybe program advocates like Silberman (1963) were over optimistic when they predicted that programmed instruction promised dramatic improvements in educational technology, which would lead to improved learning among students. On the other hand, there can be no doubt that traditional teaching models have improved as a result of advances in educational technology. Certainly, we do not view programmed instruction and traditional instruction as being in competition with one another. Experienced teachers do take refresher courses, and new teachers bring with them to the classroom many of the principles which underlie programmed instruction. It is not as though the principles of programmed instruction do not work. They do work, and they work well; the job of future educators is to make them work better and to find ways of incorporating these programs into the school program where they fit best. The purpose of this new technology is to make teachers more productive, not to replace them with machines. Machines should be used to strengthen the teaching process.

BIBLIOGRAPHY

Barlow, J. A. Programmed instruction in perspective: Yesterday, today and tomorrow. In R. T. Filep (Ed.), *Prospectives in programming*. New York: Macmillan, 1963.

Basescu, B. On frames and on editing and revising programmed instruction. In R. T. Filep (Ed.), *Prospectives in programming*. New York: Macmillan, 1963.

Blyth, J. B. Teaching machines and human beings. In A. A. Lunsdaine & S. R. Glaser (Eds.), *Teaching machines and programmed learning*. Washington, D.C.: Department of Audio-Visual Instruction, National Education Association, 1960.

Coolagan, R. B. Programming primer. *School, Science and Mathematics*, 1976, *76*, 381–91.

Costello, J. *Designing programmed instruction*. Houston, Tex.: Short Course, American Speech and Hearing Convention, 1976.

Costello, J. Programmed instruction. *Journal of Speech and Hearing Disorders*, 1977, *42*, 3–28.

Coulson, J. E. (Ed.) *Programmed learning and computer-based instruction*. New York: John Wiley & Sons, 1962.

Crowder, N. A. Automatic tutoring by intrinsic programming. In A. A. Lumsdaine & R. Glaser (Ed.), *Teaching machines and programmed learning*. Washington, D.C.: Department of Audio-visual Instruction, National Education Association, 1960.

Descartes, R. Philosophical works of Descartes (E. Haldone & G. Ross, trans.). New York: Dover, 1955.

Ebbinghaus, H. E. *Memory: A contribution of experimental psychology*. Translated by H. A. Ruger & C. E. Bussehius from *Uber das Gedächtnis: Untersuchungen zur experimentellen Psychologie* (1885). New York: Teachers College Educational Reprint Services, 1913.

Evans, J. L. *Multiple-choice discrimination programming*. Paper read at the meeting of the American Psychological Association, New York, September 1961.

Evans, J. L., Glaser, R., & Homme, L. E. *A preliminary investigation of variations in the properties of verbal sequence of the "Teaching Machine" type*. Paper read at the meeting of the Eastern Psychological Association, Atlantic City, N.J., 1959.

Fine, B. *The modern family guide to education*. New York: Doubleday, 1962.

Gilbert, T. F. Mathematics: The technology of education. *Journal of Mathematics*, 1962, *1*, 7–73.

Goldbeck, R. A., & Biggs, L. J. *An analysis of response mode and feedback in automated instruction* (Tech. Rep. 2). Santa Barbara, Ca.: American Institute for Research, 1960.

Jamison, D., Suppes, P., & Wells, S. The effectiveness of alternative instructional media: A survey. *Review of Educational Research*, 1974, *44*, 1–59.

Lange, P. C. Today's education. *National Education Association*, 1972, *61*, 59.

Pressey, S. L. A simple apparatus which gives tests and scores—and teaches. *School and Society*, 1926, *23*, 373–376.

Pressey, S. L. A third and fourth contribution toward the coming industrial revolution in education. *School and Society*, 1932, *36*, 668–672.

Roe, A. Five teaching methods tested at UCLA Department of Engineering, Research note, AID, I 1961.

Schramm, W. *The research on programmed instruction: An annotated bibliography*. Washington, D.C.: U.S. Department of Health, Education and Welfare, 1964.

Sidman, M. *Tactics in scientific research*. New York: Basic Books, 1960.

Silberman, H. F. Trends in programmed instruction—an improvement in educational technology. In R. T. Filep (Ed.), *Prospectives in programming*. New York: Macmillan, 1963.

Skinner, B. F. The science of learning and the art of teaching. *Harvard Educational Review*, 1954, *24*, 86–97.

Skinner, B. F. Teaching Machines. *Science*, 1958, *128*, 969–977.

Spencer, H. *Education: Intellectual, Moral, Physical*. New York: Appleton-Century-Crofts, 1861.

Thoresen, C. E. Relevance and research in counseling. *Review of Educational Research*, 1969, *39*, 263–281.

Whaley, D. L., & Malott, R. W. *Elementary principles of behavior*. Englewood Cliffs, N.J.: Prentice-Hall, 1971.

Williams, C. M. Information disseminator or guide of learning?—training the teacher for the classroom of the '70's. In R. T. Filep (Ed.), *Prospectives in programming*. New York: Macmillan, 1963.

9

Instructional Programming in Speech Pathology

A discussion of programmed instruction is presented here to show how principles of operant conditioning have been applied in the speech therapy setting, and because there have been quite a few instructional programs written for speech clinicians to use with their clients. Many clinicians do not have the necessary skills to evaluate these programs. Still others would like to write instructional programs but lack the knowledge required to develop them. Although it is not the purpose of this chapter to provide a short course in programming, perhaps the clinician will be able to develop some critical attitudes about programming and may even be able to construct short, workable programs as a result of studying this chapter.

I recall seeing at an American Speech and Hearing Association (ASHA) convention around the mid-1950s a computer program designed to teach students audiology. The course followed a text written by Hayes Newby. That was my initial introduction to programmed instruction in our field. Some 6 or 7 years later while studying under Robert Baker and Richard Schutz, two educational psychologists at Arizona State University, I conceived the idea of writing an instructional program to correct lisping behavior in young children. This project gave rise to my doctorate dissertation (Mowrer, 1964) in which I wrote a three-part lisp correction program. Using this lisp program as a standardized instrument, I attempted to determine the effects of three variables on the amount of correct /s/ responses produced on a criterion test following administration of the program. The variables were (1) reinforcement, (2) overt responding, and (3) mode of stimulus presentation. The instructional program was revised slightly, and a parent transfer program was added, and further testing was completed during 1965. Several instructional programs aimed at problems involving articulation, stuttering, voice, aphasia, and language have been developed. The bulk of these programs have been linear or extrinsic, as opposed to the intrinsic branching type programs developed by Crowder.

Basic Features
of an Instructional
Program in Speech Therapy

One way to explain the use of principles of programming found in speech therapy instructional programs is to present an overview of one program which clearly demonstrates these principles. Since these principles were used in the development of the S Programmed Articulation Control Kit (S-PACK) (Mowrer, Baker, & Schutz, 1968b), I will analyze it in detail. It should be noted that a variety of other instructional programs used in speech pathology also follow this basic design.

Design of Steps

The first task in designing a program is to decide the terminal objective, or what it is the program should accomplish. Next, a number of skills which are required in order to obtain the objective are identified. In the case of lisp correction, the terminal objective would be to produce /s/ correctly 100% of the time in all contexts and in all speaking situations. Van Riper (1964) has outlined a series of steps one might follow in reaching such an objective. Basically, these steps include the following subgoals:

1. ear training
2. sound in isolation
3. sound in nonsense syllables
4. sound in words
5. sounds in phrases and sentences
6. sound in conversational speech

The basic taxonomy was adopted for programming /s/ with the exception of the ear training section, which was omitted. A flow chart specifying the progressive order of presentation of each new task was constructed according to this model and is presented in Figure 9–1. Each response module represents a subobjective, which is prerequisite to the next subobjective. This process continues until the terminal objective is reached. As you can see, this is analogous to Skinner's small-step concept of programming. At the right-hand side of Figure 9–1, the actual response units subjects are required to say are shown. At the left are noted three divisions

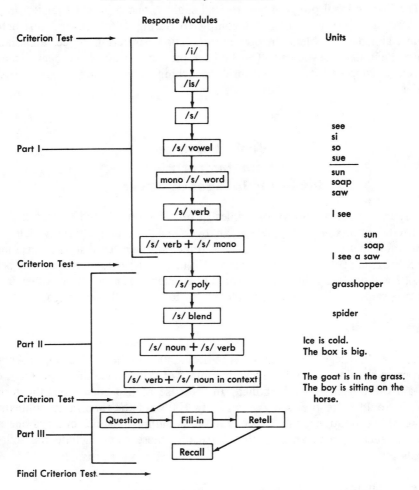

FIGURE 9-1. Flow Chart For Three-Part Lisp Correction Program Used in S-PACK

indicating three instructional sessions, each requiring approximately 15 minutes of instruction time (Parts I, II, and III).

Instructional Cues

In Figure 9–2, a flow chart outlining the sequence of cues is presented. These cues include three basic forms: those which evoke (1) sounds, (2) single words, and (3) those designed to evoke phrases or sentences. Naturally, sound cues were used exclusively during the initial stages of the program, followed by the introduction of word and sentence type cues.

The cues used can also be viewed in terms of various types. In Figure 9–3, six cue types are listed and comprise those used in the construction of S-PACK. These simple cue types plus the objectives found in the flow chart in Figure 9–1 were all that were required to build the basic program. Many redundant items were included to

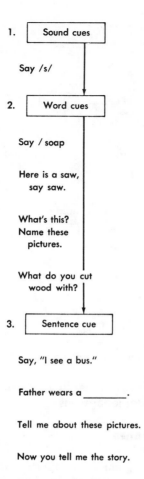

1. | Sound cues |

Say /s/

2. | Word cues |

Say / soap

Here is a saw,
say saw.

What's this?
Name these
pictures.

What do you cut
wood with?

3. | Sentence cue |

Say, "I see a bus."

Father wears a _____.

Tell me about these pictures.

Now you tell me the story.

FIGURE 9-2. Examples Of Specific Cues Used In S-PACK To Evoke Sounds, Words, And Sentences

insure that subjects obtained sufficient practice. Once a basic word list was selected, it was a simple matter to construct the actual program using the steps outlined in the flow chart plus the variety of cues.

Successive Approximation

There was no attempt to shape the /s/ sound through evoking successive approximations of /s/ in this program. One approximation used was the early introduction of the /i/ sound. This sound was chosen as the first target because (1) it is already in the repertoire of the subjects, and (2) it shares many of the same features with /s/, i.e. teeth closed and tongue in approximate position for /s/ production. The first request is, therefore, "Say /i/." This could be considered an approximation of /s/. The next request is, "Close your teeth and say /s/." In many cases, the resultant response will be an approximation of /s/, but the /s/ may be somewhat distorted, excessive air may be present, there may be a lack of stridency, or some similar distortion. No attempt is made to modify this /s/ distortion unless it results from

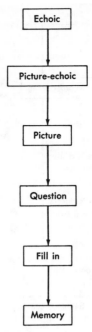

FIGURE 9-3. Six General Cue Type Formats Used In S-PACK

improper teeth closure. I have found that in most cases, this distortion is no longer present following 20 or 30 additional trials.

Definition of Correct Response

In any type of instructional program, it is important that the correct and incorrect response be clearly defined. It must be observable, countable, and manipulatable. If correctness depends on subjective judgment, then response correctness will differ according to who administers the program. Thus, the program's effectiveness depends on how accurately the response is defined. Ideally, an instructional program should be independent of variations among administrators. Any program administrator, given they meet certain requirements like age, prerequisite training, adequate hearing, or whatever, should be able to achieve similar results, providing the same program is used. But if administrators differ with respect to the feedback they provide, you can readily see how this would affect results.

Rather than rely on the acoustic qualities of the /s/, which would necessitate some subjective evaluation, the correct response in S-PACK was defined in terms of teeth closure. If an /s/ approximation was produced while the teeth were closed, providing the rear molars, not the central incissors, were touching, the response was to be judged as correct although the /s/ sounded like a distortion. If the tongue protruded between the teeth during /s/ production, the response was to be judged wrong no matter how well the /s/ sounded. Of course, as the program proceeded, it became difficult to determine whether or not the teeth were closed during /s/ production in rapid, conversational speech. In this case, as long as the tongue did not protrude, the /s/ was judged correct.

Now suppose the teeth were closed but according to the judgment of several clinicians, the /s/ was distorted. Possibly the tongue tip placement was incorrect or airstream flow was misdirected. This particular program was not designed to cope with this condition. This fact presents one limitation of programs. They cannot be all things to all people. There is no "universal" program to fit the needs of everyone.

Fading Cues

The cues listed in Figure 9–3 can be arranged to provide very strong support or little support to the individual. During early tryouts of the program, it was found that the cue "Close your teeth" was more influential in prompting the correct response than the cue "Say S." Theoretically, both position cues and model cues together offered the greatest likelihood that a correct response would be produced. Therefore, this combination of strong cues was incorporated in the program. As the correct response was emitted more frequently, these cues were eliminated and weaker cues such as, "Say it again," or, "Say it softly," were substituted. When a new task such as producing /s/ in words was introduced, the stronger cues were re-introduced again and faded as the task was practiced.

It was also felt that allowing children to look at themselves in a mirror would provide strong cues regarding teeth closure. The mirror was used during the first stages of the program in addition to the position and modeling cues. The cue fading technique used in the first part of **S-PACK** will serve as an example of this procedure.

Cue type	Instruction
Strong cues	Close your teeth and say *E.*
	Close your teeth and say *EEEsss.*
	Look in the mirror and say *EEEsss.*
Faded cue	Say *EEEsss*
Strong cues	Keep your teeth closed and say *EEESSS*
	Look in the mirror. Say *EEEsss*
	Close your teeth. Say, *EEEsss*
	Now say it like this; *Essssss*
Weaker cue	Look in the mirror and try it again
Strong cue	Close your teeth and say *s*
Weaker cue	Say *s*
Strong cue	Close your teeth and say it softly
Weaker cue	Look in the mirror. Say *s* louder
Weaker cue	Say a long *sssss*
	Say a short one, *s*

As you can see, several strong cues are introduced initially when the task is difficult, and gradually, weaker cue types are added until only the cue, "Say it again," is provided. Picture cues are also considered weak cues. Memoric cues are even weaker. An example of a memoric cue is, "What do you cut with a lawnmower?"

or "Father wears a suit and mother wears a _____." The following action illustrates how pictorial cues are introduced.

Comment	Instruction
Echoic nonsense syllables	Sue
	Si
Strong cue because of introduction of a word	Close your teeth and say, *saw*.
Picture cue plus model	Here is a picture of a saw. Say *saw*.
Memoric cues	What was the name of that picture?
	What do you cut wood with?
	Say so.
	Here is a picture of soap, say *soap*.
Picture cue alone	What is this? (Saw)
	What is this? (Soap)
Model cues	Say *saw*.
	Say *soap*.
Memoric cues	What do you wash your hands with?
	What do you cut wood with?
Pictorial cues	What's this? (saw)
	What's this? (soap)

Note the high level of redundancy in response type. The words *saw* and *soap* are used 14 consecutive times once they are introduced. The cues are gradually faded until more dependence is placed on memoric cues alone. Then three more words, *suit, soap,* and *seen,* are introduced as the cues are again strengthened and weakened. The strategy, therefore, consists of providing strong, supportive cues when a task is first introduced and gradually weakening these cues as the response is practiced. Finally, during the last part of the three-part program, the subject is simply asked, "Tell me the story while you look at these pictures." This cue alone is sufficient to generate a large number of /s/ responses in connected speech. Had this type of cue been employed during the first part of the program, the subject would almost certainly produce incorrect /s/ responses. The nature of the cues, the time of their introduction, and the fading process play an important role in response correctness. This entire area of cues is what Costello (1977) referred to as the antecedent event in programming.

Management of the Consequent Event

As you recall from chapter 7, the consequences of a response play an important role in determining the frequency with which that response recurs in the future. Also, the frequency of occurrence of this consequence (schedule of reinforcement) plays an important role in determining the likelihood that the response will continue to occur, even when it is not reinforced (resistance to extinction). Since newly learned behaviors tend to be somewhat unstable, we decided it was best to use continuous reinforcement during the early phases of the subject's program, shifting gradually to an intermittent schedule after establishing the behavior, i.e., after it was subjected to a high level of reinforcement. Thus, the subjects will be required to say more and more correct /s/'s to receive the same amount of reinforcement as they progress through the program.

The administrator's role in the consequent event is quite simple. The response is judged as either correct (teeth closure) or incorrect (tongue protrusion). It was felt that providing the subject with a redeemable token following each correct response was an effective technique for maintaining motivation during program administration. At the end of a 15-minute session, the subject could exchange his tokens for a prize or privilege.

If a response was incorrect, the administrator simply said "No" and continued to the next item. Second tries were allowed only during the first 50 items of Part I.

Criterion Measures

Three types of criterion measures were used to evaluate the subject's performance. They were classified as criteria for (1) entering into the program, (2) remaining in the program, and (3) exiting from the program. The entering and exiting criterion instruments were the same. Twenty-five items sampled various /s/ tasks presented in the program, from /s/ in monosyllabic words to /s/ in connected speech. Five items at the end which were not included in the program were designed to test generalization of the response. The criterion measures for determining whether a subject should remain in the program consisted of four tests. The first test considered the number of errors made during the first 50 items of Part I. If 30 or more errors are made, the program is terminated since it is almost certain that the subject will not succeed through the remainder of the program. Following the first 94 items, a 10-item criterion test is presented. This test includes the skills taught in Part I, /s/ in the initial position in monosyllabic words. If the subject scores eight, nine or ten items correctly, she may advance to the next part. If seven or less responses are correct, she either is terminated in the program or that part is repeated.

The same procedure is followed in Parts II and III. As you can see, the criterion tests play a vital role in a program as far as helping the administrator know the program is successful in teaching what it is suppose to teach. In traditional teaching, it is often assumed subjects have learned the material. Program criterion tests offer verification that learning has occurred. One of the basic characteristics of programmed instruction is to insure that each task is mastered before the student advances.

Shifting Stimulus Control

This subject was discussed extensively in chapter 7. We are interested in shifting the stimulus control the speech clinician exercises over the subject's correct response to other stimulus conditions, chiefly, speaking in the home situation. In this way, the correct response is reinforced in more common speaking situations and "carry-over" of the new response is achieved. As I mentioned before, although subjects produce the response correctly in the presence of the speech clinician in the training environment, the incorrect response will likely be used when speaking in the home environment. The reason, of course, is that the correct response is still under control of stimuli associated with the speech clinician, whereas the incorrect response is evoked in the presence of other stimulus conditions. One solution to this problem involved writing a parent-administered program which would essentially extend stimulus control of the newly acquired response to speaking situations in the home. This parent program was quite similar to the three-part instructional program administered by the speech clinician. Cue fading, immediate reinforcement for correct responses, gradual increase of more difficult tasks, and token redemption were all included in the program. It was to be administered by the parent in the home situation shortly following the start of the three-part, clinician-administered program. In order to insure success during initial stages of the parent program, the identical pictures used in the three-part program were also included in the parent program. Gradually, new items and stories were introduced until the parent program became an enlarged extension of the three-part program. The parent was to report to the clinician at the end of each week how many correct responses were made.

If the level of correct responses fell below 80%, the clinician scheduled the child for several lessons to determine the nature of the problem or checked the parent's criterion for a correct response. At the end of the 3-week parent program (one lesson daily Monday through Friday), the clinician sampled the first 20 /s/ productions as the child was engaged in conversational speech. If 90% of the /s/ sounds were correct, the child was dismissed as corrected and scheduled for recheck 6 months to 1 year later.

Editing and Validating the Program

One of the final stages of program construction involves the editing and validation of the program. As you will recall, it was advised that someone other than the program writer should edit and validate the program since the program writer is likely to be biased. Fortunately, two of my professors assisted me with the editing process and eliminated some of my "pet" notions. I administered the program to approximately 25 first-grade children in a series of pilot studies. Some changes were added like the use of the mirror practice with a few nonsense syllables, and certain items were clarified.

The next step consisted of field testing the three-part program with 75 children. Three variables were studied during the field-test project: the importance of (1) reinforcement, (2) mode of response, and (3) mode of stimulus presentation. From the data gathered in this study, it was concluded that it is important to provide reinforcement for correct responses, that the subject actively participate by making oral responses to program items, but it does not matter whether the stimuli are presented live or through tape recordings. For a more extensive discussion of these findings, see chapter 15 in *Operant Procedures in Remedial Speech and Language Training* (Mowrer, Baker & Schutz, 1968a).

The parent program was tested using a sample of 20 parents whose children were enrolled in a public school. No changes were made in this program. It was found again that reinforcement was an important variable and its use was retained.

A final test of both the three-part program and parent program was conducted in a rural school district in Arizona (Mowrer, 1967). Ten children who lisped were selected as subjects. A substitute teacher was selected as the administrator and provided with about two hours of training in delivering the material. After 1 month when both programs were completed, all children were given the conversational speech test. The program was effective in eliminating the lisp in eight out of ten cases.

Several other investigators have tested the effectiveness of S-PACK and consequently, offer an unbiased validation of the program. One of the first of these was conducted by Ryan (1971b). Six speech clinicians administered S-PACK to 18 third-grade children who demonstrated frontal lisping. In addition to the 30-item criterion test used in S-PACK, he administered three additional articulation tests both before and after the program was administered. He found that 50% of the children produced over 90% correct /s/ sounds in a 2-minute conversational speech sample, and 50% scored 89% or lower, suggesting the S-PACK program may not be enough to aid these children in correct use of the /s/ phoneme in conversational speech. Results of the other three tests showed significant gain beyond the .01 level of confidence in every case. Ryan's results also indicated that programmed instructional methods can be very effective. The fact that Ryan used third-grade students while I used first-grade students might help account for the discrepancy in the results.

Other validation tests of S-PACK were conducted by Clark (1974) and Evans and Potter (1974). Clark conducted a series of studies using only the three-part S-PACK with public school children who lisped. She found that 77% of the children in grades 1–7 (319 subjects) were corrected without further help. Failure of the remaining group was attributed to dentition problems, not completing the entire program, or identifiable learning disabilities. Evans and Potter compared the effectiveness of having sixth graders administer the three-part S-PACK. They used two additional test measures in addition to the 30 item S-PACK criterion test. Results of the McDonald Deep Test (72 items) showed a mean percentage correct of three before administration of the program and 93% correct when the program was terminated. Similar results were shown for the other two tests.

Validation tests are an important aspect of program development. Just because instructional material is written in a program format does not mean that it will be effective. The speech clinician who wishes to use an instructional program in therapy should carefully review the validation measures used in checking out the program before adopting it.

So far, I have reviewed in-depth procedures I used in developing an instructional program for use in speech therapy. This should help the reader understand how components from the operant conditioning paradigm can be incorporated into the instructional process. A number of other writers have also developed programmed instructional packages not only for articulation, but for other communication disorders as well. To acquaint the reader with the wide variety of current programs, I will briefly discuss programs available in each area.

Instructional Programs
for Articulation Disorders

I am aware of approximately 20 instructional programs available for use in correcting problems of articulation. Some are especially designed for correcting only one sound, while others can be adapted for any consonant sound. Also, the format of the programs differ considerably. Some are extremely detailed down to the exact words the clinician should say. They may include all necessary pictorial stimuli, plus a description of the type of reward system to be used. Others are more general in nature allowing the clinician more freedom in choosing what is to be said or what stimuli are to be used. I will attempt to group these programs according to similarities. Although some of the programs may not rigidly adhere to all criteria for program development, the basic characteristic they all share is that they are, for the most part, replicable.

Programs to Improve Auditory Discrimination

Three programs have been constructed for helping children improve their sound discrimination. One early program developed by Holland and Matthews (1963) focused on teaching /s/ discrimination to children who had defective /s/ articulation. A teaching machine was designed to present auditory stimuli consisting of tape recorded single words, pairs of words, and isolated sounds. Children could press one of three buttons to indicate their response choice. A correct choice advanced the tape to the next item, while an incorrect choice resulted in a tape review and re-presentation of the item. Thus, the machine presentation met qualifications of a Skinnerian program in that it advanced in small steps, required the student to respond, and provided immediate feedback.

Three instructional programs were tested using 27 children from second through third grade. Program 1 was found to be the most effective for teaching discrimination of /s/. It consisted of four phases. The first phase, containing 62 items, was designed to teach presence or absence of /s/ in isolation. In phase two, the first 83 items required the child to identify which one of a pair of words began with /s/, 81 items for discrimination of the final /s/ in words, and about the same number of items to teach /s/ discrimination in the medial position. Finally, 30 words were presented and the child had to determine how many /s/ sounds were contained in each word. To show how the task increased in difficulty, the early items contained one or two obvious /s/ sounds, but the final words contained sounds similar to /s/ like /z/ and /ʃ/. Phase three contained 95 items which required the child to identify the position of the /s/ within a word. Again, the first items were easy to identify, but as the program progressed, finer discriminations were required. The last phase trained the child to discriminate misarticulated sounds from correctly articulated /s/ sounds. This phase consisted of 168 items. Average time to complete the program was 2 hours, 15 minutes. Five pretests were administered before the program began and were again administered within 3 days following completion of the program.

One of the reasons Program 1 was found to be more successful than the other two programs in improving /s/ discrimination scores was because it made better use of good programming principles. All three programs were comprised of short items to which the child responded overtly and was reinforced if correct; all insured reinforcement would occur frequently; all moved in small steps from easy tasks to more difficult ones; and all attempted to control the student's observing behavior. A big advantage was that children only needed about 10 minutes of instruction with the tape recorder, and from that point on, each child could operate the program unassisted by the clinician. In addition, the entire program was replicable so that other clinicians would be able to use the program and obtain identical results. This program constitutes an excellent example of programmed instruction applied to speech therapy.

Based on Holland's (1960) earlier work relating to the use of programming procedures for teaching /s/ discrimination, Garrett (1963) developed an automated speech correction program teaching machine. It was designed to teach auditory discrimination and self-correction of the following sounds: /s/, /ʃ/, /ɛ/, and /ʊ/. A pilot study using this program was first conducted with 16 college students who had functional misarticulations, four subjects being assigned to each program. Preliminary results indicated response accuracy was just under 90%.

The program was then administered to 80 school children between the ages of 7 years, 9 months and 12 years of age. Although several variables were tested, the main program consisted of Phase one, the auditory discrimination part, and Phase two, a self-correction part. During Phase one, a correct response resulted in a brief 600-cycle pure tone, presented in the subject's earphones. An incorrect response resulted in a "sawtooth" tone and repeat of the item. The materials included in the program followed the Skinnerian intrinsic format. Garrett (1965) concluded from a second study that much of the clinician's time could be saved in teaching sound discrimination to children using his automated speech correction program.

Garrett (1973) refined his original program even more, including an automated stimulus control system. The interested reader may wish to consult this reference for additional details about Garrett's program. He concludes that the public school clinician could handle the majority of functional misarticulation cases with an automated system of therapy. Since nonprofessionals could be taught to administer the program, this would enable the speech clinician to devote more time to severe cases. Finally, the potential savings in money using this type of programmed instruction would be substantial.

A third program by Leonard and Webb (1971) was developed to test the feasibility of administering a tape recorded automated therapy program for teaching sound discrimination and production of /ɝ/, /ɚ/, plus five vowel-r combinations. A set of five tape recordings were prepared to teach the child /ɝ/ discriminations and also to allow the child practice in matching his speech to the sample. A speech clinician monitored the child's responses and made corrections when necessary. Ten half-hour sessions were provided over a 2-week period. All children heard all tapes, regardless of their performance. A total of eight children participated in the study.

Upon completion of the study, a 30-word imitation test was given, plus a discrimination test. Significantly fewer errors were made with practice words than on nonpracticed words containing the same sounds. One interesting point of this study was that successive approximation procedures were not used, nor were tongue placement cues provided. Reinforcement was given only for correct "terminal" /ɝ/ responses. It was suggested that once accurate correct-incorrect discrimination is established, the clinician's role may be one of supervision rather than of active participation.

Fully Written Instructional Programs

Programs in this section are characterized by including all instructions the program administrator is to say to the child, even down to "Say," "No, that's not right," "Close your teeth and try it again." Nothing is left to the imagination of the administrator as far as what is to be said. In fact, some programs have been prerecorded and simply played to the child.

Most programs, especially those in this section, follow a traditional treatment of teaching sounds by beginning with sound production in isolation, followed by its use in nonsense syllables, words, phrases, sentences, and connected speech. Van Riper (1939) suggested this general procedure some forty years ago and still does in current revisions of his book; but many of his suggestions are open to varying interpretation, such as specifically how many stimulus presentations should be made, when and how often to provide reinforcement, how to keep data, when to branch, what criterion standards should be used, and the like. Also, there were no data presented to indicate what degree of success a clinician should expect. Programs written since the 1960s tighten up the vagueness found in Van Riper's methods, others developed different strategies altogether.

The S-PACK program represents an attempt to tighten up traditional procedures. The articulation programs developed by Southwest Regional Laboratory (SWRL) are very similar to the S-PACK format. As a consultant for SWRL, I helped write several of these programs under the direction of Robert Baker. The programs were produced and distributed by the American Book Company in 1973 and are now public domain.

Four SWRL programs were designed to treat problems involving the misarticulation of the following four sounds: /l/, /s/, /r/, and /θ/. Each program consists of two parts: the first part to be administered by the clinician is designed to establish the target sound in the child's repertoire. It is called the Articulation Modification Program (AMP) and requires 3 to 5 days to administer. It is comparable to the three-part S-PACK program. The second part, called the Articulation Extension Program (AEP), is analogous to the parent program of S-PACK and is designed to extend and maintain the new speech behavior. A parent or speech aide can administer this section. As in S-PACK, criterion tests are used throughout, small steps of increasing difficulty are presented, cues are systematically faded, and schedules of reinforcement are varied. One member of the SWRL staff added several games in the program as a means of making the program more acceptable to game-oriented speech clinicians as well as to provide motivation for young children. Also, sound position was emphasized.

Lyn Ausberger (1976b) followed the S-PACK format in developing a program designed to correct the /w/ for /r/ substitution. This program relies almost exclusively on parent involvement. The speech clinician's role is one of evoking /ɝ/,

/ɛɚ/, and /r/ to the criterion of 10 successive correct productions. Following this preprogram criterion, the clinician trains the parent in how to administer the remainder of the program which consists of seven parts, each part requiring 1 week to administer. The parent is encouraged to give two lessons a day for a total of 70 parent-child contacts. They are also encouraged to keep accurate data regarding correct and incorrect responses, plus attach appropriate consequences, such as verbal statement like "Good," or "No," to the child's responses.

The clinician then schedules weekly meetings with the parent and child to administer a criterion test depending on what level the child is practicing. Branching steps for the first 3 weeks are provided if the child fails to meet the criterion; otherwise, lessons are simply repeated until the criterion is met. The nature of the stimulus items involves moving from echoic to picture, to question, then to memoric type responses using ample amounts of review items. No data were presented regarding the effectiveness of this articulation program.

Two other articulation programs, which also follow a strategy similar to the S-PACK format, were written by several speech clinicians in Las Vegas, Nevada, shortly following a workshop I presented there. Dorothy Bokelman (Lundquist, 1972) obtained a school-supported grant to develop, with the aid of five school clinicians, five transfer programs for the following sounds: /θ/, /r/, /ʃ/, /l/, and /tʃ/. Those programs were designed to be used after the clinician had stabilized the target sound in the child's repertoire. They were called *transfer programs* because they helped the child use the newly learned sound in a variety of speaking situations outside the therapy room setting. They were also designed to be used by a trained speech aide such as a volunteer parent or an upper class student.

The stimulus items, like those used in the parent program of S-PACK, included naming words and pictures, filling in missing words to questions, answering questions, and telling stories from picture cues. The unique aspect common to all programs was the fact that the child was gradually moved to speech settings outside the therapy room, such as in the hallway, playground, school office, and the like. Each speaking task was slightly more difficult than the previous one.

Criterion for entering the program was that the speech student be able to produce the target sound correctly during a 10-minute sample of connected speech. Fifteen steps are included in each program, each step including 50 items. The student must produce 48 of the 50 items correctly before advancing to the next step. Failure of two items refers the child back to the clinician. Several tangible reinforcers are available to the child once he earns a sufficient number of points. Data are kept regarding the accuracy of responses. Two follow-up tests are given after program completion, one 2 weeks later and another 6 weeks later. All materials are included in each program to make them repeatable in other school settings.

One of the clinicians who worked on this project developed an /r/ correction program (Jackson, 1973), and a /ʃ/ correction program (Jackson, 1976), both of which follow the same patterns as the three-part S-PACK program. The /r/ correction program presents suggestions for evoking the /r/ and proceeds with four successive lessons to incorporate /ɚ/ and /r/ in words and sentences of the child's speech. Pre- and posttests of 14 items each are included along with four other criterion tests, one of which follows each lesson. The /ʃ/ correction program follows a similar format. Reinforcement in the form of social praise is suggested throughout the programs. No home training program was designed.

Programs That Include Only Outlines

A departure from the S-PACK programming format was presented by Baker and Ryan (1971) in a system entitled, Programmed Conditioning for Articulation. This program was developed as a "universal" type program to deal with any misarticulated consonant sound. One of the differences from programs already mentioned is that it contains branch programs in case the student fails to meet a certain criterion. If failure occurs in the other programs, they are either repeated or terminated. Failure in Baker and Ryan's program results in administration of a different instructional section bypassed by more successful students. Another basic difference is that the administrator is not told specifically what to say. For example, under a stimulus column, the clinician is instructed, "Word with x in initial position appearing randomly in 2-3 word phrase." Clinicians may all present the same words, but they may also interject various comments like, "All right, now we're going to say some words," or "Let's say these words," and the like.

This program consists of three parts. The establishment part contains 17 steps plus 91 branching steps. It directs the subject through a series of tasks, beginning with sound production in isolation, with nonsense syllables, words, phrases, sentences, and finally, conversational speech. This progression has been a very standard one commonly found in most procedures designed to correct misarticulation. All of this work is done in the speech clinic setting, either with small groups or individually.

The second part begins at the word level progressing through phrases and sentences and conversational speaking situations with the parent at home as well as with the teacher and classmates at school. This transfer program includes 15 steps but no branching sections.

Finally, the maintenance program, including five steps, was designed to see that the target sound was used consistently over a 2-month period. Extensive use is made of testing the student at various points within the program. A pretest consists of evoking 10 target sounds in conversational speech. A score of less than 80% accuracy indicates the subject should enter the program. Over 80% allows the subject to go on to the next part. Each part has its own pre- and posttest, and each step must be passed at a certain criterion level before the next step can be entered.

Reinforcement schedules are specified at each step, such as reinforcement for every correct response or every other correct response. Redeemable tokens, plus social reinforcement, are used with the first part while only social reinforcement is used with the other two parts.

Another feature which departs from the S-PACK format is the way in which the clinician's stimuli are presented. Whereas the exact words the clinician is expected to say are printed in the S-PACK, Baker and Ryan present goals such as, "Word with x in initial position appearing randomly in 2-3 word phrase." Also, the expected response, while printed in S-PACK, is referred to as *sound, phrase,* or *con-*

versation in the latter program style. Finally, Baker and Ryan use a placement procedure in that a subject can be entered at any level in the program according to test performance, whereas in the S-PACK, everyone starts at the same entry spot.

A considerable amount of testing has been completed on this program involving some 1,096 children in three test sites: in an eastern, a midwestern, and a western state (Gray, 1974). A total of 176 speech clinicians administered the programs. The results of this research, conducted primarily at the public school level, suggest public school clinicians can expect to achieve about the same improvement in articulation skills using Baker and Ryan's instructional program as the authors achieved under laboratory conditions.

This type of research strategy employed by Gray, i.e., large scale field testing of laboratory developed procedures, is seldom encountered when one investigates validity data of instructional programs available in articulation. More frequently, authors develop programs, test them using a small number of students, and make their programs available for use by thousands of speech clinicians who may alter the program instructions, misinterpret these instructions, and hence, fail to achieve the expected results. Nothing can do more harm to the programmed instruction movement than the premature introduction of instructional materials. Hopefully future programmers will follow Gray's research-based model.

Once a particular programming model has been introduced to speech clinicians, this model is used by other program writers. It has been seen that the S-PACK model was influential as a style of programming in the development of the SWRL programs, the transfer programs developed in Las Vegas, and several other program formats. The programming style of Baker and Ryan can be seen in several other articulation programs as well.

One program which closely resembles Baker and Ryan's format is an articulation program designed by Lubbert et al. (1972), to be administered by speech aides. The general presentation of instructions, stimulus cues, responses, schedule of reinforcement, and criterion levels are almost identical to the style used by Baker and Ryan. But instead of three major divisions, Lubbert et al. divided their program into only two major sections. Their General Articulation Program contained six series or phases and 23 steps. Some branch steps were included, but the clinician is encouraged to make up her own branches for the aides. The second part, the carry-over section, consists of six series and 19 steps. This part would be similar to Baker and Ryan's transfer stage. It is suggested as a maintenance procedure that the final criterion test consisting of a 30-item Speech Production Task (SPT) test, a 3-minute conversational speech test, and a 3-minute reading sample, be collected once a month for 3 months. An appendix includes all words, phrases, and story materials for correction of the following sounds: /s/, /l/, /r/, /k/, /θ/, /ð/, /ʃ/, /tʃ/, /f/, and /z/. The authors stress the need for keeping accurate data throughout the program. The program was initially standardized using 96 children and later tested using a larger subject sample with a slightly revised version of the program.

A lesser known articulation program following this same programming format was written by Waters (1974) with the aid of her graduate students. Program booklets for several consonant sounds are designed to move the child through a series of steps from sound production in isolation, through using the sound in conversation speech while telling short stories. Four steps are presented with suggestions for constructing branch steps. It is also suggested that some sort of transfer program be used after the base program is completed. This program is quite similar in scope to Jackson's two programs previously mentioned.

Stimulus Shift Programs

A third programming style was created by McLean (1965) as a result of his doctoral dissertation at a time when programming work in speech therapy was just getting under way. McLean constructed an instructional program to teach articulation skills to mentally retarded subjects through a procedure he called *stimulus shift*. First, he evoked the correct target phoneme response in words through teaching the subject to imitate his model. Then he "shifted" the correct response to three other types of stimuli which had not previously evoked the correct response. He then presented a picture stimulus, next a printed word, and finally, intraverbal chains.

Each program consisted of 10 words containing the target phoneme. In the first condition, subjects simply repeated the words until 50% of them were produced correctly during four successive trials. The second condition consisted of pairing the clinician's verbal model of the word with a picture of the word held closely to the clinician's mouth as it was spoken. When 20 consecutive correct responses were uttered by the subject, the clinician presented the picture alone. When 38 out of 40 responses were correct, the word was presented without picture or verbal cues until 38 out of 40 responses were correct. Then, phrasal settings were employed to evoke the word within phrase units. McLean found generalization from trained words to untrained words within the same position boundaries. Additional practice was required before the target phoneme generalized to connected speech. The program was completed after 78 training blocks (each containing 10 words) were presented during a 2½-week period. McLean's purpose in using this type of program was to investigate the application of operant procedures to articulation learning, rather than to develop wide application of instructional programs; consequently, his population sample size was very small.

Based on McLean's original work, Garrett (1973) adapted this general programming format into what he called a *microunit*. Altering the criterion McLean had established, eliminating the pairing condition, and including a fifth step which he called a *functional condition,* Garrett tested his microunits with 10 public school children and again with 41 others. He found that all 41 children in the second study achieved criterion (10 out of 10 successive correct productions) under all four conditions after 23 minutes of individual therapy, and all generalized to untrained words.

Garrett then combined the microunit program with Phase two of his Automated Stimulus Control System described previously. He developed a decision-making flow chart which enabled the speech clinician to decide which of the two programs to administer to children who were able to produce the target sound correctly upon command. Research results involving 152 children placed in one or both of the two instructional programs led Garrett to conclude that the public school speech clinician could handle the majority of functional articulation problems with automated programmed therapy procedures. Furthermore, much of this therapy could be conducted by nonprofessionals. Garrett was somewhat pessimistic regarding the impact his type of automated program would have on the public school delivery system. "After years of positive reports found from research studies," he stated, "only a few scattered instances can be found of classroom instruction being carried out solely by teaching machine or computer, to say nothing of programmed instruction in other forms".

Expanding on McLean's concept of stimulus control, Delbridge and Larrigan (1973) prepared a thorough treatment program for the treatment of the /s/ and /z/ phonemes. It consisted of two levels. Level 1 included echo, picture, and intra-verbal words, whereas level 2 included two and four word combinations. A transfer section was included as a final part of level 2 activities in which stories were presented, designed to evoke conversational speech. Although the programming format is much more complete than either McLean's program or Garrett's microunit, no data were presented concerning the effectiveness of the program. This is also the case with the programs developed by Jackson and Waters mentioned earlier.

Still another adaptation of McLean's stimulus-shift approach was devised by Carrier (1970), who wrote a program to be conducted by mothers of children who had articulation problems. After the clinician taught the sound in isolation, Carrier's program could be used to teach any of the consonants or blends, one at a time. Six lessons were presented, each representing a different objective. Lesson 1 consisted of 20 picture cards, 10 containing words in the initial position, and 10 representing words in the final position. As the child correctly echoed the words back to the mother, he was given poker chips and praised. When the child produced 20 consecutive correct responses, he moved on to lesson 2. Criteria for advancing to other lessons was the same. In lesson 3, the mother showed the pictures but did not name them. Pictures were paired with questions about the pictures in lesson 4. Pictures were dropped in lesson 5, and in lesson 6, objects around the house were used as stimuli. Two sessions were given daily, each evoking 60 responses.

Ten children age 4 to 7 years received the program as written by Carrier. Ten other children received a different treatment. Each child was taught the correct sound production in the clinic situation. They were given a battery of four articulation tests to determine the effectiveness of each of the programs. Results indicated that children who completed the program tended to show improvement on scores of each of the tests administered. Carrier indicated these children may use the target sound correctly in conversational speech. Each of the 10 children received less than 3 weeks total time with the parent program. It was argued that supportive personnel like mothers can help the speech clinician reduce her case load through the use of programmed materials.

Another variation of McLean's idea of pairing one stimulus with another is the Paired-Stimuli Technique by Weston and Irwin (1971). It was based on the assumption that specific, phonemic responses within a subject's repertoire could be generalized to other phonemic contexts by pairing the subject's correct production of a word with other words containing that sound. Once the subject is taught to say one word correctly, this word is then paired alternately with 10 other words until eight of the 10 words are repeated correctly during two successive sessions. A new key word with the target sound in a different position is selected and the process is repeated until both initial and final positions are corrected. This procedure has been designed to be used for correcting /s/, /r/, /ʃ/, /tʃ/, /t/, /d/, /g/, /v/, /θ/, /dʒ/, /l/, /f/, and /k/, 13 consonant sounds in the initial and final positions, as well as /z/ in the final position. The same basic program format is used for teaching all sounds.

Although there is no provision for including use of the correct target sounds in conversational speech settings, Irwin and Griffith (1973), in a follow-up study of the Paired-Stimuli Technique, stated they were confident that generalization to spontaneous speech will occur as a result of using the paired-stimuli procedures. The program was tested using 126 public school children who were trained on one target phoneme. Sixteen speech clinicians provide the therapy. A mean of 79 minutes was required to reach criterion standards on both initial and final positions for each target sound. A Screening Deep Test of Articulation and a communicative-handicappingness scale were used to evaluate the effectiveness of this procedure. The tests were administered before teaching, immediately after teaching, and 2 weeks after termination of teaching. Results indicated that the percent of acceptable productions increased from preteaching to postteaching and were maintained 2 weeks later. Improvement on the other eight nontaught phonemes did not occur.

Specific Sound-Evoking Program

Shriberg (1975) wrote an eight-step program for the sole purpose of evoking /ɝ/. His program writing style is simple to follow and consists of three objectives, the exact instructions to be given by the clinician, a response definition, exact verbal statements which serve as reinforcers, and termination criteria. The program was delivered to 65 children from 4 to 12 years of age by 19 clinicians. Seventy percent of the children progressed through the program in a mean time of 6 minutes of instruction and attained correct /ɝ/ productions. Shriberg concluded that his systematic procedure greatly increased the speech clinician's effectiveness in evoking /ɝ/. He felt once the /ɝ/ was evoked and adequately stabilized, other instructional programs which begin at this level could then be administered in order to incorporate the sound in words as well as conversational speech.

Distinctive Feature Programs

A more recent advent in articulation programming, a departure from the traditional content discussed so far, is the use of programming in distinctive feature therapy. One of the earliest adaptations of distinctive feature therapy was suggested by McReynolds and Bennett (1972). Unfortunately, the article reporting their investigation of feature generalization did not include a complete description of their program, hence, it is not possible to duplicate their work. The description presented indicated that the program consisted of two phases. Phase 1 taught the child to produce the feature as contained in a phoneme in the initial position in a nonsense syllable, while Phase 2 taught production in the final position. Each phase could consist of five steps each requiring the child to perform a more complex task. Continuous reinforcement was provided during imitation training. When a 90% correct criterion was reached, pictures were used to evoke responses. Reinforcement was on an FR-3 schedule; although program description was sketchy, this represented a first attempt at programming this type of therapy.

It was not until some four years later that Costello and Onstine (1976) published a replicable distinctive feature program they used to remediate /t/, /θ/, and /s/. In actuality, their program amounted to an extension of the work done by McReynolds and Bennett (1972). Two children just past the age of 4 years were selected as subjects to whom the program was administered. Both children used the continuant feature only partially and since stops were substituted for continuants, /t/, the sound substituted for /θ/ and /s/, was selected as a step which could be contrasted with continuants /θ/ and /s/. Each child was scheduled individually for 30-minute sessions 4 days a week until the program was completed. One child required 32 sessions; the other required 50 sessions. The authors point out that their purpose in presenting this program was only to demonstrate the feasibility of adapting programming techniques to feature therapy, not to present a thoroughly tested, standardized program.

Their programming techniques were based on the Skinnerian model in that it comprises a series of small steps, each increasing in difficulty. Nine phases representing nine major goals were written, along with a series of 21 steps designed to accomplish these goals. The general format resembles the one designed by Baker and Ryan (1971) in that general stimulus events are identified, rather than specific verbal statements to be read; general responses are indicated as well as the reinforcement schedule and criterion levels. Branch steps are provided if the child does not reach criterion levels.

The authors present a detailed description of administration procedures which include definition of correct responses, consequence alternatives, use of different schedules of reinforcement, the token economy system, criterion levels, branching, data recording system, and control of off-task behavior. The conclusion reached after administering this program to the two children studied was that it was an effective device to use in teaching correct articulation to the two children studied.

Several other programs such as *Programmed Articulation Therapy,* developed by Psaltis and Spallato (1973), have been written in a programmed format but will not be reviewed here because of space limitations.

A summary of articulation programs reviewed in this chapter which were designed during the 15-year period between 1961 and 1976, is presented in Figure 9–4. Note that an attempt has been made to group these programs according to the general format each follows. As can be seen in Figure 9–4, the boom years in articulation programming were 1970–74. This is about 10 years after a large group of programs were written for classroom instruction in mathematics, social studies, and language arts. It is difficult to predict what future developments may transpire in articulation programming.

Program Development in Articulation

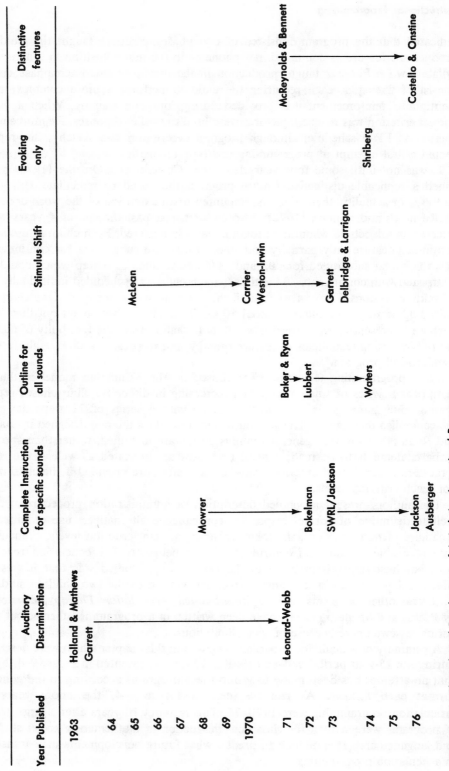

FIGURE 9-4. *Chronological Development of Articulation Instructional Programs*

It would be interesting to find out how many working clinicians presently make use of these programs.

The trend in programming in articulation seems to be as follows: first research-oriented individuals develop programming strategies designed to test out certain hypotheses. The more successful or promising program strategies are adopted by a few practicing speech clinicians or others interested in research application. They, in turn, modify the programs somewhat, and eventually, some of these programs find their way to the market place where they are bought and used by other practicing speech clinicians seeking more effective procedures. These programs, some of which have never been field-tested, undergo further modification in the hands of the practicing clinicians. Certainly, the clinician who administers programs should be in a much better position to individualize instruction than could be expected from using a "prepackaged" program. However, by the time an instructional program is delivered to a child in whatever form, one can expect that many modifications will have been made on the original design. Hopefully, these modifications will result in an improvement of the program's effectiveness.

Instructional Programs for Stuttering

Instructional programs for the treatment of stuttering have lagged behind those written for the treatment of articulation disorders. Only within the past few years have several instructional programs in stuttering been offered commercially. At present, there are less than a dozen such programs reported in the literature, although there are many "neo-programs." This is because for many years, therapeutic emphasis has been placed on changing the stutterer's attitudes and feelings, thus making clinicians reluctant to adopt tight, programming techniques for such elusive concepts as attitudes, self-concepts, and anxiety feelings. Each stutterer was considered as having a unique set of needs, and these needs could be met best through an individualistic counseling approach. Nevertheless, a wide variety of procedures for the treatment of stuttering have been proposed.

Delayed Auditory Feedback

One of the first attempts at programming therapy for stutterers was reported by Goldiamond (1965). He took the position that stuttering, like any other verbal behavior, was an operant behavior that could be modified by systematically manipulating its consequences. Following a sizeable number of research projects which began in 1958, Goldiamond developed a standardized procedure using delayed auditory feedback at varying delay settings. The first step is establishment of a baseline of initial speaking performance, followed by three or four sessions in which the stutterer learns to correctly identify instances of stuttering. Then, about three sessions are devoted to the use of delayed auditory feedback beginning with 250 milliseconds delay. The stutterer learns to prolong vowels and slow down speech rate during this phase. Next, about five sessions are conducted during which the auditory delayed feedback is gradually faded out in 50 millisecond steps, while speech rate is increased during and following termination of the feedback. Finally, home-reading assignments were provided to insure fluency. Fluency was thus maintained in home-speaking situations.

A large number of studies were conducted between 1959 and 1969 to study the effects of delayed auditory feedback as a treatment procedure to reduce stuttering. Several of these studies reported "programs" which were successful in establishing fluency. One of the more sophisticated programs using this procedure was developed by Ryan and Van Kirk (1971). A basic outline of the steps in this program is presented in Figure 9-5.

Step	Stimulus	Response
1–3	Identification of stuttered words.	Identify stuttered words.
4	Instructions to read slowly. Set DAF at 250.	Read slowly in prolonged manner with DAF earphones.
5	Instructions to read slowly. Set DAF at 200.	Read slowly in prolonged manner with DAF earphones.
6	Instructions to read slowly. Set DAF at 150.	Read slowly in prolonged manner with DAF earphones.
7	Instructions to read. Set DAF at 100.	Read slowly in slightly prolonged manner with DAF earphones.
8	Instructions to read. Set DAF at 50.	Read with DAF earphones.
9	Instructions to read. Set DAF at 0.	Read with DAF earphones.
10	Instructions to read.	Read
11–30	Recycle with monologue and conversation.	Monologue or conversation.

FIGURE 9-5. Steps In Ryan's Delayed Auditory Feedback (DAF) Program (From Homans, John, A Textbook of Surgery 6th ed., 1945.
Courtesy of Charles C Thomas, Publisher, Springfield, Illinois.)

Branch programs were also written. After the stutterer completes the delayed auditory feedback program, a transfer program is presented followed by a rate control program.

This type of treatment procedure lends itself very nicely to programming techniques since the steps in delayed auditory feedback are clearly definitive as in the response class, i.e., stuttering behavior. One merely has to specify the size of the steps, set a criterion for moving from one step to the next, and attach a positive consequent event to correct responses. There is no direct attempt to alter the individual's feelings or attitudes.

A program patterned after Goldiamond's DAF program called Conversational Rate Control Therapy was written by Curlee and Perkins (1969). Phase 1 of this program consisted of two steps. Step one included the five parts of the DAF sequence designed to establish a slow rate of fluent speaking. The DAF is first set at 250 milliseconds delay at maximum intensity. The stutterer is instructed to talk until she can converse for two consecutive 15-minute periods with no stuttering. The same criterion is used for the second sequence at 200 milliseconds delay. During the third sequence, DAF is reduced to 50 millisecond steps using the same criterion until no delay is used. If two instances of stuttering occur within a 5-minute period, the stutterer is returned to the previous DAF step. It is not entirely clear to me why the DAF reduction sequence is repeated in sequences four and five of this program, but evidently, a repetition is required, beginning again at 200 millisecond delay, working down through 150, 100, 50, and 0 millisecond delay periods.

Step two involves a time-out procedure wherein 30 seconds of silence plus extinction of a room light is contingent on stuttering. Gradually, the length of time, light extinction, plus silence, is reduced by 5-second time intervals until the stutterer can speak fluently for two 15-minute periods. Phase 2 consists of two steps designed to extend fluent speaking to everyday speaking situations. The author's report data of 14 adolescent and adult stutterers which indicate that about 30 hours of therapy are required to complete this program. The average rate of stuttering was reduced to 1.3 times per 30 minutes of speaking time upon program completion. Clients observed their stuttering decreased from 75% to 95% in situations outside the clinic in which clinicians were not present to observe them.

Several other delayed auditory feedback programs have been reported and reviewed (Soderberg, 1969; Ryan, 1974).

"Traditional" Therapy Programming

A great deal of what has been labeled *symptomatic treatment* in stuttering as part of the treatment suggested by Van Riper (1964) and several other clinicians was adapted to a program type format by Ryan (1964) and reported subsequently in his book (Ryan, 1974). In its present form, it consists of 10 steps to establish fluency in reading using identification, cancellations, pullouts, and prolongation procedures; 10 steps using the same procedures during monologue speaking conditions; and 10 steps for establishing fluency in conversation—a total of 30 steps. Branch steps are provided should the individual fail at any step. Ryan (1974) reported results with 19 stutterers ranging in age from 10 to 43, totaling some 247 hours of therapy time. All subjects but one decreased rate of stuttering under this program. Ryan was not entirely satisfied with these results, primarily because while stuttering decreased significantly, what might be considered "normal" fluency was not achieved. His work represents one of the few attempts to place traditional type therapy procedures in a programmed format. Shames (1970) outlines a program similar to the one suggested by Ryan.

Increasing Mean Length of Utterance

Several investigators have developed instructional programs which consist of establishing fluency by requesting the stutterer to first say one-word utterances until a criterion of fluency is met, then two-word utterances, followed by three-word utter-

Year Published	DAF	Increase Utterance Length	Traditional
1964			Ryan
1965	Goldiamond	Rickard & Mundy	
1966			
1967	Perkins		
1968			
1969	Perkins	Leach	
1970			
1971	Ryan & Van Kirk Ingham & Andrews	Ryan & Van Kirk Mowrer	
1972			
1973			
1974			
1975			
1976			
1977			
1978		Mowrer	
1979			
1980			

ances, and so on until the stutterer is able to speak fluently in conversation. One of the first such programs was developed by Rickard and Mundy (1965), who reported using this sequence of increasing utterance length from single words to phrases and sentences. Fluent speech was successfully established. Later, both Leach (1969) and Shaw and Shrum (1972) reported successful results using essentially this same type of program.

I also constructed a program based on increasing the mean length of utterance which was quite similar to those developed earlier. This program (Mowrer, 1971) contains nine parts, each divided into four to nine steps. Each step consists of the following:

Program Developments in Stuttering

Thematic Content Desensitization & Relaxation	Home Program	Punishment	Controlled Speech
	Emery		
		Haroldson, Martin & Star	
Lanyon			
Shames			
	McGough, Peins & Lee	Martin & Gaviser	
Calatta & Rubin			
Tyre, Marsto, Companik, Zenner			Webster
		Costello	
			Shames & Florance

1. Instructions to be read to the stutterer by the clinician about specifically what the stutterer is to do during that step.

2. Instructions to the clinician concerning special features about the particular activities during that step.

3. How long the speaking time should be.

4. Nature of the consequent event.

5. How to score the responses.

6. Criterion for moving to the next step.

7. What to do if the criterion is not met. A sample of one of the steps is presented in Figure 9–6.

Step A-5 Word List 2

> *Subject's Instructions:* "Now we'll change the loudness of the signal." (If the light is used say, "We'll use the light signal this time.") "Read from List 2 in order."
>
> *Clinician's Instructions:* Use the light timer, set at 6 on and off per minute, if available. If using the beep tape, reduce the volume of the recorder until it can just barely be heard.
>
> *Cycle:* 10-minute period or if light is used, stop after 120 two-word combinations have been read.
>
> *CES:* 1 "good" to each fluent 2 word combination.
>
> *Score:* x = 2 words
>
> *JUMP:* Go to Step A-6 when 3 consecutive cycles have been completed each containing no more than 6 disfluencies.
>
> *Stop:* If JUMP criteria is not met within 6 cycle attempts go to Branch Step A-5BR. If 5 and 6 are successful, then do a 7th cycle.

FIGURE 9-6. Step A-5 Of The S-1 Fluency Program

The first six parts of the program deal with stabilizing fluency in situations in which word lists and paragraphs are read and conversations are held with the clinician. Two parts are designed to transfer fluency to school, home, and telephone situations, and the last part deals with maintaining fluency. The program is designed so it can be duplicated with little or no training on the part of the clinician who administers it.

Data from 20 subjects age 8 to 43 years who completed part or all of the nine programs indicated that the further the subjects went through the program parts, the greater the degree of fluency (Mowrer, 1975). A mean of 5½ hours was required to complete at least 75% of the program parts.

Mowrer (1979) revised the S-1 program to make it more adaptable for students in the elementary school setting. Materials also are included for use with adult stutterers. A reading level of at least second grade is required to complete the program. Six program parts are included, designed to establish fluent speech under a wide variety of speaking situations. As the final objective of this program, the client will speak to the speech pathologist for 5 minutes about selected topics while maintaining 98% fluency. There is no attempt to transfer the fluent speech established in the clinic or school setting to other speaking situations outside these settings. The speech pathologist must devise the assignments necessary to make the transition with each client. Procedures are expected to differ greatly, depending upon the nature of the speech problem and the age of the client. This program is self contained and could be delivered by an aide. A minimum of about 7 hours of therapy time is required to administer all six programs.

Ryan and Van Kirk (1971) also used the principle of increasing mean length of utterance in a 54-step program, beginning with reading single words, and proceeding through the steps until 5-minute sessions of fluent, conversational speech are evoked. Branch programs were constructed to be used if criterion was not met within specified time or accuracy standards. Data are presented for nine stutterers ranging in age from 7 to 35 years, representing 207 hours of therapy. Ryan (1974) reports these programs, designed to gradually increase utterance length, are highly successful in producing fluent speech. He also noted a saving in therapy time since much of the attention given to the stuttering behavior itself, found in many traditional treatments, is omitted.

Other versions of this type of program reported in an article by Ryan (1971a) were designed to be used with young children, including preschool children who were unable to read. These programs began by presenting very simple tasks which required utterance of one word, and by altering the stimulus conditions, required longer and longer utterances. Ryan strongly recommends this type of program as an excellent treatment procedure for child stutterers.

Thematic Content and Desensitization Procedures

There have been some attempts to modify stuttering frequency simply by attaching positive or negative statements to certain types of remarks made by stutterers about their speech or speaking situations. This procedure is one which is easily programmed. Williams (1957) discussed a basic rationale for this type of therapy. In a discussion of programs designed to modify the stutterer's basic attitude about his speech, Shames (1970) lists three such program formats.

In the first program, the clinician engages in conversation with the stutterer and reacts favorably to the stutterer's positive statements about his speech or speaking situations. The stutterer might say, "I stuttered less today," to which the clinician might say, "Good, I'm glad to hear that." Negative statements by the stutterer are reacted to by such comments as, "I don't understand," or "I don't agree." The stutterer receives no instructions as to what the intent of the sessions are. Frequently, the clinician may interject noncontingent comments to encourage conversation like, "Now let's talk about your job."

A second program requires the clinician to respond encouragingly to positive statements made by the stutterer, but no reply is provided to negative statements. Finally, the third program is similar to the first program with the exception that noncontingent responses are not made by the clinician. These are the types of responses which are necessary to keep conversation flowing. If the stutterer does not say anything, the clinician remains silent.

Data of four subjects are presented by Shames, and in all cases, stuttering behavior was reduced during the 12 to 14 sessions of the therapy period. Although these programs cannot be considered "true" programs in the sense that no criterion levels are established and there is no progression in task difficulty, it would be impossible to tighten the format into a more formalized program structure. It would be difficult to anticipate exactly what the clinician should say in terms of antecedent and consequent event statements since each stutterer would have different feelings to express. There seems to be little attempt on the part of clinicians to devise other thematic content programs, partly because of these problems, plus the fact that high levels of fluency have not been obtained using the procedures described above. Additional work in this area is presented by Shames and Egolf (1976).

Another stuttering treatment currently receiving considerable attention in the literature is the use of desensitization procedures as a way of dealing with the stutterer's attitudes.

The literature in this area is far too broad to be covered in this section; consequently, only a few references will be selected as examples of programming. Here again, "clean-cut" programs have not been written in these areas, but the procedures reported approach what might be considered a program format.

Drawing from the work of Rachman (1967) and Wolpe (1959) regarding systematic desensitization, Lanyon (1969) adapted these procedures to a programmed approach in the treatment of an adult stutterer using a manual he and others developed (Lanyon et al., 1968). The first few sessions were spent practicing muscle relaxation exercises, accompanied by 15–20 minute daily home practice periods for the first 2 weeks.

A 29-item fear hierarchy of selected speaking situations was then constructed. The stutterer was asked to signal when anxiety feelings were aroused by picturing the feared speaking situations. Desensitization consisted of first getting the stutterer in a relaxed state, then requesting her to imagine the first item on the fear hierarchy. When the stutterer had succeeded in imagining an item for two 10-second intervals without anxiety, the next item was again presented. Following the sessions, the subject in this experiment showed considerable improvement.

A follow up of Lanyon's procedure was reported by Tyre et al. (1973), who used essentially the same type of program with another adult stutterer. Two types of fear hierarchies were developed: one for an academic speaking environment, and one for speaking in social settings. Again, the stutterer was first presented with relaxation exercises, followed by the same desensitization process used by Lanyon during the sessions. Improvement in fluent speech of the stutterer reported by Tyre et al. was much the same as Lanyon reported. While each subject's fear hierarchy may be different, the program format for all cases is essentially the same; most important is the fact that these procedures are replicable, a basic prerequisite for programmed instruction. It would be impossible, though, to devise a program of this type specifying specific words to be spoken by both the clinician and subject or identifying fear situations common to all stutterers.

Another type of program that falls into this category of changing attitudes about fluency is one devised by Culatta and Rubin (1973). Their point of view is that the stutterer must be taught to take responsibility for his own speech behavior. The task of the clinician is to structure and direct conversational topics so the stutterer gives certain critical responses. The success of the program depends on the clinician's skill in asking relevant questions and evoking responses from the stutterer which reflect changes in the attitudes about his fluency.

Culatta and Rubin's program actually consists of two sections. The first six objectives deal with what the authors classify as the cognitive area, or changing the way in which the stutterer feels about his stuttering. During this portion of the program, the objective is to help the stutterer understand that he is capable of speaking fluently, and if he wishes to become fluent, he must accept the responsibility for doing so. Obviously, it would be difficult to specify the exact statements to be made by the clinician since much of what the clinician says depends on the responses of the stutterer.

Following progression through the first six objectives, five additional objectives concentrate on speech performance characteristics, or what the authors call *manner of production*. It is during this section of the program that fluent speech is practiced. Each objective has one criterion which must be reached before moving to the next objective.

Data were presented for six male subjects from 19 to 33 years of age. Following baseline measurements, the 11-step program was completed by all subjects in two to four sessions, separated by intervals of 2 to 5 days. Maximum completion time was 11 days. Fluency was assessed immediately after program completion. A chi-square analysis revealed that reduction in stuttering was significant for all six subjects according to words spoken on the pre- and posttest. With regard to attitude change, three subjects changed their attitude as measured by five changes out of six questions, while two subjects showed little attitude change. One subject altered half of his initial responses on the six-item test.

Here again, it is not possible to replicate this program completely, first, because complete instructions were not provided by the authors, and second, due to the unique individuality of each stutterer, it would be impossible to completely program this type of treatment procedure.

Finally, Zenner (1976) reports of work he has done in the cognitive and performance areas as well as in the intellectual area to treat stuttering. He uses desensitization procedures described by Lanyon, but again, it is not possible to build a formal program using his procedures.

Learning Controlled Speech Patterns

Two recent programs have been developed that focus upon teaching the client a new way of talking. This newly learned controlled speech pattern is then used in daily speaking situations. Webster's (1975) Precision Fluency Shaping Program (PFSP) uses a standardized procedure of teaching five target behaviors: prolonging the syllable, blending syllables together, motorplanning syllable change, taking a full breath, and initiating syllables with gentle onset. He maintains that the stutterer must meet exacting standards when learning to produce these target behaviors. He uses the Voice Monitor, a measurement device, to assist stutterers in determining exact loudness levels of voice onset curves. Webster feels we should approach the therapeutic process as an exact science, not as an art. Therefore, procedures used in counseling designed to alter attitudes are not employed in his program. The program is designed to be given during an intensive 3 week, daily therapy period. Webster also wants the person who administers this program to be thoroughly trained in using the procedures so that the target behaviors are mastered to exacting criterion standards.

Webster (1980) presented data about 200 subjects who were randomly selected from over 1,000 stutterers who had completed his program. The mean of disfluent words taken from reading and spontaneous speaking samples was 15.2% during pretreatment and 1.3% during posttreatment, 19 days later. Disfluent speech rose to only 3.2% when follow-up speech samples were taken from the same individuals, 10 months later.

The Perceptions of Stuttering Inventory (PSI), a self-report inventory developed by Woolf (1967), was also administered during the same test periods. The PSI proportedly measures how satisfied one is with her speech. The mean pretreatment score was 30.4 while the mean posttreatment score, 10 months later, was 5.7 and 9.2. Nonstuttering speakers obtain scores of 10 or under.

According to another subjective rating questionnaire administered after treatment, most clients reported they no longer stuttered except for an occasional repetition. Eighty-three percent of the subjects reported their fluency was adequate.

A few clients show little or no change in fluency as a result of attending Webster's program. He explains that some people are not skilled in obtaining new motor skills. They may be reinforced for stuttering in the social environment. Some of the clinicians may fail to deliver the program with required precision. Also, the technology of program procedures has not been perfected. Nevertheless, the data reported by Webster are impressive.

D. Schwartz and L. Webster (1977) designed a variation of Webster's program. Instead of intensive therapy, clients were seen three times a week for 2-hour sessions during 3 months. The total hours of therapy amounted to about the same as Webster's Roanoke clinic program. They report that 97% of the 29 subjects studied showed a positive change in fluency. About 70% of the subjects attained fluency levels of 94% or better compared with Webster's (1975) report that 80% achieved a fluency level of 97% or better. D. Schwartz and L. Webster conclude that although their results were not quite as impressive as Webster's, their program was less expensive and required neither extensive travel nor absence from school or work.

The important feature about D. Schwartz and L. Webster's data is that Webster's program can be replicated with comparable results.

One of the most recent programs developed is called Stutter-Free Speech written by Shames and Florence (1980). In this program, the client learns a system of behavioral tactics and rules to help her either move progressively toward stutter-free speech, or back up to speaking in a more systematic manner. The program is divided into five phases. In phase one, the client learns to develop volitional control over speech using delayed auditory feedback. Self reinforcement and monitoring stutter-free volitional control over speech is the goal of phase two. In phase three, the newly learned speech pattern is transferred to other speaking situations outside the clinic environment, and during phase four monitored speech is replaced with unmonitored speech. Finally, phase five involves follow-up of stutterers who have completed the program.

The authors present a program outline of each phase of the program including the following features: step, training task, conditions, time, target behavior, contingency for off-target responses, and reinforcement. Results of seven clients who successfully completed this program are discussed.

Punishment Programs

Fortunately for the stutterer, at least, there have been no total programs which feature severe punishment as the sole treatment method. Parts of some programs include punishment phases, or they have been used only on a short-term experimental basis. Martin (1968) described several different experiments in which punishment procedures were used to establish fluency. It would be difficult to classify these isolated studies as "programs" since criterion standards and program steps as such were not identified. Punishment programs of this nature could be developed, but because of the temporary effects punishment has on reducing stuttering, plus the undesirable side effects resulting from punishment procedures, it is doubtful if any clinicians will pursue such treatment procedures which utilize shock or other types of strongly aversive stimuli.

Time-out procedures which are a milder form of punishment have been successfully used in reducing stuttering behavior by a number of clinicians (Martin & Gaviser, 1971; Haroldson et al., 1968). Costello (1975) outlines the basics of this simple procedure in a format that could easily be programmed. The procedure consists of simply attending to fluent utterances with smiles, positive remarks, and the like, and following occasions of stuttering with the word *stop*, plus withdrawal of attention for a period of 10 seconds during which time the stutterer is not permitted to speak. The stutterer resumes speaking and continues to receive positive feedback for fluent speech until another occasion of stuttering. Reports of three cases were presented, all showing drastic reduction of stuttering behavior in reading, monologue, and conversational speaking situations. Although Costello points out that the procedures are replicable, an instructional program as such was not presented. More information regarding specific stimulus events and criterion levels would be required before this procedure could be used as a "program."

Home Study Programs

There have been a few attempts to create home study programs to enable the stutterer to monitor her own progress through a series of written or tape recorded lessons. Ted Emery developed a correspondence course for stutterers from his office in Florida and has collected an impressive list of testimonials from stutterers attesting to the fact that their speech as been helped through home study* Basically, Emery uses the approach of helping the stutterer develop self-confidence and good speech habits through a series of correspondence lessons mailed to the stutterer's home. Here again, this would not be considered a true instructional program since criterion levels for advancement are not established, there is no immediate feedback, and small, sequential steps are not developed.

In an attempt to find more efficient and effective ways of treating stuttering, McGough, Peins, and Lee (1971) compared a home-based, tape-recorded centered therapy program with traditional therapy and no therapy at all. Their findings, involving a sample of 36 stutterers, indicated that the home-based program utilizing programmed cassette tape lessons was more effective in reducing stuttering than were the other two conditions. The tape series consisted of 12 highly structured 30-minute tape recordings which the stutterer listened to over a 6-month period. One tape-recorded lesson is sent to the stutterer every 2 weeks, which he listens to daily. The stutterer records vocal exercises on the tape as well. Every 2 weeks the stutterer meets with the speech clinician to discuss his progress. Each taped lesson

---

* Personal communication. For more information write: The Emery Institute, Box 867, Winter Park, Fla. 32789.

includes structured practice in oral reading, conversational speaking, telephone work, stressful and nonstressful speaking situations, practice on difficult words and phrases, introductions, impromptu and extemporaneous speaking situations. Peins, McGough, and Lee (1971) pointed out several advantages of this type of self-improvement program. This program could be viewed as being similar to other home-study programs available in so many academic areas, one difference being that the subject must provide his own positive or negative feedback rather than depend solely on a "key" or a clinician's feedback. Support for self-administered feedback is provided from results of a study by Cross and Cooper (1976). They found that the least amount of stuttering occurred in therapy sessions with stutterers in which subjects were made responsible for reinforcing their own fluent speech. This datum suggests that program writers may not always be required to "build-in" external feedback into their instructional program.

Another clinician who also utilized cassette tape lessons as a follow up to his therapy is Martin Schwartz as reported by Lee (1976). Once the stutterer has had a few weeks of intensive therapy in the clinical setting, he returns home where he is contacted frequently via instructional taped cassettes. Since each stutterer is dealt with differently with regard to information contained in the cassette tapes, these tapes could hardly be viewed as programmed lessons.

Miscellaneous Programs

I reserved this section for program formats which do not exactly fit under the above categories. One is a telephone program I developed (Mowrer, 1969). It was a very simple program and has been used with only a few stutterers. It was designed to increase fluency in the home environment once fluency was established in the clinic setting. The clinician listened to the stutterer read from a magazine for a period of 15 minutes or until five disfluencies were uttered—whichever came first. Criterion was reached when five consecutive 15-minute readings were accumulated with no disfluencies. This program is outlined in Figure 9–7.

Biofeedback is a recent addition to stuttering therapy; it allows the stutterer to view his state of tension or relaxation on an oscilloscope which displays EMG signals. Lanyon et al. (1976) attached electrodes to the stutterer's face and jaw area where tension was high during stuttering. Their program consisted of asking the stutterer to say words keeping the oscilloscope wave form, which indicated tension, as small as possible.

They were also asked to count from 1 to 100 while watching the wave form. On each alternate 100 word series, the feedback was turned off. Six complete on-off alternations were collected for each subject. Other subjects were given several lists of 100 common one-syllable words to read, followed by two-syllable words, three-syllable phrases, and four-syllable sentences. A 95% criterion level of fluency was used for passing each step. Lanyon et al. found stuttering was greatly reduced or absent during the controlled experiments.

There are two other recent programs, both commercially available, for the treatment of stuttering. One is called the Personal Fluency Kit developed by Cooper (1976). One part of this kit includes a fluency control program involving procedures to reduce speech rate through a series of steps involving production of single syl-

Telephone Program for Stutterers

1. Dial stutterer's phone number.

2. "Hello. This is _____."
"Are you ready?" If answer is "No," wait until he returns to the phone with the appropriate reading material.
When answer is "Yes," continue to step 3.

3. "Turn to page _____." (pause)

4. "Begin reading at the top of page _____."
(Begin timing now)

5. When a stuttered word is uttered, count it aloud. ("One" for first stuttered word, "Two" for second, etc.)
After saying the number, say "Stop. 1–1000, 2–1000, 3–1000, 4–1000, 5–1000. Begin reading." The subject must be silent until the clinician says ". . . Begin reading."

6. After saying "5" for the fifth stuttered word, draw a ring around that word, note the exact time and say, "Your time is up. Goodbye." After the stutterer says "Goodbye", hang up.

7. Scoring. You will record two bits of information on the 3-cycle graph, (1) the total number of words read aloud from the reading material, and (2) the total number of words he could have spoken in the time recorded for that session (150 × minutes).

FIGURE 9-7. *Experimental Program To Increase Fluency During Telephone Conversations*

lables: one-, two-, and three-syllable words, sentences, and paragraphs. Easy speech onset is practiced in words and paragraphs. Deep breathing is learned as words and sentences, then paragraphs are produced. The same type of sequence is followed in teaching loudness control, easy contact speech, and syllable stress. Three other parts of this kit deal with other aspects of stuttering, such as identification of the problem, attitudes, and examination of the problem. The entire kit is reported to be a highly structured program with explicit guides and therapy procedures.

Eclectic Approach

Finally, one other treatment program will be presented because it represents an eclectic approach to the programming of remedial procedures. Developed by Boberg (1976), it features an intensive type therapy in which stutterers reside at the treatment center for 3 weeks, similar to the Ingham and Andrews program (1971). Treatment procedures feature teaching prolongation and cancellation procedures within a behavior modification framework. Five phases of treatment are outlined, most of which employ clinician-operated counters, clock timers and discrete consequent events. Criterion level for continuing from one phase to the next is 98% fluency on a specified task. Data are presented describing the performance of 21 stutterers who completed the program (1973–74). Although no difficulty was experienced in establishing a high level of fluency, follow-up investigation revealed the high level of fluency is not maintained once the client leaves the treatment environment.

Summary of Stuttering Programs

It has already been mentioned that effective, clean-cut programs have been difficult to devise for the treatment of stuttering. Perhaps the nature of the stuttering problem does not lend itself to remediation through programmed type instructional methods. On the other hand, certain aspects of the stuttering problem can be effectively dealt with using programming techniques. It may be that programmed materials could best be applied to establish fluency, whereas other individually tailored counseling techniques would be more appropriate for dealing with attitudes and feelings held by stutterers.

Instructional
Programs for Voice Training

Very little work has been reported regarding the development of instructional programs for the treatment of voice disorders. The few attempts reported deal with problems associated with vocal nodules, which result from vocal abuse. Tom Johnson at Utah State University has been primarily responsible for the development of several programmed treatment approaches to voice disorders, the first of which appeared in 1969 (Johnson, 1974). This led to the development of a vocal abuse modification program written by Hunsaker (1970), and later refined by Johnson (1975).

This program contained a detailed outline of eight therapy sessions, each session consisting of from seven to ten steps. Basically, the first session was designed to explain the nature and cause of vocal abuse to the parent and child through the use of pictures and verbal description. The purpose of the program and its operation was also explained, i.e., target behaviors, using the wrist counter, data collection periods, situations in which counting will occur, and the like. The child was given an assignment for the following week. The remaining sessions consisted of checking on the child's progress, charting behaviors, providing reinforcement, and evaluating voice quality. Periodic rechecks were scheduled as necessary. Johnson (1975) reported that the success of the program has been high (over 90%) in reducing vocal nodules.

A pitch-change program, designed by two students under Johnson's direction, Coachbuilder (1972) and Greiner (1973), consisted of a comprehensive program for changing pitch which incorporated traditional pitch-change procedures. Their program had 14 steps designed to raise pitch in a step-by-step manner. They contained all necessary clinician instructions, specific stimulus events, response specification, consequence specifications including schedule changes, criterion levels for moving to the next program step, as well as branch programs. Data for only a few subjects completing this program have been reported.

Another program for the modification of hoarse voice quality resulting from vocal abuse was presented by Drudge and Philips (1976). Their program was aimed at shaping the client's voice quality through a series of steps which serve to gradually increase the duration and complexity of tasks until the goal of clear voice quality in spontaneous conversation is reached. Each step of the 31-step program was designed to accomplish one of four major goals: (1) elimination of vocal abuse, (2) easy initiation of phonation, (3) increase clear phonation time, and (4) increase in loudness without increase in laryngeal tension. Self-evaluation, which leads to elimination of hard glottal attacks, is verbally reinforcing on a variable schedule. Criterion levels for each step in the program are also identified. Data for three subjects are presented, indicating that the criterion of 80% success was met on each step by all subjects, although time required to meet each requirement differed greatly among subjects.

Bensen (1978) designed a program to change habits resulting in vocal abuse, for use with children six years of age and older who can read at the first grade level. This program is divided into three parts. The goal of the first section, Program A, is the systematic reduction of vocal intensity levels as measured by a sound level meter in the clinic setting. Criterion measures required to advance from one step of the program to another are stated in decibel ranges, indicated by sound level meter readings. Program B is designed to establish control over vocal abuse in situations outside the clinic, such as at home and at school. The third section, Program C, is administered by trained siblings at home in an attempt to permanently change vocal abuse habits that occur in specific situations. Two other, optional, programs are available: one to establish correct vocal behavior in the playground, and a parent management program used in the home. Programs A and B also can be used with adults who abuse their voice through loud talking. Bensen's program is fully self-contained including visual stimuli, record forms, and referral forms. One need only purchase an inexpensive sound level meter (under $50.00) from a local electronics shop. Unfortunately, no data have been published regarding the effectiveness of Bensen's program.

In view of the fact that the prevalence of children who have voice disorders range from estimates of 6% (James & Cooper, 1966) to 23% (Silverman & Zimmer, 1975), it is surprising that there has not been more activity in developing instructional programs for the treatment of voice disorders. Results of several surveys indicate that voice disorder cases make up only from 2 to 4% of the clinician's caseload (Black, 1964; Bingham et al., 1961). Deal et al. (1976) suggest that the lack of instructional programs in the area of voice disorders may account for the reason why so few voice cases are selected for therapy. They feel many clinicians simply are not aware of specific procedures which can be used to alter voice quality. This fact may be ample justification in support of developing instructional programs. They offer the clinician very specific types of guidance in planning and therapy. Of course, a clinician's individual therapy procedures may vary widely from program formats depending on individual cases, but nevertheless, the general instructional strategy remains intact.

Newly developed programs such as the one by Wilson (1977) may help remedy the lack of instructional materials available for the treatment of voice disorders.

Instructional
Programs for Aphasia

Whereas Johnson was responsible for much of the work done in programming therapy for the treatment of voice disorders, Holland (1969) was responsible for initiating the use of instructional program techniques aimed at rehabilitating aphasic patients. Taylor (1964) also was very influential in devising programmed materials for aphasic patients. Other earlier efforts employing principles of programming with aphasics included the work of Filby and Edwards (1963), and Rosenberg (1965), who programmed specific tasks for aphasics such as form and perceptual discrimination tasks.

Holland and Harris (1968) present one of the more complete discussions of their use of programming with aphasics in a book edited by Sloane and MacAulay, *Operant Procedures in Remedial Speech and Language Training*. They describe a 10-month project using programmed instruction almost exclusively as a technique for teaching language skills to an adult aphasic. Needless to say, the programs used in this training were all tailored to meet the specific needs of the 23-year-old patient being studied. Programs were developed to teach (1) language usage, (2) repetition and auditory memory span, (3) retention span, (4) writing description of sense, (5) spelling, and (6) special language difficulties.

The program format of most of the material closely followed the traditional type of program item developed by Skinner, more so than programs which have been written for articulation, voice, and stuttering therapy. For example, the items for the sense-training task consisted of 200 written frames for which the subject was to furnish a written response. After writing his response, the next item was presented on a card and the correct answer to the previous item was presented in the upper corner of the card. The following is an example of one of the items:

> You smell with your nose. You smell odors with your nose. You use your nose to smell _____ .

This 200-item program was completed during three successive clinical sessions during which time he independently worked through the program. He was then asked to complete the program again, this time tape recording his reading of the items plus his answers. An illustration of one of the spelling task program items is as follows:

> I can't _____ his name.

The subject then had to choose one word from these items: *remember, remembre, remeber, remebmer,* and *remembre.* As you can see, these types of tasks lend themselves perfectly to Skinner's form of programming.

Holland and Harris (1968) were very pleased with the progress they achieved using programmed instructional techniques, not only in terms of the benefits derived on the part of the patient, but also in terms of what the programming experience meant to the clinicians. It forced them to carefully define their goals and to break learning activities down into small components. The program also provided measurable effects of their therapy strategy plus insight into further instructional designs. The savings in the clinician's actual therapy time was also great, not so much for this one case, but when many aphasics are involved, the savings can be substantial. The aphasic to whom the program was administered was particularly pleased that he was able to see daily progress using programmed instructions. He liked the fact that he knew exactly what was expected of him and that he obtained immediate feedback to each item.

A subsequent report of the use of programmed instructional techniques with seven aphasic patients, all over 50 years of age, was reported by Holland (1970). She pointed out some special features about programming for aphasic patients. Reinforcement consisted of either verbal feedback (correct or incorrect), or simple, forward progression in the program. Error rate, typically held to 10% or less in most programs, was not viewed as a critical factor for aphasics. Due to perseverence and extreme response variability, it was unrealistic to expect error rate not to go beyond the 10% level. Also, when errors were made, the aphasic was moved ahead in the program once a correct response was made, rather than routing the individual back through a previous item. The subjects appeared to learn through making errors.

Holland further recommended that writing instructional programs can result in the creation of excellent therapy materials which are extremely effective in rehabilitation. She also felt it was wise for the clinician to devote time to the experimental development of personalized programmed materials, rather than to depend solely on programs written by others. Once the principles of program construction are clearly understood, i.e., reinforcement, shaping, fading, and so on, writing programs for individuals is a simple task. It is also a very time-consuming task, and time is one commodity most clinicians are very short of.

As a result of a thorough system of diagnosing and classifying aphasic symptoms, Porch (1971) has suggested some treatment procedures which are taught to clinicians who attend workshops in the use of his aphasia tests.

Programmed Instruction for
Tongue Thrust Therapy

Fletcher and Peterson (1974) developed what they viewed as "a complete, programmed approach to tongue thrust remediation." It was made commercially available in 1974. This program, designed for all ages, consists of carefully planned, step-by-step procedures which can be replicated easily. Mandibular stabilization is first established, followed by procedures to establish tongue seal and finally, hyoid movement patterns. Criterion levels are established at each step, which must be met before an individual can proceed to following steps. Evidently, remediation of tongue thrust patterns lend themselves nicely to programming techniques.

One other program for correcting incorrect swallowing habits which result in tongue thrust was presented by Pierce and Warvi (1976). This program consists of a series of exercises and drills incorporated into a 12-lesson package for use with children 4 to 10 years of age. Although I have not seen this program, it is advertised as a progression of exercises presumably in programmed fashion. This particular program has come under rather severe criticism by Pannbacker (1977) on the basis of several questionable assumptions made by the authors. The interested reader may wish to refer to Pannbacker's article.

Instructional Program for
Cerebral Palsied Children

McDonald et al. (1976) describe an adaptation of the System 80 teaching machine for use with intellectually "normal" cerebral palsied children. Little else has been mentioned in the literature which would pertain specifically to programming materials for cerebral palsied children. Of course, it would be possible to adapt most of the articulation programs for use with these children, but generally, no specific reference is made to the cerebral palsy condition.

Instructional Programs for Language Therapy

There is no doubt the programming movement has strongly influenced instructional materials designed to remediate various language skills. More programs have been written for language instruction than for any other single area in speech therapy.

Fristoe (1974) sent questionnaires to authors and publishers of over 200 language programs in an effort to identify key components of each program. The results of this study were published in a descriptive catalogue in which three pages of information are devoted to a description of each program. One reason why so many language programs are available is because a large number of professionals are engaged in language remediation, many of them coming from the fields of special education and psychology. To put it simply, language instruction has not been dominated by speech pathologists as has areas such as articulation, voice, and stuttering. Educators have long realized that a key factor to training many handicapped children lies in providing more effective language instruction. Indeed every public school teacher is expected to provide certain language instruction to all children through what has been referred to as a *language arts curriculum*.

It was during the mid-1960s when language programs were first introduced. The Peabody Language Kit developed by two educators, Dunn and Smith (1965–68), was one of the first attempts at providing an organized structure to language instruction. The original instructional package has been revised and now consists of four parts developed to meet the needs of four age groups of children from 3 to 9½ years of age. Each of the four kits consist of 180 lessons composed of a wide variety of activities and materials for stimulating receptive, associative, and expressive linguistic and cognitive processes. No specialized training is required to use the materials. Overall language development is stressed rather than particular psycholinguistic skills. But reported research regarding the effectiveness of these materials seems meager. Available research reports only that overall scholastic improvement is greater using the materials at least 30 minutes daily than if the materials are not used. Concerning the use of criterion tests, reinforcement schedules, and the like, this instructional kit could not be considered as a "program" and was not intended to be one.

Bereiter and Engelmann (1966) produced a beginning and advanced language training program for culturally disadvantaged children in the preschool environment. This program was later modified and titled the *Distar Language Program,* (Engelmann et al., 1969; Engelmann & Osborn, 1970). This program was a highly organized sequential program which could easily be replicated.

While programs were emerging for socially and culturally handicapped children, Lovaas (1966) was developing a procedure for establishing speech and language

skills with psychotic children. MacAulay (1968) worked out some effective programming procedures to teach certain language skills to nonverbal retarded children.
Risley and Wolfe (1968) were piloting work in teaching certain language skills to
severely retarded echolalic children. Language skills of autistic children was a target
for concern by Hewett (1965). All of the professionals mentioned above had little
or no training in speech pathology but were well aware of programming procedures.

It was not until the early 1970s that efforts appeared among speech pathologists
that could be regarded as language programs. Among the first such programs designed by and written primarily for speech pathologists was one by Gray and Ryan
(1971). This program was highly structured and included all of the basic features
of programmed instruction, such as exact words to be spoken, criterion levels,
branch steps, detailed data recording system, and so on. A number of carefully
planned workshops conducted in several states were designed to teach speech clinicians proper program delivery. Clinicians were instructed not to deviate from the
programmed material. Data regarding the effectiveness of their program, which
was basically concerned with the syntactic development of language skills, were
reported in a text by Gray and Ryan (1973), a few years after field testing was
completed. There are few instructional programs available which are as detailed
and specific as the one developed by these two speech pathologists.

There were other speech pathologists who felt a more functional approach to
language acquisition should be taken. Emphasis was placed on teaching language
as an ongoing communication process. Attention was given not only to syntax,
but to developing concepts, increasing vocabulary, widening semantic horizons,
and the like. The work of Miller and Yoder (1972, 1974) clearly illustrates stress
which was placed on the functional characteristics of language instruction. The work
of these two authors represent what might be better classified as instructional guidelines, rather than strict programming procedures in the sense of exact instructions
to be followed. They maintain that teaching procedures will vary greatly depending
on the individual nature of the child, the personality of the teacher, and the instructional situation. It would be impossible, according to this philosophy, to specify
exactly what the teacher should say or do. Tight programming procedures might
stifle creativity and spontaneity. While it would be quite possible to specify objectives and criterion performance levels in program fashion, a large number of speech
pathologists strongly object to "packaged programs" which specify exact words the
clinician and child should say. Several programs in addition to the two developed
by Miller and Yoder which provide guideline formats have been written by Bricker
and Bricker (1974), Stremel and Waryas (1974), and Marshall and Hegrenes (1972).

Not all speech pathologists would agree that functional aspects of language cannot be programmed according to a more rigid format, similar to the one devised by
Gray and Ryan (1971). Although some programs provide more specific instructions
regarding the exact nature of the antecedent and consequent events, all of the following programs provide enough information to enable the clinician to deliver
the program in a similar manner. These programs include those developed by
Kent (1974), Tawney and Hipsher (1972), Carrier (1974), Dunn and Smith
(1965–68), Bereiter and Engelmann (1966), and Ausberger (1976a).

Program	Specifically Described	Content	Sequence	Entry Behaviors	Exit Behaviors	Training Methods	Generalization Intra	Generalization Extra	Production and Comprehension
Bricker & Bricker (1974)	No	Functional	Functional	Infants, Prelanguage	Simple Sentences	Prompting & Fading	+	+	Both
Carrier (1974)	Yes	Functional	Functional	Minimal Language	Simple Sentences	Prompting & Fading	Yes	No	Both*
Dunn & Smith (1965–1968)	Yes	Functional	Functional	Sophisticated Language	Complex Sentences	++	No	No	Both
Engelmann, Osborn & Engelmann (1969)	Yes	Functional	Functional	Some Language	Simple Sentences	++	Yes	No	Both
Engelmann & Osborn (1970)	Yes	Functional	Functional	Sophisticated Language	Complex Sentences	++	Yes	No	Both
Gray & Ryan (1971)	Yes	Syntactic	Developmental	Sophisticated Language	Complex Sentences	Imitation	Yes	Yes	Prod.
Guess, Sailor & Baer (1976)	+++	Functional	Functional	Minimal Language	Simple Sentences	Prompting & Fading	Yes	Yes	Both
Kent (1974)	Yes	Functional	Functional	Minimal Language	Simple Sentences	Prompting & Fading	Yes	Yes	Both
Lovaas (1966)	Yes	Functional	Functional	Minimal Language	Simple Sentences	Prompting & Fading	No	No	Both
Marshall & Hegrenes (1970)	No	Functional	Functional	Some Comprehension, Imitation	Simple Sentences	Prompting & Fading	No	No	Both*
Marshall & Hegrenes (1972)	No	Functional	Functional	Some Comprehension, No Production	Simple Sentences	Prompting & Fading	No	No	Both
Miller & Yoder (1972)	No	Syntactic & Semantic	Developmental	Some Comprehension, No Production	Simple Sentences	Imitation, Expansion, Modelling	+	+	Both
Miller & Yoder (1974)	No	Semantic	Developmental	Verbal Imitation, Cognitive Awareness	Two Word Level	Imitation, Fading	+	+	Both
Risley & Wolfe (1968)	Yes	Functional	Functional	Echolalic Behavior	Simple Sentences	Imitation, Fading	No	No	Prod.
Stremel & Waryas (1974)	No	Syntactic & Semantic	Developmental	Comprehension of Commands and Labels	Complex Sentences	Imitation	Yes	Yes	Both
Tawney & Hipsher (1972)	Yes	Functional	Functional	Minimal Language	Simple Sentences	Prompting & Fading	Yes	Yes	Comp.

* Nonspeech programs

+ Program was not described in sufficient detail to ascertain.

++ Programs use complex training methods which are not easily categorized.

+++ Program is in preparation.

FIGURE 9-8. Analysis Of 16 Instructional Programs For Remediation Of Certain Language Skills (Reprinted By Permission Of P. J. Connell, University of Wisconsin)

An excellent review of 16 language programs currently available is presented by Connell et al. (1977). They list some of the essential characteristics of these programs, a summary of which has been reproduced in Figure 9–8. Connell et al. provide information about these instructional programs designed to aid the practicing clinician in selecting the proper instructional materials for their clients.

One program by Ausberger (1976a), not reviewed by Connell et al., is a clear-cut example of the use of a programmed format in teaching certain aspects of syntax. It was specifically designed for use with children whose syntactic skills lag from one to five years behind those skills found among other children. The program consists of 12 goals sequentially arranged beginning with *the* and *noun*, and ending with *the + noun + will + verb + (anything else)*. Each goal contains four steps representing individual session activities. Step A of Goal 1 is reproduced in Figure 9–9.

GOAL 1

OBJECTIVE	The child will learn to use the construction. The + Noun such as the horse or the pig.
	STEP A
MATERIALS	Syntax Wheel 1
PREPARATION	Place Syntax Wheel 1 in front of the child so that he can easily see the pictures. Rotate the wheel to picture 1.
INSTRUCTION	Ask the child to name the picture in the "window."
EVALUATION	If the response is correct, say "yes" or "good" and rotate the wheel to the next picture. If the response is incorrect, say the right name and ask the child to repeat it. Then rotate the wheel to the next picture.
DATA	Mark an "X" when the child names the picture correctly. Mark an "O" with an "X" in the center when the child repeats the name correctly. Mark an "O" when the child gives an incorrect name or is unable to repeat the name correctly.
CRITERION	Remain at this step until the child can name all eight pictures in a row without any prompting from you.
INTENDED RESPONSES	1. pony 2. mouse 3. car 4. ball 5. table 6. girl 7. boy 8. dog

FIGURE 9-9. Step A Of Goal 1 Of Ausberger's Syntax One *Program (Reprinted By Permission Of Communication Skill Builders, Tucson, Arizona)*

Note that all antecedent and consequent events, criterion levels, and data requirements are clearly specified. Monthly check-up tests are provided to follow up on
correct syntax usage once the program is completed. This provides but one example
of the use of a programmed technique for one aspect of language therapy.

There are, of course, many other language programs which have recently become
available commercially. Examples of two such programs, intended for use with
severely handicapped children, are *Non-SLIP* by Carrier and Peak (1975), and
another by Guess et al. (1976), which is a 60-step program to help develop functional language. Navakovich and Zaslow (1973) structured 700 activities designed
to improve language skills based on deficiencies found on ITPA Tests. A *Developmental Syntax Program* written by Coughran and Liles (1974) consists of structural drills covering use of articles, pronouns, possessives, objectives, and verbs.
Other language programs are tied in with university projects as part of student
training programs. One such program is in operation at the University of Tennessee
Department of Audiology and Speech Pathology in Knoxville, Tennessee. It is described by Adler et al. (1976) in a guide which expands on an eclectic, pragmatic
approach to training preschool children who have language handicaps. McDonald
and Blott (1974) and McDonald et al. (1974) presented an outline of a language
program used at Ohio State University based on a behavioral contingency model
which specified antecedent stimuli designed to evoke certain language responses
which were to be followed by specific consequences.

It is far beyond the scope of this text to provide a comprehensive review of the
wide variety of language instructional materials which have been developed during
the past 20 years. While many of the materials mentioned here are not programs
in the strict sense of the word, there appears to be ample evidence of a movement
in this direction. This is especially true with specific language skill areas, such as
instructional goals. A total programmed approach to language instruction appears
to be inappropriate since the area of instructional needs is so vast and complex.
At the present time, it seems as though speech clinicians must be satisfied with a
piece-meal approach to programmed language instruction.

Evaluating
Instructional
Programs

When you consider how many programmed materials are available for correcting
communication disorders, the task of evaluating these programs seems overwhelming unless some specific criteria are used to aid in the evaluation process. When
teaching students how to evaluate instructional programs, I advise them to consider the following guideline.

Guidelines for Program Evaluation

I. General Features

    A. Manual

        Is an instruction manual included? If so, is it written clearly, and does it
        provide sufficient information to give an accurate description of the program
        in terms of the points listed under internal organization?

B. Administration

    1. Ease of administration: Is program administration simple or is special training required to administer it?

    2. Administrator: Who may administer the program—clinician, aides, parents, teachers?

    3. Additional materials: Are any other materials needed, such as pictures, tokens, toys, games, etc.?

    4. Setting: Is the program administered to one person at a time or to a group?

C. Target Behavior

Specifically what behaviors are identified for change—disfluency, misarticulation, language, voice? If for misarticulation, specifically, what sounds?

D. Target Population

What age group is identified? Are any cultural or intellectual restrictions identified or taken into consideration?

E. Cost and Availability

What is the cost of the program? Can certain parts be purchased separately? Is the program available to anyone? Or is it restricted to those who possess certain qualifications?

F. Data

Are data presented to demonstrate effectiveness of the program? If not available in the manual, are any other published data referring to it published? Where?

G. Time Required

How many hours are required to complete the program? How long is each session?

II.   Internal Organization

A. Baseline

Is a pretest included for establishing a baseline of the behavior? Is the same test used as a posttest measure?

B. Record Keeping

Is some procedure suggested for keeping a record of the number of correct and incorrect responses? Are forms provided? Is any procedure offered for graphing the data?

C. Criterion Tests

Are criterion tests included at certain points in the program which enable the administrator to determine when to advance to the next unit? How many?

D. Branch Program

Are branch programs provided which can be followed if the subject is unable progress through a particular step or unit?

E. Reward System

What kind of reward system is provided, i.e., social praise, tokens, toys, or what? Is there any evidence of an attempt to control the schedule of reinforcement? If so, how is this schedule manipulated?

F. Generalization

Does the program contain a section which will enable the new response to generalize to other speaking situations? Are these suggestions or actual steps to be followed by someone? Who? How long does this follow-up program last?

G. Special Features

What special features does the program contain which have not been covered by other sections in these guidelines?

Answers to the questions contained in this guideline should help the speech clinician decide the merits and limitations of a particular program. Questions that are answered negatively or that are unanswerable point out weaknesses in the program. It is not uncommon for some speech clinicians to send questionnaires to publishers of programs. Much can be learned at the program evaluation stage that could assist the clinician in her efforts to get top quality instructional materials. Nothing is more disappointing to the speech clinician than to invest money for instructional materials which do little more for them than collect dust on the shelf because the material is inappropriate, inadequate, or totally useless.

As an example of program evaluation, several students in one of my classes prepared an evaluation of ten programs available in the areas of articulation, stuttering, and voice (see Figure 9–10).

You may wish to follow this general format in evaluating other programs. Supervisors in school districts employing several clinicians might find it very helpful if each clinician would evaluate one program in a specific area. The combined results could be shared with other clinicians to help them make decisions about the appropriateness of programmed materials.

Growth of the Programming Movement in Speech Pathology

There can be no doubt that the educational movement started in the 1960s has had a tremendous effect on instructional methodology used by speech clinicians since then. Evidence of continued efforts to develop and use programmed materials seem to be increasing at the present time. Current workshops designed to teach principles of programming to speech clinicians are also popular, as illustrated by a recent ASHA convention short course given by Costello (1976). This continued growth may be explained by the fact that programmed materials fulfill several important functions for the practicing speech clinician.

Recently, there has been a major thrust in speech pathology to become more accountable for the effectiveness of services provided. This has lead many speech clinicians to search for more effective materials and educational strategies which offer promise of improving instruction. Field-test data from several instructional programs specifying predictable results offered speech clinicians hopes that by using

FIGURE 9-10. Evaluation Of Ten Instructional Programs

Features	S-1 Program to Increase Fluency	Stimulus Shift Articulation Kit	SWRL Articulation Program	Articulation Control Program
cost	$10.00	$16.95	$8.00	$8.00
manual	yes	yes-kit	yes and parent's book	yes-stories-word list
materials	beep tape, stop watch, counter, tape recorder	stop watch, reinforcers, tape recorder, hand counter	games	reinforcers
administration	technician	technician after target phoneme evoked & stable	aides for AMP parents-peers for AEP	aides after sound stabilized in isolation
behavior	disfluency	/s/, /z/	/θ/, /s/, /r/, /l/	/s/, /r/, /l/, /k/, /θ/, /z/ /tʃ/, /t/, /f/, /g/
population	individuals with at least 3rd grade reading level	anyone—including physical disabilities	individually 5 yrs. up	individually 4 yrs. up
available data	IDEAS in manual	IDEAS no	American Book Co. not published	IDEAS
time	1-3 wks. intensive	no	3 wks. of 15-20 minute sessions 3-5 times weekly	yes 4 times a week for 8 wks. 15-20 min. sessions 3 min. conversation & SPT
baseline	yes	1 min. session @ each level baseline overview	yes	80% accuracy
posttest records	same after 1st 6 programs score sheets cycles	score sheet provided, may use 6 cycle graph	same as baseline forms provided for AEP	baseline weekly recording sheet per session-3 cycle log
criterion	98% fluency	as many correct words as possible in one minute	50% acc. to move to next step	3-30 min. SPT 3 branch criteria
branch rewards	yes social-money for young children	yes—smaller steps written in social-token economy from CRF to VR	social praise-game playing at end of good sessions	yes social-token economy from CRF to 10% VR
generalization	transfer to school phone, classmates	5 transfer activities, one for each level	Artic. Extention Program	home carry-over with intermittent reinforcement
special features	jump criterion			no pictures

Features	Articulation Base Program	R Correction Program	Las Vegas Articulation Transfer Program
cost	$3.00 per sound	$6.00	$3.00 per book
manual	yes-procedures and definitions		
materials	tokens	tokens	other people to talk to
administration	therapist	aide	aide after sound evoked
behavior	all common misarticulated sounds	r, vocalic and consonantal	most common articulation errors
population	5–8 years-individually	elementary through jr. hi individually	school age children individually
available	DeKalb University	IDEAS	Las Vegas School System
data	none	little	yes
time	a few weeks	95 minutes 1–15 min. and 4–20 min.	15 steps-one month if daily
baseline	conversation sample SPT	pretest	pretest
posttest	same as baseline	posttest	yes
records	correct and incorrect graphed on 3 cycle log graph	forms provided use + and −	yes
criterion	when finish program	at end of each unit	48 out of 50 items correct on each of 15 steps
rewards	start with CRF change to VR when pictures used	social-tokens from small VR to large suggests using one	limited reinforcement menu
branch	no	no	no
generalization	transfer to school and home after program completed	no	steps done in different environments
special features	no	no	no

Features	Vocal Node Reduction Program	Irwin-Weston Paired Stimuli Memphis State Univ.	Vocal Intensity Abuse Reduction Program
cost	$4.00	$30.00	$25.00
manual	yes	yes	yes
materials	tape recorder, tape, model of larynx, wrist counter, index cards, pictures of vocal nodules, reinforcers, graph paper	tokens and rewards	sound level meter
administration	clinician	technician	clinician
behavior	vocal abuse	articulation errors	vocal abuse
population	individually-anyone	group or individual 5 yrs.+	individual 5 yrs. +
available	IDEAS	National Educator Service	IDEAS
data	85–90% success	yes	no
time	till nodules gone	differs	not specified
baseline	voice recorded and hearing test given	paired stimuli kit	sound level readings
posttest	voice sample	McDonald Deep test	voice sample
records	individual keeps index cards	McDonald Deep test / yes	voice sample / record forms included
criterion	remove nodules	socially acceptable production of target sound w/no reinforcement on 8 out of 10 words in 2 successive sessions	voice at specified level
rewards	reinforcement menu	token economy	reinforcement schedule specified
branch	no	no	no

these programs, they too might obtain similar results. The fact that many programs were replicable, that is, one merely had to read the instructions to a client, was especially appealing to those clinicians who were using paraprofessionals to help provide services. Since many programs contained all necessary stimulus materials, the clinician no longer was required to cut out pictures and spend time designing speech activities. By using prepared instructional materials, the speech clinician was freed from much time-consuming lesson preparation.

The fact that most programs contained built-in pre- and posttests provided an additional advantage of providing the necessary accountability measures often required of them by their supervisors and administrators. The use of instructional programs in speech pathology also seemed to be the "in thing" among educational circles since programmed materials are used to some extent by almost every classroom teacher throughout the country. Upon entering most modern classrooms one is confronted with a wide assortment of educational kits, reading programs, instructional cassettes, science learning packages, and self-teaching films. These are appropriately boxed and shelved according to skill levels, interest levels, age levels, and ability levels. Providing educational supplies has become a leading business venture of some manufacturers. Many college professors are eagerly preparing sellable instructional materials, rather than writing theory-oriented textbooks. The potential market among prospective teacher consumers far outweighs the student textbook buyer, and publishing firms were quick to discover this fact. Selling all four levels of the *Peabody Language Development Kit* grosses the manufacturer some $420.00, while the *Non-SLIP* language program retails for $238.00. Some programs like those designed by the Monterey Learning Systems and the Hollins Communications Research Institute require the potential program user to attend special training sessions at a tuition of from $250 to $500 for each participant. One can easily see that instructional programs will be well advertised and marketed enthusiastically when such large sums of money are involved. This fact is not meant to be a criticism of the program movement, just an observation with respect to explaining its growth.

Finally, instructional programs offer the speech clinician who has not had the benefit of training in some areas an immediate solution to instructional problems. If, for example, the clinician was not exposed to treatment procedures for vocal nodule reduction during her training, she is able to provide effective services to children who develop voice problems due to vocal misuse simply by following a prewritten instructional program. But this use of programs could turn out to be detrimental. If the program writer fails to provide the necessary information regarding adequate diagnosis of the problem, or if the clinician fails to provide an adequate diagnostic evaluation, a program might be administered to a person to whom it should not be administered. In fact, such indiscriminate program administration may actually harm the client, not to speak of the valuable loss of time and discouragement encountered. The burden of responsibility rests with the clinician who administers the program.

The widespread use of instructional programs could greatly alter the role the speech clinician has had in the past. There can be no doubt that many self-contained programs can be administered by paraprofessionals who have had little training in speech pathology. With the increased use of instructional programs by paraprofessionals, the speech clinician may be forced into supervision type activities that requires her to oversee therapy, rather than provide it. More emphasis might be placed on diagnostic activities, developing community relations, and administrating total programs than on simple service delivery. The fact that many speech clinicians are unprepared for this activity and indeed, may not even be interested in administrating programs, may discourage them from using instructional programs of any type as a protective measure of their present job definition.

Frankly, I think the average speech clinician will have little choice with respect to whether or not programs will be used. Pressure from publishing houses, other teachers, colleagues, and the current educational movement will cause them to be swept up with the times. Of course, new instructional developments may supplement or supercede instructional programming and thus alter the present course of instructional strategy; but this has yet to come. For the present, we can look forward to an increasing amount of programmed materials to flow from the publishing houses.

I truly believe that the programmed instruction movement in speech pathology has been, and will continue to be, a beneficial contribution to the improvement of instruction in speech pathology. Although the concept of what constitutes a program has changed since its original description some 20 years ago, the basic aspects tied to a scientific methodology remain unchanged. The practicing clinician should make every effort to keep abreast of new instructional materials and demand data from field test results. We must dig deeper than the label on the package!

BIBLIOGRAPHY

Adler, S., Nolan, D., Sinclair, S., Thomas, A., & Wallace, S. *An interdisciplinary language intervention program*. Knoxville, Tenn.: University of Tennessee, 1976.

Ausberger, C. *Syntax one*. Tucson, Ariz.: Communication Skill Builders, 1976a.

Ausberger, C. *Here's how to handle /r/*. Tucson, Ariz.: Communication Skill Builders, 1976b.

Baker, R. D., & Ryan, B. P. *Programmed conditioning for articulation*. Monterey, Ca.: Monterey Learning Systems, 1971.

Bensen, C. *Vocal intensity abuse reduction program*. Tempe, Ariz.: Ideas, 1978.

Bereiter, C., & Engelmann, S. *Teaching disadvantaged children in the preschool*. Englewood Cliffs, N.J.: Prentice-Hall, 1966.

Bingham, D. S., Van Hattum, R. J., Faulk, M. E., & Taussig, E. Program organization and management. *Journal of Speech and Hearing Disorders Monograph Supplement*, 1961, *8*, 33–49.

Black, J. W. Relationships among fundamental frequency, vocal sound pressure, and rate of speaking. *Language and Speech*, 1964, *4*, 196–199.

Blyth, J. B. Teaching machines and human beings. In A. A. Lumsdaine & R. Glaser (Eds.), *Teaching machines and programmed learning*. Washington, D.C.: Department of Audio-visual Instruction, National Education Association, 1960.

Boberg, E. Intensive group therapy program for stutterers. *Human Communication*, 1976, *1*, 29–42.

Bricker, W., & Bricker, D. An early language training strategy. In R. Schiefelbusch & L. Lloyd (Eds.) *Language perspectives*. Baltimore: University Park Press, 1974.

Carrier, Jr., J. Application of functional analysis and a nonspeech response to teaching language. In L. McReynolds (Ed.), *Developing systematic procedures for training children's language, ASHA Monograph Number 18*. Washington, D.C.: American Speech and Hearing Association, 1974.

Carrier, Jr., J. A program of articulation therapy administered by mothers. *Journal of Speech and Hearing Disorders*, 1970, *35*, 344–353.

Carrier, Jr., J. K. & Peak, T. *Non-SLIP*. Lawrence, Kan.: H & H Enterprises, 1975.

Clark, B. J. Using a short-term lisp correction program for more effective distribution of clinicians' time. *Language, Speech and Hearing Services in Schools*, 1974, *5*, 152–155.

Coachbuilder, D. *Programmed approach to the remediation of pitch disorders of the voice*. Unpublished masters thesis, Utah State University, 1972.

Connell, P. J., Spradlin, J. E., & McReynolds, L. V. Some suggested criteria for evaluation of language programs. *Journal of Speech and Hearing Disorders*, 1977, *42*, 563–567.

Cooper, E. *Stuttering therapy: A total approach*. Austin, Tex.: Learning Concepts, 1976.

Costello, J. The establishment of fluency with time-out procedures: Three case studies. *Journal of Speech and Hearing Disorders*, 1975, *40*, 216–231.

Costello, J. *Designing programmed instruction.* Houston, Tex.: Short Course, American Speech and Hearing Convention, 1976.

Costello, J. Programmed instruction. *Journal of Speech and Hearing Disorders*, 1977, *42*, 3–28.

Costello, J., & Onstine, J. M. The modification of multiple articulation errors based on distinction feature theory. *Journal of Speech and Hearing Disorders*, 1976, *41*, 199–215.

Coughran, L., & Liles, B. *Developmental syntax program.* Austin, Tex.: Learning Concepts, 1974.

Cross, D. E., & Cooper, E. B. Self- versus investigator-administered presumed fluency reinforcing stimuli. *Journal of Speech and Hearing Research*, 1976, *19*, 241–246.

Culatta, R. A., & Rubin, H. A program for the initial stages of fluency therapy. *Journal of Speech and Hearing Research*, 1973, *16*, 556–568.

Curlee, R. F., & Perkins, W. H. Conversational rate control therapy for stuttering. *Journal of Speech and Hearing Disorders*, 1969, *34*, 245–250.

Deal, R. E., McClain, B., & Sudderth, J. F. Identification, evaluation, therapy, and follow-up for children with vocal nodules in a public school setting. *Journal of Speech and Hearing Disorders*, 1976, *41*, 390–397.

Delbridge, L. & Larrigan, L. *Stimulus shift articulation kit.* Tempe, Ariz.: Ideas, 1973.

Drudge, M. K., & Philips, B. J. Shaping behavior in voice therapy. *Journal of Speech and Hearing Disorders*, 1976, *41*, 398–411.

Dunn, L., & Smith, J. *Manual for the Peabody language developmental kit, level p, 1, 2, and 3.* Minneapolis: American Guidance Service, 1965–1968.

Engelmann, S., Osborn, J., & Engelmann, T. *Distar language I, teacher's guide.* Chicago: Science Research Associates, 1969.

Engelmann, S., & Osborn, J. *Distar language II, teacher's guide.* Chicago: Science Research Associates, 1970.

Evans, C., & Potter, R. The effectiveness of the S-Pack when administered by sixth-grade children to primary-grade children. *Language, Speech and Hearing Services in Schools*, 1974, *5*, 85–90.

Filby, Y., & Edwards, A. E. An application of automated teaching methods to test and teach form discrimination to aphasics. *Journal of Programmed Instruction*, 1963, *2*, 25–33.

Fletcher, S. G., & Peterson, D. D. *Tongue thrust therapy program.* Austin, Tex.: Learning Concepts, 1974.

Fristoe, M. (Ed.), *Language intervention system for the retarded: A catalogue of original language structured programs in the U.S.* Montgomery, Ala.: State of Alabama Dept. of Education, 1974.

Garrett, E. R. Programmed articulation therapy. In W. Wolfe & D. Goulding (Eds.), *Articulation and learning.* Springfield, Ill.: Charles C Thomas, 1973.

Garrett, E. R. Correction of functional misarticulation under an automated self-correction system: Summary report, submitted to the U.S. Office of Education, Project No. 2749, 1965.

Garrett, E. R. *An automated speech correction: A pilot study.* Paper read at the American Speech and Hearing Association 1963 National Convention. *Asha*, 1963, *5*, 796 (Abstract.)

Goldiamond, I. Stuttering and fluency as manipulatable operant response classes. In L. Krasner & L. P. Ullmann (Eds.), *Research in behavior modification*. New York.: Holt, Rinehart & Winston, 1965.

Gray, B., & Ryan, B. *A language program for the nonlanguage child*. Champaign, Ill.: Research Press, 1973.

Gray, B., & Ryan, B. *Programmed conditioning for language: Program book*. Monterey, Ca.: Monterey Learning Systems, 1971.

Gray, B. A field study on programmed articulation therapy. *Language, Speech, and Hearing Services in Schools*, 1974, *5*, 119–131.

Greiner, G. *A programmed therapy approach to mutational voice disturbances*. Unpublished masters thesis, Utah State University, 1973.

Guess, D., Sailor, W., & Baer, D. M. *Functional speech and language training for the severely handicapped, part I and part II*. Lawrence, Kan.: H & H Enterprises, 1976.

Haroldson, S., Martin, R., & Starr, C. Time-out as a punishment for stuttering. *Journal of Speech and Hearing Research*, 1968, *11*, 560–566.

Hewett, P. M. Teaching speech to an autistic child through operant conditioning. *American Journal of Orthopsychiatry*, 1965, *35*, 927–936.

Holland, A. L. *The development and evaluation of teaching machine procedures for increasing auditory discrimination skill in children with auditory disorders*. Unpublished doctoral dissertation, University of Pittsburgh, 1960.

Holland, A. L. *The development and evaluation of programmed instruction techniques for aphasia rehabilitation*. Final report, Social and Rehabilitation Service, Department of Health, Education, and Welfare, Washington, D.C., 1969.

Holland, A. L. Case studies in aphasia rehabilitation using programmed instruction. *Journal of Speech and Hearing Disorders*, 1970, *35*, 377–390.

Holland, A. L., & Harris, A. B. Aphasia rehabilitation using programmed instruction. In H. Sloane & B. MacAulay (Eds.), *Operant procedures in remedial speech and language training*. Boston: Houghton Mifflin, 1968.

Holland, A. L., & Matthews, J. Application of teaching machine concepts to speech pathology and audiology. *Asha*, 1963, *5*, 474–482.

Hunsaker, J. C. *Behavioral management approach to vocal disorders*. Unpublished masters thesis, Utah State University, 1970.

Ingham, R., & Andrews, G. *Stuttering: A description and analysis of a token economy in an adult therapy program*. Paper presented at the American Speech and Hearing Association Convention. Chicago: November 1971.

Irwin, J. V., & Griffith, F. A. A theoretical and operational analysis of the paired stimuli technique. In W. Wolfe & D. Goulding (Eds.), *Articulation and learning*. Springfield, Ill.: Charles C Thomas, 1973.

Jackson, M. *Programmed articulation therapy for the modification of /r/*. Tempe, Ariz.: Ideas, 1973.

Jackson, M. *Programmed articulation therapy for the modification of sh*. Tempe, Ariz.: Ideas, 1976.

James, H. D., & Cooper, E. B. Accuracy of teacher referrals of speech handicapped children. *Exceptional Children*, 1966, *33*, 29–33.

Johnson, T. A behavioral research approach to the clinical treatment of voice disorders. *Iowa Speech and Hearing Association Journal*, Fall/Winter 1974.

Johnson, T. *A precision approach to hyperfunctional voice disorders*. Logan, Utah: Utah State University, 1975.

Kent, L. *Language acquisition program for the retarded or multiply impaired*. Champaign, Ill.: Research Press, 1974.

Knox, J. *Knox articulation correction program*. Tempe, Ariz: Ideas, 1972.

Lanyon, R. Behavior change in stuttering through systematic desensitization. *Journal of Speech and Hearing Disorders*, 1969, *34*, 253–260.

Lanyon, R., Barrington, C., & Newman, A. C. Modification of stuttering through EMG biofeedback: A preliminary study. *Behavior Therapy*, 1976, *7*, 96–103.

Lanyon, R., Manosevitz, M., & Imber, R. Systematic desensitization: Distribution of practice and symptom substitution. *Behavior Research Therapy*, 1968, *6*, 323–329.

Leach, E. Stuttering: Clinical application of response-contingent procedures. In B. Gray & G. England (Eds.), *Stuttering and the conditioning therapies*. Monterey, Ca.: Monterey Institute for Speech and Hearing, 1969.

Lee, J. Application and justification of Martin Schwartz's airflow technique in the treatment of stuttering. *Asha*, 1976, *18*, 601.

Leonard, L. B., & Webb, C. E. An automated therapy program for articulatory correction. *Journal of Speech and Hearing Research*, 1971, *14*, 338–344.

Lovaas, O. I. A program for the establishment of speech in psychotic children. In J. K. King (Ed.), *Childhood autism*. Oxford: Pergamon Press, 1966.

Lubbert, L., Johnson, K., Brenner, C., & Alderson, A. *Behavior modification articulation program for speech aides*. Tempe, Ariz.: Ideas, 1972.

Lundquist, R. L. (Project Director), *Speech therapy transfer program*. Las Vegas: Clark County School District, 1972.

MacAulay, B. D. A program for teaching speech and beginning reading in nonverbal retardates. In H. Sloane & B. MacAulay (Eds.), *Operant procedures in remedial speech and language training*. Boston: Houghton Mifflin, 1968.

Marshall, N., & Hegrenes, J. A communication therapy model for cognitively disorganized children. In J. McLean, D. Yoder & R. Schiefelbusch (Eds.), *Language intervention with the retarded*. Baltimore: University Park Press, 1972.

Martin, R. The experimental manipulation of stuttering behaviors. In H. Sloane & B. MacAulay (Eds.), *Operant procedures in remedial speech and language training*. Boston: Houghton Mifflin, 1968.

Martin, R., & Gaviser, J. Time-out as a punishment for button pushing. *Journal of Speech and Hearing Research*, 1971, *14*, 144–148.

McDonald, J. D., & Blott, J. P. Environmental language intervention: The rationale for a diagnostic and training strategy through rules, context, and generalization. *Journal of Speech and Hearing Disorders*, 1974, *39*, 244–256.

McDonald, J. D., Blott, J. P., Gordon, K., Spiegel, B., & Hartmann, M. An experimental parent-assisted treatment program for preschool language-delayed children. *Journal of Speech and Hearing Disorders*, 1974, *39*, 395–415.

McDonald, E., Carling, A., Maier, C., & Richards, W. D. *The use of system 80 instructional programs with cerebral palsied children*. Philadelphia: Home of the Merciful Savior for Crippled Children, 1976.

McGough, W. E., Peins, M., & Lee, B. S. A home-based tape recorder approach to rehabilitating the stutterers: Evaluation of an economic treatment. Final report. Research and Demonstration Project No. 2932-S, U.S.S.R.S. New Brunswick, NJ.; Rutgers Medical School, 1971.

McLean, J. E. *Shifting stimulus control of articulation response by operant techniques*. Unpublished doctoral dissertation, University of Kansas, 1965.

McReynolds, L. V., & Bennett, S. Distinctive feature generalization in articulation training. *Journal of Speech and Hearing Disorders*, 1972, *37*, 462–470.

Miller, J., & Yoder, D. A syntax teaching program. In J. McLeon, D. Yoder & R. Schiefelbusch (Eds.), *Language intervention with the retarded*. Baltimore: University Park Press, 1972.

Miller, J., & Yoder, D. A ontogenetic language teaching strategy for retarded children. In R. Schiefelbusch & L. Lloyd (Eds.), *Language perspectives*. Baltimore: University Park Press, 1974.

Mowrer, D. *An experimental analysis of variables controlling lisping responses of children*. Unpublished doctoral dissertation, 1964.

Mowrer, D. Programmed speech therapy—a field test. *Asha*, 1967, *9*, 369.

Mowrer, D. *Modification of speech behaviors: Ideas and strategies for students*. Tempe, Ariz.: Ideas, 1969.

Mowrer, D. *Technical research report S-1: Reduction of stuttering behavior*. Tempe, Ariz.: Ideas, 1971.

Mowrer, D. An instructional program to increase fluent speech of stutterers. *Journal of Fluency Disorders*, 1975, *1* (2), 25–35.

Mowrer, D. *A program to establish fluent speech*. Columbus: Charles E. Merrill, 1979.

Mowrer, D., Baker, R., & Schutz, R. Operant procedures in the control of speech articulation. In H. Sloane & B. MacAulay (Eds.), *Operant procedures in the control of speech and language training*. New York: Houghton Mifflin, 1968a.

Mowrer, D. Baker, R., & Schutz, R. *S programmed articulation control kit*. Tempe, Ariz.: Educational Psychological Research Associates, 1968b.

Navakovich, E., & Zaslow, E. *Target on language*. Bethesda, Md.: Christ Church Child Center, 1973.

Pannbacker, M. Don't like, won't buy. *Asha*, 1977, *19*, 58–59.

Peins, M., McGough, W. E., & Lee, B. S. Tape recorder therapy for the rehabiltiation of the stuttering handicapped. *Language Speech and Hearing Services in Schools*, 1972, *3*, 2, 30–35.

Pierce, R. B., & Warvi, V. *Swallow right*, rev. ed. Huntsville, Ala.: Swallow Right, 1976.

Porch, B. E. Multidimensional scoring in aphasia testing. *Journal of Speech and Hearing Research*, 1971, *14*, 776–792.

Psaltis, C. D., & Spallato, S. L. *Programmed articulation therapy: Time to modify*. Springfield, Ill.: Charles C Thomas, 1973.

Rachman, S. Systematic desensitization. *Psychological Bulletin*, 1967, *67*, 93–103.

Rickard, H., & Mundy, M. Direct manipulation of stuttering behavior, an experimental-clinical approach. In L. P. Ullman & L. Krasner (Eds.), *Case studies in behavior modification*. New York: Holt, Rinehart & Winston, 1965.

Risley, T., & Wolfe, M. Stimulus factors in training echolalic children. In H. Sloane & B. MacAulay (eds.), *Operant procedures in remedial speech and language training*. Boston: Houghton Mifflin, 1968.

Rosenberg, B. The performance of aphasics on automated visual-perceptual discrimination, training, and transfer tasks. *Journal of Speech and Hearing Research*, 1965, *8*, 165–181.

Ryan, B. *The construction and evaluation of a program for modifying stuttering behavior*. Unpublished doctoral dissertation, University of Pittsburgh, 1964.

Ryan, B. Operant procedures applied to stuttering therapy for children. *Journal of Speech and Hearing Disorders*, 1971a, *36*, 264–280.

Ryan, B. A study of the effectiveness of the S-Pack program in the elimination of frontal lisping behavior in third-grade children. *Journal of Speech and Hearing Disorders,* 1971b, *36,* 390–396.

Ryan, B. *Programmed therapy for stuttering in children and adults.* Springfield, Ill.: Charles C Thomas, 1974.

Ryan, B., & Van Kirk, B. *Programmed conditioning for fluency: Program book.* Monterey, Ca.: Monterey Learning Systems, 1971.

Shames, G. Operant conditioning and therapy for stuttering. In M. Fraiser (Ed.). *Conditioning in stuttering therapy: Applications and limitations.* Speech Foundation of America, 1970, *7,* 17–35.

Shames, G. H., & Egolf, D. B. *Operant conditioning and the management of stuttering: A book for clinicians.* Englewood Cliffs, N.J.: Prentice-Hall, 1976.

Shames, G. H. and Florence, C. L. *Stutter-free speech: A goal for therapy.* Columbus: Charles E. Merrill, 1980.

Shaw, C. K., & Shrum, W. F. The effects of response-contingent reward on the connected speech of children who stutter. *Journal of Speech and Hearing Disorders,* 1972, *37,* 75–88.

Shriberg, L. D. A response evocation program for /ɝ/ *Journal of Speech and Hearing Disorders,* 1975, *40,* 92–105.

Schwartz, D., and Webster, L. M. More of the efficiency of a protracted precision fluency shaping program. *Journal of Fluency Disorders,* 1977, *2,* 205–216.

Silverman, E., & Zimmer, C. H. Incidence of chronic hoarseness among school-age children. *Journal of Speech and Hearing Disorders,* 1975, *40,* 211–215.

Soderberg, G. A. Delayed auditory feedback and the speech of stutterers: A review of studies. *Journal of Speech and Hearing Disorders,* 1969, *34,* 20–29.

Stremel, K., & Waryas, C. A behavioral-psycholinguistic approach to language training. In L. McReynolds (Ed.), *Developing systematic procedures for training children's language. ASHA Monograph, 18.* Washington, D.C.: American Speech and Hearing Association, 1974.

Taylor, M. L. Language therapy. In H. C. Burr (Ed.), *The aphasic adult: Evaluation and rehabilitation.* Charlottesville, Va.; Wayside Press, 1964.

Tawney, J., & Hipsher, L. *Part II, systematic language instruction: The Illinois program.* Danville, Ill.: Interstate Printers & Publishers, Inc., 1972.

Tyre, T., Stephen, M., & Companik, P. The use of systematic desensitization in the treatment of chronic stuttering behavior. *Journal of Speech and Hearing Disorders,* 1973, *38,* 514–519.

Van Riper, C. *Speech correction: Principles and methods,* 1st ed. Englewood Cliffs, N.J.; Prentice-Hall, 1939.

Van Riper, C. *Speech correction: Principles and methods,* 4th ed. Englewood Cliffs, N.J.: Prentice-Hall, 1964.

Waters, B. *Articulation base program.* DeKalb, Ill.: Department of Communication Disorders, Northern Illinois University, 1974.

Webster, R. L. *Precision fluency shaping program.* Roanoke, Va.; Communications Development Corporation, 1975.

Webster, R. L. Evolution of a target-based behavioral therapy for stuttering. *Journal of Fluency Disorders,* 1980, *5,* 303–320.

Weston, A. J., & Irwin, J. V. Use of paired-stimuli in modification of articulation. *Perceptual Motor Skills,* 1971, *32,* 947–957.

Williams, D. A point of view about 'stuttering.' *Journal of Speech and Hearing Disorders,* 1957, *22,* 390–397.

Wilson, F. B. *Voice disorders.* Austin, Tex.: Learning Concepts, 1977.

Wolpe, J. *Psychotherapy by reciprocal inhibitation.* Stanford, Ca.; Stanford University Press, 1959.

Woolf, G. The assessment of stuttering as struggle, avoidance, and expectancy. *The British Journal of Disorders of Communication,* 1967, *2,* 158–171.

Zenner, A. Philosophy and treatment of stuttering, Cassette tape. Tempe, Ariz.: Ideas, 1976.

Assignment 6

Administering Antecedent and Consequent Events

Overview

A variety of programmed instructional materials are available for pathologists to use in the treatment of articulation, stuttering, and language disorders. One such program designed for the correction of frontal lisping is the S-PACK program. The basic principles of programmed instruction are well illustrated in the construction and use of this program. Once the pathologist has a clear understanding of these principles, construction and administration of other instructional programs will be easier.

During this exercise you will provide both the instructions (which have been written for you) and the consequent event, following a child's response that has been pre-recorded on the tape. Sometimes incorrect responses will occur. If you make a mistake in judging a response, you will be informed by the narrator on the tape. This experience approximates as closely as possible the delivery of articulation therapy without the actual presence of a client.

Objective: To practice administering antecedent and consequent events using a structured, pre-written articulation correction program, S-PACK (Mowrer et al., 1967).

Materials: Assignment 6, Selections A–D.

Description of the Session: The first therapy session presented consists of a college student administering a portion of the S-PACK to a boy who has a frontal lisp. It is used as a demonstration to provide you with an understanding of this type of program delivery. The remaining three portions of the tape consist of a girl's responses to items in the S-PACK. You are to provide the antecedent and consequent events as you read portions of S-PACK from your workbook. At times, the girl will lisp and you are to provide the appropriate consequences.

Procedure: One way you can gain experience in learning how to administer a speech therapy session is to practice providing antecedent and consequent events to a client. The purpose of this instructional tape is to provide you with this type of practice in a highly structured programmed format. The S-PACK (Mowrer et al., 1967), an instructional program for the correction of a frontal lisp, is an instrument well suited to provide this practice. The S-PACK is divided into three parts, each requiring about 10 to 15 minutes to administer. Part I focuses upon establishing /s/ in isolation and in words. Part II teaches /s/ in different positions, in blends, polysyllabic words, and phrases. Part III focuses upon production of /s/ in connected speech. You will practice administering only a few items from each of the three parts.

But first, it would be helpful to listen to someone administer these antecedent and consequent events to a client so you can get an idea of what will be expected of you during this training session. You will hear a college student administer the first 28 items of S-PACK to a third grade boy who lisps. The student's rate of delivery is much faster than what I would consider normal delivery speed. She seems to be so rushed that she forgets to tell the child to close his teeth when he errs on an item. Nevertheless, listening to the tape will give you an idea of how this particular program is administered. Follow the script of the session, Table 6–1 as you listen.

Play Assignment 6, Selection A.

SELECTION A

Table 6–1. *Script for Selection A.*

Antecedent Event	Response	Consequent Event
1. Close your teeth and say, /i/.	/i/	Good
2. Close your teeth and say, /is/.	/is/	Good.
3. Look in the mirror and say, /is/; /is/.	/iθ/	No. (She should have said, "Close your teeth and try it again.")
Again.	/is/	Good.
		Good.
4. Say, /is/.	/is/	Good.
5. Keep your teeth closed and say, /is/.	/is/	Good.
6. Look in the mirror. Say, /is/.	/is/	Good.
7. Close your teeth. Say, /is/.	/is/	Good.
8. Now say it like this: /is/.	/is/	Good.
9. Look in the mirror and try it again.	/is/	Good.
10. Close your teeth and say, /s/.	/s/	Good.
11. Say, /s/.	/s/	——— (Should always follow a response
Again.	/s/	——— with a consequence.)
12. Close your teeth and say it softly.	/s/	Good.
13. Look in the mirror. Say, /s/ louder.	/s/	Good.

Table 6–1, cont.

Antecedent Event	Response	Consequent Event
14. Say a long /s/.	/s/	Good.
15. Say a short one, /s/.	/s/	Good.
16. Say /s/ two times.	/s,s/	Good.
17. Close your teeth and say, /s/.	/s/	Good.
18. Look in the mirror and say, /s/.	/s/	Good.
19. Say it softly.	/s/	Good.
20. Say it loudly.	/s/	Good.
21. Say it quickly.	/s/	Good.
22. Say, /sɔ/.	/sɔ/	Good.
23. Look in the mirror. Say, /sɔ/.	/sɔ/	Good.
Open your mouth when you say it.		
Like this.	/sɔ/	Good.
Again.	/sɔ/	Good.
24. Close your teeth and say, /si/.	/si/	Good.
25. Say, /o/.	/o/	Good.
26. Say, /so/.	/so/	Good.
27. Say, /aɪ/.	/aɪ/	Good.
28. Say, /saɪ/.	/saɪ/	Good.

Now that you have heard how the S-PACK is delivered, you should be able to provide the consequent and antecedent events yourself. The next three selections on the tape will give you practice in administering a few items of each part of this three-part program. Part I, designed to evoke /s/ in isolation and in monosyllabic words, will be presented first, followed by Parts II and III. Actually, each part is designed to be administered over a 3-day period; but because we are only interested in practice administering a program, much of the program will be omitted.

SELECTION B

Selection B will provide you with practice using Part I of S-PACK. During this first part, the number of each instructional item will be announced. You will read aloud the instruction printed immediately beside that number. Then you will hear a child respond. Decide whether the response is correct or not. Then, provide a consequence. You'll provide one type of consequence if the child's response is *correct* (a correct /s/) and another if the response is *incorrect* (lisp).

If the child's first try is correct, say *good* and place an imaginary token in front of you. This action might seem unnecessary because there is no child in front of you to receive the imaginary token. I suggest you do it simply to get into the feel of a real session.

If the child's first try is wrong, say, "No, close your teeth and try it again."

If the child's second try is correct, say "Good" but do not give a token.

If the child's second try is wrong, say, "No, you didn't close your teeth," and go on to the next item.

When you play the tape, the narrator will say *'one.'* Then read aloud the first item in Table 6–2 while the tape player continues to run. After a pause, you will hear a child say /i/. You will say *good* and place an imaginary token in front of you. Then the narrator will say *two.* Read the second item aloud. You will hear the child respond. Attach a consequence and proceed in this fashion through item 30. You may wish to review the consequences you will be attaching to the child's correct and incorrect responses before continuing. Find Table 6–2 below.

When you are ready, play Assignment 6, Selection B, Part I, and follow the script on Table 6–2.

Table 6–2. *Script for Selection B, Part I.*

1. Close your teeth and say, /i/.
2. Close your teeth and say, /is/.
3. Look in the mirror and say, /is/.
4. Say, /is/.
5. Keep your teeth closed and say, /is/.
6. Look in the mirror. Say, /is/.
7. Close your teeth. Say, /is/.
8. Now say it like this: /is/. (Prolong /s/.)
9. Look in the mirror and try it again.
10. Close your teeth and say, /s/.
11. Say, /s/.
12. Close your teeth and say it softly.
13. Look in the mirror. Say, /s/ louder.
14. Say a long /s/. (Prolong /s/.)
15. Say a short one, /s/.
16. Say /s/ two times.
17. Close your teeth and say, /s/.
18. Look in the mirror and say, /s/.
19. Say it softly.
20. Say it loudly.
21. Say it quickly.
22. Say, /sɔ/.
23. Look in the mirror. Say /sɔ//. Open your mouth when you say *ah,* like this, /sɔ/.
24. Close your teeth and say, /si/.
25. Say, /o/.
26. Say, /so/.
27. Say, /aɪ/.
28. Say, /saɪ/.
29. Say, /sɔ/.
30. Say this word: say.

SELECTION C

Selection C involves the administration of Part II. It does not include second attempts on items as the first 30 items of Part I did. In Part II, the task changes from teaching /s/ in isolation to teaching it as well as /z/ in a variety of positions in monosyllabic and polysyllabic words. Later in this section, short phrases are introduced.

Start the tape at Assignment 6, Selection C. Read aloud the directions to the child, given in the script of Part II (Table 6–3). Do not read aloud phrases in parentheses—but imagine you are doing these things.

Table 6–3. *Script for Selection C, Part II.*

1. Close your teeth and say /s/.
2. Keep your teeth closed and say, /s/.
3. What is this? (*Point to a picture of soap.*)
4. Where do you wash your hands?
5. Look in the mirror and say, soap.
6. Name these pictures. (*Point to a picture of a saddle.*)
7. (*Point to a picture of a saw.*)
8. (*Point to picture of sun.*)
9. Where do people keep money?
10. Close your teeth and say, /is/.
11. Look in the mirror and say, /os/.
12. Say, /aɪs/.
13. Say, ice.
14. What is this: (*Point to a picture of ice.*)
15. Close your teeth and say, yes.
16. Say, yes.
17. Is ice cold?
18. What do you put on a horse?
19. Yes or no, is this where you wash your hands? (*Point to a picture of a sink.*)
20. What is this? (*Point to a picture of ice.*)
21. Is it cold?
22. You wash your hands with _____.
23. Say yes if you want to say some more words.
24. What's this? (*Point to ice.*)
25. What's this? (*Point to bus.*)
26. What's this picture? (*Point to dress.*)

SELECTION D

Selection D presents Part III, a review of Parts I and II, and introduces a story sequence about Sam and his sailboat. Follow the same procedure as you did in Parts I and II: say *good* and give a token following each correct response; say *no* and give no token following each incorrect response.

You will note that in Part III, the schedule of reinforcement begins to change from a FR-1 to a VR-2.* For example, the response "I *see* a chicken in the gra*ss*" has two /s/ sounds but only one token is presented. In item 25, two /s/ responses are made for one reward. Later in the program, and especially in the parent program (which you won't administer during this training session), the schedule of reinforcement changes to VR-5. Gradually, reinforcement is faded out altogether. Only during early stages of training it is important to provide frequent and immediate reinforcement following correct responses.

Listen now to Assignment 6, Selection D as you follow the script in Table 6–4.

There are several instructional programs that follow a format similar to the S-PACK. They are designed to correct misarticulation; a few programs have also been written to remediate stuttering.

In review, the important point of this training session was to demonstrate to you the effectiveness of presenting highly structured antecedent events plus accurate consequences in a preplanned, systematic manner. Once you master this format, you can devise similar instructional programs to meet the specific needs of different individuals.

---

*An FR-1 schedule means a positive consequence follows every correct response. A VR-2 schedule means a positive consequence follows an average of every two correct responses.

Table 6–4. *Script for Selection D, Part III.*

1. Name these pictures. (*Point to saw.*)
2. (*Point to soap.*)
3. (*Point to saddle.*)
4. (*Point to grasshopper.*)
5. (*Point to zipper.*)
6. (*Point to ice cream cone.*)
7. Where is the book? (*Point to book on table.*)
8. (*Point to goat in grass.*)
9. Say, I see a girl eating a banana.
10. Say, I see _____.
11. Here's a picture of a boy named Sam. Say his name.
12. He has a _____.
13. Sam wants to sail his _____.
14. What does Sam want to do?
15. One day, Sam went to a pond to sail his sailboat. What did he want to do at the pond?
16. Who went to the pond?
17. He put his sailboat in the water and it sailed away. What did he put in the water?
18. What happened to Sam's sailboat?
19. Sam tried to reach his sailboat with a _____.
20. The sailboat sailed away too fast and Sam couldn't reach it with his _____.
21. Why couldn't Sam reach his sailboat?
22. What did Sam try to do?
23. Sam told his dog Spot to go in the water and get his _____.
24. Spot the dog jumped into the water and got Sam's _____. I'm going to tell part of the story but I want you to fill in some words for me when I stop. Ready?
25. One day _____ took his _____ to the pond so
26. he could _____ it.
27. The boat sailed away and _____ tried to reach it with a _____.

UNIT 5 STUDY QUESTIONS

1. Define programmed instruction.
2. Why was Pressey unsuccessful in his attempt to initiate programmed instruction?
3. How did Skinner's work on programmed instruction differ from Pressey's?
4. Differentiate between intrinsic and extrinsic programs.
5. What is the major problem in using the test-retest method of determining which of two methods is best?
6. Describe Skinner's three components of programmed instruction.
7. List some criticisms of Skinner's approach to programmed instruction.
8. Describe Costello's four components of a programmed instructional package.
9. List some common faults in writing instructional programs.
10. What is the future outlook for the use of programmed instruction techniques in education?
11. What types of problems are most instructional programs in speech therapy designed to correct?
12. What is the first task in developing instructional program?
13. What is a flow chart?
14. Why was /i/ used to evoke the /s/ sound in the S-PACK?
15. Why is it so important to clearly state the difference between correct and incorrect responses when writing a program?
16. As you progress through an instructional program, how is the schedule of reinforcement usually changed?
17. What three types of criterion measures are used in the S-PACK?
18. How is stimulus shift accomplished using the S-PACK?
19. Briefly describe the extent of programs available for correction of articulation.
20. How is the stimulus shift concept utilized in McLean's instructional program?
21. Describe what Ryan accomplished in adapting therapy methods in stuttering.
22. Why might it be difficult to develop an instructional program designed to change attitudes of stutterers?
23. For what type of voice disorders are programmed instructions available?
24. Is it possible to formulate and execute pre-written instructional programs for aphasics?
25. How comprehensive are instructional programs in language instruction?
26. What characteristics would you look for in a good language instructional program?
27. What is the outlook for the use of instructional programs in speech therapy?

Unit 6

Use of Counseling and Psychotherapy as a Means of Modifying Behavior

Objectives

The objectives of this unit are to enable you to: identify at least six procedures counselors use to help people in distress or in need of information; illustrate two uses of the psychoanalytic approach in speech therapy; outline the rationale of the phenomenological approach; define and illustrate the use of behavioral counseling; define five counseling skills used by speech clinicians; define the three steps of the grief process; and identify four ways speech clinicians can facilitate the grieving process.

Suggested Assignments

Your assignment for this unit will include reading chapter 10 in order to gain an overview of basic counseling and psychotherapeutic techniques and how these techniques are used by speech/language pathologists.

In addition, you are to select and read three recent articles about counseling and prepare a one-page summary of each article. Consult the *Reader's Guide to Periodical Literature* under subject-title Counseling, where you will locate articles about this subject. You may wish to review current issues of *Counselor Education and Supervision, Personnel and Guidance Journal,* and *Journal of Counseling Psychology*.

Finally, study questions are provided at the end of this unit to help you review important information presented here.

10

Basics of Counseling and Psychotherapy in Speech Pathology

The individual whose sole task is modifying articulation behaviors could be thought of as a technician. A number of school districts presently employ speech aides or paraprofessionals whose job description is just that—to provide remedial services to children who have speech problems. But the speech pathologist fulfills a much larger role than just correcting speech. One of these roles consists of helping people who have problems which relate to their communication difficulties. Frequently, the clinician must consult parents, husbands or wives, relatives, peers, teachers, or other individuals who are directly or indirectly concerned with those who have communication problems. Our purposes in interacting with these individuals are varied. We may advise the wife of an aphasic patient how to cope with the many problems experienced by stroke patients during their recovery period. We may be called upon to counsel with an individual who will soon have his larynx surgically removed. Certainly in this case, a good deal of counseling will be required during the course of speech training. The parent who asks why her child stutters, the high school boy who resists therapy attempts, and the stutterer who feels inadequate all require consultation from speech clinicians.

The fact that counseling is an important part of the speech clinician's job is well recognized by those who define and describe the responsibilities of the clinician. Johnson (1946) described a number of counseling procedures speech clinicians could follow in helping speech-handicapped individuals better understand themselves and the world about them. Stutterers and college students who had various types of adjustment problems were helped by Bryngelson's (1966) course in speech hygiene using a group therapy approach. Van Riper (1947) devoted an entire chapter of his book to the speech clinician's role as a counselor in helping people solve personal problems. Parents of young children require considerable counseling from speech clinicians, as Luper and Mulder (1964) point out. Williams (1957) relies heavily on counseling procedures to help stutterers better understand the semantical aspects of their speech problems, as well as the feelings they harbor about stuttering. Frequently, much of what we do in voice therapy entails counseling, especially when emotional disturbances are closely associated with the voice problem (Moncur & Brackett, 1974). Speech clinicians are encouraged to assist teachers in providing counseling and guidance to children in their classes who have speech problems (Anderson & Newby, 1973). A form of psychotherapy, or mental hygiene, is frequently indicated in all cases of dysphemia and in many cases of dylalia, departhria, dsyphonia, and aphasia (West et al., 1957).

These are but a few of the many examples found in speech pathology textbooks which mention the importance of counseling in speech therapy. Some speech clinicians have developed therapeutic systems which rely almost entirely on counseling procedures. Hejna (1960) and Backus and Beasley (1951) present an approach to the correction of articulation disorders based chiefly on a counseling model. Procedures for determining whether direct, nondirect, or indirect therapy techniques were discussed by Hahn (1961). Low et al. (1959) describe a method of therapy which utilizes the speech clinician as a type of counselor who organizes communication experiences designed to develop speaking success in interpersonal relationships. Although most of the methods listed above present an adequate model for clinicians to follow in conducting speech therapy, direct, supervised training is usually required before a clinician can develop skill in administering this type of therapy.

It has also been recommended that speech clinicians use psychotherapy as a tool in speech therapy (Van Riper, 1947). West et al. (1957) discuss psychotherapy in terms of mental hygiene or *organized common sense*. As a treatment for stuttering, Van Riper (1963) stated psychotherapy may be valuable as a therapeutic method for reducing anxiety, guilt, and hostility. Psychodrama, a special technique of psychotherapy, was employed with stutterers by Lemert and Van Riper (1944). Honig (1947) found marked improvement with groups of stutterers at the end of an experiment using psychodrama. Trogan (1965) described a psychotherapeutic method for treating stuttering known as *kinetic discharge therapy*. A lengthy description of the psychoanalysis of stutterers is presented by the psychiatrist Glauber (1958). Stutterers have been treated by various forms of neo-Freudian types of psychoanalysis, group psychotherapy, nondirective therapy, and psychodrama.

As one reviews the literature in speech pathology regarding the use of counseling and psychotherapy, there can be no doubt about the importance of these procedures as a potential means of altering behaviors directly or indirectly associated with some communication problems. Yet, each author seems to have his or her own interpretation of just what constitutes counseling and psychotherapy. Therapy procedures incorporating counseling or psychotherapy are often sketchy, to say the least. It is difficult for the speech clinician to comprehend and to use counseling techniques without some basic understanding of the principles underlying counseling and psychotherapeutic procedures. Frequently, speech clinicians overlook potentially useful procedures simply because of their unfamiliarity with effective counseling techniques. This chapter outlines a basic rationale for the use of several types of counseling procedures and presents suggestions for their use.

Definitions

First of all, it is important to define *counseling, guidance,* and *psychotherapy.* This is not an easy task since there appears to be much debate in the field of guidance and counseling itself with regard to roles, definitions, and goals of the profession.

Guidance

In the broad sense, guidance influences the ideas, thoughts, or behaviors of another person, whether the information be written or spoken. It can be provided by essentially anyone professionally trained or untrained, child or adult. Used within the framework of the school system, it consists of services from educators who have an understanding of the psychoeducational development and behavior of children (Woody, 1969). Any educator is a potential source of guidance in this sense. Much of what we call *guidance* occurs in the classroom between the teacher and an individual child about specific problems, or as informal group sessions in which information is presented. It can consist of dispensing information, giving advice, offering suggestions, persuading or any other type of service designed to influence the individual in her best interests. It may be limited to information-giving types of academic or vocational advisement. The individual should have complete freedom to accept or to reject the advice.

A somewhat different concept of guidance is held by some schools which refer to guidance as a *program,* a component of pupil personnel services. Counseling is a *process* within the guidance program. Counselors provide student assistance in the guidance program.

By association, guidance and counseling have come to be virtually synonymous terms, overlapping if not interchangeable. You will hear the terms *guidance counselors* and *counselors* used quite indiscriminately to refer to practitioners. In most cases, counseling is perceived to be more extensive than guidance. We generally associate counseling with modifiers such as vocational, educational, academic, developmental, behavioral, adjustment, social, ethical, and financial. Those same adjectives are almost as frequently associated with guidance. It is usually thought that anyone can provide guidance, but professional training is required to provide counseling and psychotherapy.

In essence, a nondefinition of guidance is, "Guidance is education, and education is guidance." Reacting to this position, Katz (1967) suggests that guidance and counseling be reserved for professional intervention in the choices open to a student. This means guidance is primarily concerned with "alternatives," or choices, between competing values, as opposed to teaching "universals" such as good reading, good health, mathematics, and the like.

Just what is the difference between counseling and guidance from the speech clinician's point of view? Your answer is as good as mine; it depends on how you prefer to define the terms. If you inform a school counselor you are providing counseling services to a student, he may be offended because you are not a licensed counselor. But if you tell him you are providing guidance to the student, no questions will be asked. We have the same sort of conflict in attempting to distinguish between speech therapy and speech improvement. We generally contend that to practice speech therapy, professional training and in some cases a license is required; but anyone can engage in speech improvement activities whether they have a college degree or a high school diploma.

We can only conclude that there is no standardized, universally agreed upon definition of guidance. Its definition depends upon the context in which it is used, whether in reference to a program, as a facet of instruction, or as simply one person giving another person advice.

Counseling

As has been mentioned, counseling usually refers to an interaction between individuals where one person, the counselor, has had extensive training in the process of helping others cope with problems. Definitions of counseling are about as numerous as writers who attempt to define the subject. McGowan and Schmidt (1962) presented an eight-point definition of counseling. They describe counseling as a social learning interaction between two people, ranging from simple advising to long-term, intense, psychological treatment. Clients are usually "normal" individuals who have problems of one kind or another, as opposed to psychologically disabled individuals. Their function is to help clients understand and accept what they are, to realize their potential and, if necessary, to alter their attitudes, outlook, or behavior. Listening and talking are usually the primarary interactive methods. Psychological tests, social and biographical histories, outside resources, and other psychological or sociological instruments are used also.

Gustad (1953) describes counseling as a learning-oriented process in which a professionally competent counselor assists the client to learn more about himself and help him put this understanding into effect in terms of perceiving realistic goals so that the client will be a happier, more productive member of society. Brammer and Shostrom (1968) characterize counseling as educational, supportive, situational, problem solving, conscious awareness, and short term, with emphasis on the normal individual.

Finally, Fitzgerald (1965) reports that over 90% of the total membership of the American School Counselor Association approved a statement of policy defining counseling as "an accepting, non-evaluative relationship in which [a pupil] is helped to better understand himself, the environment he perceives, and the relationship between these," its purpose being "that most pupils will enhance and enrich their personal development and self-fulfillment by means of making intelligent decisions."

Sometimes, it is possible to define a term by stating the objective or goal. But the search for "the goal" of counseling is equally frustrating, especially when one considers statements like one published by Arnold (1962) in which he said that counselor educators "simply do not know what they are doing, nor how to evaluate it [counseling]." Another strong criticism comes from Stefflre (1963) who feels counselors might learn more about helping adolescents from reading Salinger's *The Catcher in the Rye* than from reading the latest counseling journals. Thoresen (1969) contends counselors are so busy counseling they have little time to consider what they are doing or how they are doing it. In regard to research in counseling he said, "Most published research is quite simply a waste—a waste of valuable time and resources." He points out that much turbulence and turmoil have been experienced in counseling theory, research, and practice. A review of the literature on counseling reveals several authors cite the confusion and ambiguity about goals, purposes, and objectives. This confusion includes school guidance, student personnel and counselor education programs, as well as specific counseling techniques.

Terminology used in counseling also tends to confuse those who struggle with a search for an adequate definition. It is extremely difficult for one to operationally define such frequently used terms as *constructive growth, therapeutic relationship, experimental syndrome, autonomous, self-realization, genuine,* and *congruently related activities.* The vague terminology used to describe the counseling process is of little help in determining goals.

Two major points emerge from the literature on counseling goals, however. One expressed by Patterson (1964) states that client-centered counselors have one goal for all clients, "essentially maximizing freedom of specific choices of behavior to allow maximum self-actualization." This view holds that the primary product of counseling is "insight," and counseling can be successful without behavioral change. Krumboltz (1966), on the other hand, said the goals should not be the same for each individual. Behaviors which constitute problems should be changed. Thoresen (1969) feels the goal of counseling is to change behavior in such a way that behavioral outcomes can be objectively measured. Counseling cannot be considered successful until the problem that brought the client to counseling is alleviated or eliminated.

Anyone realizing the complexity of human behavior can readily understand why providing definitions and goals in this area is so difficult. We have only to consider the problems that confront us when attempting to define stuttering or establish therapy goals. A universal definition or treatment program for language problems is equally difficult to agree upon. We even have difficulty attaching a name to ourselves (speech clinician, speech correctionist, speech pathologist, language clinician, or communicologist?). The point of the discussion so far is not to tint our view of the area of counseling and guidance as a confused and bewildered lot, but to make the speech clinician aware of the fact that this area is in a state of growth and development. We must be cautious about grasping one theory of counseling that we happen to be exposed to and following this procedure religiously with every individual. We must realize we are not working with a closed, explicit body of knowledge, complete with how-to-do-it kits. Rather, we are exploring an open, ambiguous collection of ideas and methods. Much of what we know comes from a wide range of activities: practical, theoretical, accidental, experimental, and even from mystics. We must not be discouraged at finding disagreement and differences among various theories of counseling. What we must be able to do is sort out as best we can what appears to fulfill the needs of the individuals we serve.

Pychotherapy

One way of defining psychotherapy is to place it on a continuum with counseling (Brammer & Shostrom, 1968). In fact, at the far end of the continuum we could place guidance activities in which simple information is provided, such as instructions on how to fill out a form or where a college catalogue can be found. On the other end would be long-term, intensive therapy designed to bring about extensive change of personality of a psychotic individual. Somewhere in the middle, counseling activities would be found. As you might guess, the amount of professional training required to perform at each level of the continuum increases as one moves from guidance to psychotherapy.

There are many theoretical approaches to psychotherapy, psychoanalysis being one of the better known models. Evolving from Freud's early works, a number of variations of his basic method have emerged, namely, neoanalytic, neo-Freudian, and social psychological theories. Another major group of theories have been developed by Rogers (1951, 1961) called *nondirective therapy* and later known as *client-centered therapy*. Procedures developed by Rogers have been extremely influential, especially in the field of counseling.

The many diverse forms of psychotherapy appear to have one common bond: they strive to help the client or patient achieve *insight* into understanding why he believes, acts, feels, or thinks the way he does. Actual behavior change is secondary. The story is told of a stutterer who traveled to New York for extensive psychotherapy as a treatment for his stuttering problem. Upon returning to his home some nine months later, he was met at the airport by his close friend.

"Well," his friend said, "How did it go?"

"J-J-J-J-Just f-f-f-f-fine," replied the stutterer.

"But gosh," said his friend, looking a bit puzzled. "You've been away nine months for treatment and you still stutter. Didn't it do you any good?"

"Oh y-y-y-yes, I k-k-k-know," he smiled. "B-B-B-But now I know wh-wh-wh-why I stutter."

This is not so much a joke as you might think. There are many stutterers who feel fluent speech is not an important goal. What is important is the way he *feels* about himself and his speech. Some feel understanding and insight can do much to alleviate and greatly reduce the severity of stuttering.

Just as it is difficult to provide one good definition for counseling, it is equally difficult to define psychotherapy. Winder (1957) identified six components of psychotherapy: (1) there must be a continued interpersonal relationship; (2) the therapist must be specially trained; (3) the client must feel dissatisfied with his personal or interpersonal adjustment; (4) psychological procedures must be used; (5) there must be an underlying psychological theory from which the therapist operates; and (6) the objective must be to ameliorate the problem that brought the participants together. It would seem that these prerequisites would serve as a basis for counseling as well.

Brammer and Shostrom (1968) view psychotherapy as supportive, reconstructive, depth emphasis, analytical, focus on the unconscious, emphasis on neurotic personalities, and long term, whereas counseling is educational, problem solving, conscious awareness, emphasis on normal individuals, and short term. Psychotherapy is associated more with psychiatry and clinical psychology, while counseling is regarded as school-oriented. Counseling implies *adjustment,* whereas psychotherapy implies *personality change.*

Therapy procedures used in psychotherapy differ widely but can be classified into three major types, according to Smith (1967): (1) Supportive procedures are designed to help clients get better control of their impulses, ego strength, and interest in the acceptance of reality. Techniques used would include giving information, persuasion, suggestion, reassurance, modifying environment, group activity, and tutoring; (2) Re-educative procedures attempt to help the client attain insight which will result in more favorable self-concepts, goals, motivation, and to some extent, behaviors. Theories such as those expounded by Rogers and adjustment-type approaches would fall into this area; (3) Reconstructive approaches strive toward helping the client achieve insight into both conscious and unconscious conflicts. The primary purpose is to restructure the personality. Theories dealing with psychoanalysis would fit here.

Play therapy for young children, as well as group therapy for adults, are two specific procedures used in psychotherapy, both of which have been employed as part of speech therapy, especially with individuals who stutter. Basic to the success of all procedures is the nature of the therapist-client relationship. This is usually a warm, accepting environment in which the client feels free to express himself.

In attempting to summarize the discussion thus far, it seems appropriate to consider guidance, counseling, and psychotherapy functions as a continuum. Figure 10–1 outlines the various aspects of all three functions, from one extreme to the other.

It might be best to think of each function as a process. The process of guidance involves information giving. Counseling is a process of helping people solve problems, which involves much more than giving information, whereas psychotherapy is reserved for those who have profound adjustment problems. Each process uses an approach or specific method of helping an individual. A variety of approaches are available. For example, a counselor might use a type of psychoanalytic approach to help an individual with a problem, or she may choose to work directly on the problem behavior. Again, she might prefer to take an approach which leads the individual into insightful thinking about himself. She may be very directive or very passive.

Similarly, the psychotherapist could make use of any of the same approaches selected by the counselor. He might be directive, nondirective, psychoanalyze the patient, or if qualified, use drug therapy. Not quite so many options are open to the guidance counselor or adviser due to the type of training she has and kind of problem encountered. For example, she would never use psychoanalysis but may choose to modify behaviors or serve as a reflective listener. Each person involved in the process has several choices of approaches which could be taken toward the treatment of the problem. These choices are presented next.

	Guidance	Counseling	Psychotherapy
Major Goal	Provide information	Solve adjustment problem	Change personality
Type of Person Served	Normal person seeking information	Normal person with personal problem	Abnormal person unable to cope with problem
Training Required	None to Bachelors	Masters to Doctorate	Masters to Doctorate
Time Required for Services	Immediate	Short term	Long term
Events Considered	Present events	Present and future events	Past events
Theory	No theory	Moderate theory	Strong theory background

FIGURE 10-1. Functions Of Guidance, Counseling, And Psychotherapy

Principal Approaches

Counselors and psychotherapists use a wide variety of procedures designed to help people who have problems. Sometimes the same procedure might be used by each to different degrees. At one time, these procedures were best known by the individuals who developed them. "Schools" developed by the name of Freudian, Neo-Freudian, Sullivanian, and Rogerian. More recently, descriptive titles are used to describe the theory or general approach being used; and schools are classified under titles such as psychoanalytic, phenomenological, and behavioral. These theories are useful because they describe and explain what is being done and why.

Because the speech clinician receives intensive training in rehabilitative procedures and because she works directly, and often intensely, with communication handicapped individuals, she is ideally suited to provide counseling. Whether counseling is provided to the client or to his associates, the speech clinician must operate from some theoretical orientation. This orientation may consist of our own intuition, developed as a result of our past experience, or we can choose from basic principles derived from the experience professionals have had in helping people with problems. Obviously, the second choice is the preferred one. Clinic supervisors, and to some extent, professors, pass on in a more or less organized fashion a viewpoint about principles of counseling, but rarely is there a formal attempt to expose student clinicians to a variety of counseling theories. Several theories and techniques used by counselors and psychotherapists to help people cope with problems will be presented. With this knowledge, you should be in a better position to select appropriate techniques to help you deal more effectively with people-type problems. At present, you may have some vague notions about what should happen during clinician-client communicative interaction but lack the repertoire of techniques and theory to feel confident in counseling someone.

Psychoanalytic Approach

When one thinks of psychotherapy, psychoanalysis immediately comes to mind. We picture the client stretched out on a long, comfortable couch at the head of which is a bearded analyst with notebook in hand, attempting to interpret the client's rambling. Today, the couch may have been replaced by a comfortable chair and the analyst may be clean-shaven, but he is still going through a process of interpreting the client's remarks. The essence of a psychoanalysis is the careful investigation of one's psychosexual life history. The unconscious is the seat of life energy which emerges through the personality. If an unresolvable conflict arises among various sources of energy, then individuals are inept or unable to solve problems that confront them. The ego, id, and superego represent some of the chief energy forces within humans. Conditions are created in which the client feels completely free to talk about anything, especially in response to the analyst's questions. From the patient's verbalizations, the analyst attempts to reconstruct the development of personality and to explain why the client behaves the way he or she does. The emphasis is on probing into past events which will explain present behaviors.

The training required of a psychotherapist using this technique is extensive. A doctorate degree is required, with specialization in psychotherapeutic methods. Frequently, an analyst is also a psychiatrist who holds a medical degree. They work in private practice and in private hospital settings, usually treating people who are considered "mentally ill." Certainly few, if any, speech clinicians have received training sufficient enough to allow them to use this technique. This technique has been a methodology employed in the treatment of stutterers.

Psychoanalysis Used in Stuttering: Psychoanalytic methods have been employed as a treatment of stuttering for some time. In fact, Freud worked with several patients who stuttered but felt the psychoanalytic approach offered neither insight nor help for stutterers (Glauber, 1958). He was quoted as saying that he gave up the treatment of stuttering since he was never successful in treating it (Froeschels, 1951). Other psychoanalysts have not been so pessimistic. Analysts seem to have a "field day" with the case history and analysis of stutterers since the problem seems focused in the oral region. This appears to be the seat of all kinds of early sex related "hang-ups."

Glauber (1953) describes a treatment of stuttering in which two analysts are assigned to each case, one for the stutterer and one for the mother, who is the center of concern. It was through the original anxieties and feelings of love and hate for her child that the seeds of stuttering were planted. The therapist for the mother is assigned to help break the bonds that hold her to her child and to provide her with necessary treatment since she is considered very neurotic. Interviews of 4 to 5 hours in length and projective testing are initiated first in order to devise a treatment plan for each case.

The first task in analysis with the mother is to convince her she needs treatment and to explore her relationship to her own mother. Next, she needs to vent her pent-up emotions and disappointments experienced when she was a child. She needs to realize how closely tied she has been to her narcissistic mother and separate herself from this unhealthy relationship.

The husband is brought into the therapeutic setting when the mother is ready to work on their relationship, which has been one of sado-masochism and frigidity. The father must learn to act more positively toward both the wife and child.

The treatment of the child is basically no different from the treatment of any neurotic child. Stuttering as the overt symptom is not treated, and speech therapy is avoided. A completely permissive atmosphere is created in which the therapist speaks freely but does not require the child to talk. The child is allowed to express his anger through play situations. It was noticed that in some cases, fluency improved after only a few weeks having expressed aggression by biting, chewing, or smearing objects in the playroom. Later, stuttering reappears during the process of resolving oedipal conflicts.

After 6 weeks of treatment, there is usually much less concern about the stutterer. In a number of instances, stuttering has disappeared before this time, but it should be emphasized that reduction of stuttering is *not* the chief goal. The aim is to normalize the psychological constellation of the entire family. Then stuttering will cease to be a family phobia, lose its excessive charge of anxiety, and the symptom (i.e., stuttering) may disappear by itself. The key to success is freeing both the mother and child from their state of unconscious fusion, by loosening the mother's ties to narcissistic love-objects and by turning toward real love-objects.

As you can well understand, this is no task for a 22-year-old speech clinician who has just finished her master's degree! And I must admit, this therapeutic approach would not be one I could handle either. Nevertheless, it is an approach we should at least know about since it is occasionally mentioned in the literature. For example, Fried (1972) reports a psychoanalytic diagnosis of an adult stutterer and felt if more treatment was indicated, he would follow up the behavior therapy applied with psychotherapy, involving psychoanalysis as the method.

Psychoanalysis has not enjoyed great success as a method of eliminating stuttering, according to many writers. It is very expensive and often requires treatment over several years. Wolpe (1961) considers psychoanalysis an ineffective way to treat stuttering after reviewing a number of follow-up studies. Van Riper (1973) drew a similar conclusion about the poor effects of psychoanalysis when used alone as a treatment of stuttering.

Psychoanalysis and Voice Problems: Psychoanalysis has been used for the treatment of individuals whose voice problems are of functional origin. Moses (1954) describes the many vocal features common to those who have been diagnosed psychotic or neurotic. He feels the same psychoanalytic technique is appropriate for both types of individuals. In advising the laryngologist who directs treatment, he recommends that physical treatment be accompanied by a psychotherapeutic approach. The laryngologist, Moses feels, should acquire the necessary knowledge to provide psychotherapy, find the underlying emotional conflicts, and help the patient become aware of how these conflicts can affect the voice.

Phenomenological Approach

This approach views each individual as having a unique perception of reality which the therapist must attempt to duplicate in order to fully understand the client. The emphasis is on the present, rather than on the past or future. The client's feelings about himself (self-concept) and the world around him are of greatest concern. The goal is to assist the individual in developing positive concepts about himself in a way that releases his full potential. The self- or client-centered theories fit best in the phenomenological approaches because they focus on the person and his perceptions about himself.

A Gestalt approach emphasizes the self as part of the reality of the larger community in which the individual participates. Honesty and openness in encounters with others, along with broadened awareness, is one of the principal goals.

The philosophy of existentialism has also influenced approaches in this area. Emphasis is placed on humanness and human potential. One of the best-known approaches in the phenomenological category is one advocated by Rogers (1951) called *client-centered counseling*. As a procedure to help individuals who, while not being severely disturbed, find it difficult to cope with their problems, Rogers (1946) feels client-centered therapy is far superior to psychoanalytic approaches. He states, "It may be said that we now know how to initiate a complex and predictable chain of events in dealing with the maladjusted individual . . . which operates effectively in problem situations of the most diverse type" (p. 394).

The chain of events Rogers refers to consists of six elements, designed to provide an experience to release the growth forces within the individual. Rogers feels no external aid or environmental manipulation is needed to unleash what he considers to be forces within the individual. The six important elements necessary to release these forces are

1. The counselor realizes that the individual is responsible for himself and that the counselor cannot change the individual or solve the problems for him.

2. The counselor relies on the individual's inner drive or force to become mature, socially adjusted, independent, and productive rather than imposing his own will upon the individual.

3. A warm, permissive atmosphere is created for the individual so he is free to discuss his attitudes or feelings no matter what they are, or he is free to withhold the expressions if he desires.

4. There are virtually no limits set on behavior other than behaviors which might result in destruction of property or those which would be illegal.

5. The counselor must be accepting, neither approving nor rejecting, of the behaviors and attitudes expressed. His deep understanding of the individual's responses is conveyed through sensitive reflection and clarification of the individual's attitudes.

6. The counselor must place no value judgments on the individual's statements or behaviors. He should not ask probing questions, blame the individual, offer advice, suggestions, offer resistance, or in any way attempt to persuade the individual.

If the above conditions are met, Rogers stated that "it can be said with assurance that in the great majority of cases the following results will take place:"

1. The individual will express attitudes and ideas which are of great concern to him.

2. He will analyze these attitudes and perceive them differently than he had perceived them previously.

3. He will acquire a clear understanding of his attitudes and behavior.

4. In the light of this new perception, he will choose new goals on his own initiative, which will be more satisfying than his maladjusted goals.

5. He will change his behavior in a way which will allow him to reach these goals. This new behavior will be more spontaneous, less tense, more in harmony with social needs of others, and will result in a better adjustment to life situations.

Rogers reports that Snyder (1945) analyzed a number of cases with "strictly objective research techniques," which verified Roger's theory and procedures. First, there is a period of catharsis, followed by a phase when insight occurs, finally resulting in a phase of increased positive choice and action. The effects sometimes may be shallow, resulting in only a new look at an immediate problem, or it may result in a profound personality change. The process is the same, Rogers claims, whether the individual requires only three or four sessions to understand how childish he has been acting, or whether the individual is on the verge of a nervous breakdown and after 20 or 30 sessions, develops deep insight which enable him to reorganize his life.

Basic to this approach is the assumption that the individual can solve his own problems and make the necessary behavioral adjustments, providing the therapist creates a suitable, psychological atmosphere. No other assistance from the therapist is necessary. Under suitable conditions, the maladjusted individual is capable of exploring and analyzing his attitudes at a comfortable rate and to a depth required for satisfactory adjustment. The individual has the capacity to follow steps without external guidance or suggestion which will lead him toward a more comfortable relationship to his reality. This concept reminds one of air-filled plastic clown figures which are weighted at the bottom with sand. If they are tipped over, they will right themselves due to the force of gravity, attracting the sand weight back to its position. A maladjusted individual might be perceived as one who is held tipped over on his side. By creating conditions which will enable him to remove the force pulling him to the side, he will right himself because of the very nature of the forces at work within himself. Rogers feels strongly that each of us have these "self-righting" forces within us. He calls it the client's *capacity*. The counselor's sole job is to help the individual release the inherent self-contained forces within us which give direction to our lives.

The full force of client-centered therapy is realized in Roger's concept of the therapy session. He feels the client knows what areas to explore, how often the interviews should be, how to lead the interview, when to cease exploring an area he is not ready to divulge, which repressions need to be uncovered to build a comfortable adjustment, how to discover and to apply insights by himself that will lead to constructive behaviors, and when therapy should be terminated. This willingness to accept the fact that the client takes the leading role in directing therapy, according to his desires, rather than those of the therapist, points out a major departure from other therapeutic approaches.

One wonders what skills the therapist must possess since the client has so much responsibility. Rogers makes it clear that creating the unique atmosphere enabling a client to make these changes is a difficult task requiring considerable training and experience. One does not say, "Okay, now I want you to feel free to tell me anything that's on your mind because I'm a very accepting person," and the client proceeds to pour out his soul! To develop qualities of empathy, understanding, acceptance, sincere interest in others, plus a strong, personal warmth often requires years of training and practice. One counselor using this technique described it as deceptively simple. Each word you choose, how it is said, and its precise timing in the conversation becomes critically important to developing the proper atmosphere. This method of counseling demands the most exhaustive, penetrating, and comprehensive consistency. He feels client-centered counseling demands discipline, utmost sensitivity, appreciative awareness, and a constant attitude of understanding.

Rogers' attitude about the value of client-centered counseling is far from passive. He states the results may sound too good to be true (that was my feeling, too), but he maintains he has research to back up his claims. He went on to say that the original hypotheses were rapidly becoming established as facts and that his case records and research gave credulity to his counseling approach. Some 30 years have passed since Rogers made these statements. Today, client-centered counseling is considered by some to be a valuable approach in some cases, but it certainly takes a back seat to behavior therapy approaches. One wonders if the lack of enthusiasm for client-centered counseling results from the fact that it is too difficult to train skills necessary to become an "ideal listener," or whether the results counselors obtain using the approach simply are not as spectacular as Rogers claims.

A rather sarcastic and morbid joke about a client-centered counseling session clearly reveals the opinion many have about the effectiveness of this approach. It seems a disturbed client constantly complained that she had an overpowering desire to commit suicide. The counselor, being very noncommittal, took the following approach:

HE: Hello, Miss Finch, how did things go this week?
SHE: Terrible.
HE: You weren't pleased with what happened?
SHE: No.

HE: Oh

SHE: I feel like jumping out the window.

HE: You really feel like jumping out the window?

SHE: Yes

She moves toward the window.

HE: Oh, I see.

SHE: I'm going to open the window.

HE: You really feel like opening the window and jumping out, don't you?

She opens the window and sits on the sill.

SHE: I feel this tremendous desire to jump out.

HE: I see, looking down in the street makes you feel like you actually want to jump out doesn't it?

SHE: I'm going to jump.

HE: You really want to jump out the window.

At this point the client leaps from the window and falls "ker-splat" on the hard pavement ten stories below. The counselor calmly walked over to the window, leaned out to look at the pavement below and said, "Ker-splat!"

As you might guess, critics of client-centered counseling do not feel reflection is always an appropriate or effective way of treating all types of problems.

Client-Centered Approaches Used in Speech Therapy.

Client-centered counseling has never enjoyed widespread popularity as an approach in speech therapy. One of the first reported uses of the approach was by Thorn (1947) as a technique for treating voice disorders. She noted that many individuals who came to speech clinics to seek help with a voice problem or inability to speak before audiences have no pathological or physiological problems which could account for their speech problem. Many complain that they have little self-confidence, feel inadequate or insecure, or voice some other related personality problem. Some clinicians refer individuals with these types of complaints directly to psychologists. Others try relaxation therapy, voice control procedures, or advise them to enroll in a course in public speaking. Typical approaches are to use advice, persuasion, praise, blame, encouragement, and to motivate the individual to work on his speech. All too often, the individual terminates therapy because of "lack of interest or motivation," "poor attendance," or "lack of progress." Thorn points out that frequently, the clinician is relieved to have terminated the case because of her own feelings of inadequacy in dealing with the case.

The client-centered therapy presents a radical departure from the traditional treatment methods. The clinician regards herself as not knowing the answers to the client's problem. There is no need for extensive diagnostic procedures other than those necessary to rule out physiological causes, no need to map out treatment strategies, to probe deeply into the client's past, or force him to interpret his remarks. The basic assumption is that the client knows what is best for him, and changes will occur when conditions are suitable.

Although Thorn's use of client-centered therapy with individuals who had speech problems was limited, she felt she was able to verify Rogers' predictions about the success of the technique. The counseling procedure was not an easy one to master, she points out, since as speech clinicians, we tend to be very directive during therapy.

One young lady who received client-centered therapy complained of feeling great panic when asked to speak in class. She would perspire, her voice would falter, and she felt very much ill-at-ease. During therapy, she reviewed experiences in high school that led to the development of inadequate speech. She then discussed problems she had at home and other areas of personal distress. After several interviews of this type, she took steps to ask her English teacher to allow her to give oral reports in class. Eventually, the panic symptoms decreased and disappeared altogether.

In another case, a college student desired to become a teacher but was discouraged from this profession because of a harsh voice quality and rapid, jerky speech rate. Following two client-centered interviews, she admitted her father was an alcoholic for which she was both ashamed and angry. She could not invite friends to her house and felt reluctant to visit others. Following several more interviews, she discussed these problems with her father and her hostility changed to sympathy. She explained her rapid speech was a protection against possible probing questions others might ask of her. After several sessions, the clinician noticed that pace of her speech slackened and the harsh quality diminished. She was able to resolve her personal problems as well as her speech problems with no formal speech therapy or suggestions from the clinician.

Thorn was quick to point out that not everyone can benefit from this type of therapy. Some cases do not respond favorably. The fact that some respond favorably to this treatment is evidence that speech clinicians probably should develop the necessary skills required to use Rogers' technique when deemed appropriate. I can recall several instances when counseling students that I should have used an approach like this one instead of trying to solve their problem for them. It is probably safe to say though that most speech clinicians under the age of 30 are familiar with this technique through name only.

Hahn (1961) outlines an approach to nondirective speech therapy based on the theories of Rogers and Axline. She suggests this approach would be best suited for the individual who must solve present personal problems before efforts toward improving communication can be effective. He must first discover for himself new behaviors which will help him better understand and adjust his attitude toward himself, his speech, and other listeners. This is accomplished by the speech clinician, who provides a situation in which the individual is perfectly free to express himself. There is no effort to correct, or in any way respond to, defective speech. As the individual freely expresses himself and begins to recognize, understand, and accept his confused feelings and atypical behaviors, the barriers which halted proper growth and development will be broken down. Improvement in communication skills will follow as the individual works through his adjustment problems.

Objects and materials are provided in the therapy room if the client is a child. He may manipulate these in any way as he talks. The clinician reflects the feelings he believes are being demonstrated. The child becomes aware of his own feelings, and thus begins the process of self-understanding. If the client is a young child, the therapy session in which toys are manipulated is called *play therapy*.

Hahn presents an example of a 7-year-old boy who does not want to attend speech therapy. His behavior was not deviant enough to warrant referral to a psychologist, and the parents would not follow such a recommendation. The case history revealed a disturbed mother-son relationship which produced the speech problem. He could not take direction, was tense and fearful, tended to destroy possessions of others, was antisocial, and verbally abusive to others. The speech clinician scheduled this child for hourly sessions in which he was told he could do what he wished (within certain limits). As he crashed one car into others, the clinician reflected:

"He wants to get the other cars out of there. He wants to hurt them." The boy hid the red car.

"He is afraid," said the clinician.

"Yes!" screamed the boy, "They will get him."

An earthquake destroyed the cars.

"You want everything destroyed," observed the clinician.

The red car came back to life. The clinician continued:

"You are alone now. This feels good."

Through the reflective and accepting process, the child gradually learns to clarify his attitudes and accept his feelings of hostility. With this growth comes a change in his manner of speaking, sometimes to the degree that formal speech therapy is not required. For others, they become adjusted sufficiently to accept correction of their speech. Hahn stresses that only a trained person should attempt to undertake nondirective play therapy.

Due to the strong emphasis on models, based on learning theory in speech therapy during the last decade, little attention has been given counseling techniques of the phenomenological type described above. These counseling procedures are seldom mentioned in the literature. We have no way of knowing to what extent these techniques are taught or even practiced in training institutions throughout the country. My guess is that these approaches have been swept out with the tide of behavior modification procedures. My guess also is that they will be "re-discovered" and redefined in another 20 years as teachers become disenchanted with some aspects of the behavior modification movement. The wise clinician should realize that client-centered counseling may be ideally suited for some clients, and the skills required for directing sessions of this type might be very useful. In fact, the traits Rogers suggests for the successful counselor are good ones to have during any interview or counseling session conducted by the speech clinician. The chief limitation of phenomenological theories is their high degree of subjectivity, which often leads to vagueness, mysticism, and an inability to verify procedures through research.

Behavioral Approaches

The influence of the behavioral movement in psychology has been strongly felt in every aspect of education, including the field of counseling. A new approach called *behavioral counseling* has been introduced by some as the way to treat many behavioral problems. The most significant departure from phenomenological approaches is that behaviorists perceive the actual behaviors of the client as the prime problem and the modification of these behaviors the chief goal of therapy. Furthermore, efforts are made to obtain direct measures of the behavior before and after treatment. Success of the counseling is judged by the amount of change which has been brought about in the behavior. Behavior therapy is based upon learning theory and principles of conditioning. Just as Rogers felt client-centered counseling is the preferred technique for minor problems as well as those which incapacitate the individual, behaviorists also believe techniques of behavior modification can be used in combating a wide variety of problem behaviors. The success of behavioral counseling techniques as an effective means of helping individuals with problems seems undeniable. Probably more research has been reported using these methods than any other approach. Entire journals are devoted to nothing more than published articles about research using behavior modification procedures.

An accurate description of four essential features of behavioral counseling is provided by Krumboltz and Thoresen (1969). First, a goal must be selected. It must be selected by the client, be agreeable to the counselor, and its attainment must be capable of being measured objectively. The goals set by other approaches such as to become self-actualized, to learn to make important personal decisions, or to become a happy person, would not be agreeable to the counselor because it would be impossible to empirically measure goal outcomes. Many counselors experience difficulty at this point because they are unable to translate the client's problem with clear, behavioral objective statements.

A second feature of behavioral counseling is tailoring techniques to meet the needs of the client. Behavioral counselors not only rely heavily upon conditioning the client through use of appropriate reinforcers, but also use techniques of modeling, role playing, cognitive structuring, simulation, confrontation, and counterconditioning, as well as variations or combinations of these techniques.

A third characteristic is a willingness to experiment with a wide variety of techniques as long as there is an attempt to assess the accomplishment of the goal. Therefore, sensitivity training could be included as part of the behavioral counselor's repertoire providing one can measure the degree to which the client's sensitivity has been altered.

Finally, there must be a constant effort to monitor feedback from counseling sessions. Research studies are an accepted means of providing evidence of success in counseling. In other words, behavioral counseling procedures must stand the test of scientific scrutiny.

Defining the Problem: Since identification of the problem and selecting behaviors to modify are frequent stumbling blocks to behavioral counselors, it would be most helpful for speech clinicians to be aware of ways to identify possible problems with which they may be confronted. Once clear behavioral objectives can be stated, the job of modifying behavior becomes much easier. Krumboltz and Thoresen (1969) identify seven such problems one is likely to encounter.

1. Complaint about someone else's problem: Occasionally, a teacher will complain to the speech clinician about a problem child in her room. The child may have a hearing loss and be inattentive or unable to complete seatwork assignments. Another child who cannot be understood by his kindergarten peers presents a discipline problem in class. Still another child who has a cleft palate is unaccepted by others in his class and causes problems on the playground. To most of us who have conducted speech therapy in the public schools, these complaints are common.

The first question to ask is "Who is my client?" In almost all cases, it is the person who brought you the problem; in the case above, it was the teacher. She has far more contact with the problem child and is in a much better position to help solve the problem than you are. Therefore, it would be best for the two of you to work on it together. Begin by visiting the classroom or situation where the child's maladaptive behavior occurs and analyze how the teacher handles the problem. Behavioral goals are identified and suggestions are given to the teacher regarding how the child's behavior could be changed. Assessments are made of the child's behavior as well as the teacher's observation of the child. The same procedure is carried out with parents who complain about the behavior of their children. The counselor remains sympathetic with the person who presents the problem but continues to discuss ways the parent can cope with the problem. Of course, the speech clinician may also be working with the child's speech problem as well, so in effect, she may have two clients.

2. Problems expressed as feelings: Frequently, stutterers say they feel inadequate, or an aphasic patient complains he is depressed. Those who work in hospital settings often listen to complaints of adults, who describe their problems in terms of feelings or attitudes, rather than behaviors. The first step is to listen carefully to the complaint and be able to reflect the problem back to the client in such a way that the client understands what is to be done. This clarification of the problem may in itself be sufficient for the client to take steps to resolve the problem. If not, one way to help the individual is to confront the client with his own behavior. For the person who complains of feeling inadequate, analyze just what behaviors he engages in to make him feel inadequate and suggest what he should do to act more independently. Williams (1957) takes this approach when he confronts the stutterer with the fact that he does certain things when he stutters. In order to change stuttering behavior, he must learn to do things which promote fluency. Another way to develop feelings of adequacy is to acquire additional skills. Enroll in courses, develop hobby interests, or build competencies in some special area. Checks are made on these achievements and used as indications of successful counseling.

Another effective way to deal with feelings is through the use of group therapy. Those who feel their problems are unique soon learn otherwise when confronted with experiences of others who have had similar problems. Group therapy is used frequently as a method of helping stutterers cope with feelings they previously felt no one else had. The Lost Cord Club, for individuals who have had their larynx removed, is an ideal setting in which problems can be discussed openly. The sharing of feelings with one another usually results in a more accurate perception of the problem. Frequently, such discussions help to diminish the importance of the problem and nothing more need be done.

3. Lack of a goal: Strange as it may seem, a number of people are unable to formulate any goal or purpose in life. This may be true especially for aphasic patients. Goals must be man-made, and each person must find his own goal in life, whether it be working at an occupation, painting, making money, or demonstrating for some cause. Most people strive toward some unattainable goal throughout their lives without ever attaining it, but just having a goal gives purpose and meaning to life. The person without a goal is encouraged to read books about others who have attained goals, join organizations that have clear-cut goals, and interact with others. This must be an active-seeking process guided carefully by the counselor.

4. The desired goal is unacceptable: Suppose the client's goal is unacceptable to the counselor. The client may wish to commit suicide or discontinue working on his speech. In cases like this, it is best to let the client know the consequences of his decision. The counselor's job is to explore with the client different, alternative goals and the advantages and disadvantages of each in terms of consequences. Often, students seek advice from their professors about dropping out of school to get married (which might be a good goal for some students, by the way), dropping a client with whom they have been unsuccessful, and so on. Identifying the problem is the first step in solving it.

5. Client does not know his behavior is inappropriate: Sometimes, the counselor only hears one side of the story, which is the client's distorted viewpoint. After further investigation, it might be found that the client blames everyone for her problems. Simple confrontation of the problem may be sufficient to make the client aware of her problem. Group therapy might be an effective means of confronting the client with her maladaptive behavior. Sociometric devices can also be used because people often will communicate opinions in writing which they would not otherwise do. Once the problem is identified, alternative behaviors can be selected and learned in appropriate situations.

I recall one young man who requested speech therapy for a mild stuttering problem. One thing I noticed was a continued head shaking as he listened to someone else talk. This was very disturbing to those who communicated with him, but no one ever said, "Say, do you know you shake your head a lot when you listen to me?" I videotaped his behavior and asked him to watch himself on the videotape replay. Once he identified the objectionable behavior, it was rather simple for him to eliminate it within a few sessions. Once he agreed what the objectionable behavior was, it was rather simple to bring it under control.

6. Problems of choice: We have all experienced occasions when we cannot decide which of two things to select. In some situations, making a choice becomes a real conflict. A man may wish to divorce his aphasic wife, yet, feels guilty about his desire because his wife requires his help. The husband needs help in investigating many alternatives so that he does not perceive the solution as an "either-or" proposition. "Brainstorming" with the clinician might prove very beneficial in this case. Once alternatives are available, the client is encouraged to engage in activities which will test the feasibility of the chosen alternatives.

7. Refusal to identify a problem: There are some individuals who just like to talk to others and are not really interested in identifying a specific problem. Perhaps you have a neighbor like that. If the counselor is unsuccessful in pinning down the problem, it may be advisable to use different approaches, such as a transactional encounter group.

Example of Behavioral Counseling: As an illustration of techniques used in behavioral counseling, Hosford (1969) reported the case of a sixth-grade girl who was unsuccessful in speaking in front of her class. Speech clinicians are frequently asked to assist with problems of this kind. In this case, the teacher asked the counselor for assistance. The counselor visited the classroom and observed the child attempting to deliver a book report. Her voice could barely be heard in the front row. Further observation gave indication that she spoke normally in all other situations. A conference with the child revealed she was aware of the problem, wanted to correct it, but was unable to do so by herself. Her parents realized there was a problem, but did not know what to do about it.

The counselor explained that learning a behavior a little at a time in a relaxed atmosphere was an effective way to build a new behavior, and the child agreed to try. The counselor met with the child once a week for 6 weeks, during which time the child role played giving an oral report. In the first session, she practiced getting out of her seat and walking to the front of the room. She also read orally from her seat. Each week she increased the length of her presentations. The counselor provided ample praise for her attempts. Also working with the teacher, the counselor gradually increased the degree to which she performed orally in class in front of the group. The teacher agreed to include her in a social studies committee which gave weekly oral reports. She was to participate only to the degree that she experienced no anxiety. Her first activity was to stand at a map and point while someone else spoke. Later, she made brief announcements or answered a few questions. The committee sat in the front of the class in a semicircle, which provided a more relaxed atmosphere. Counseling sessions were terminated when she reported she was taking an active part in class discussions while facing the class.

Soon, she was able to present oral reports while standing in front of the class. At the end of the school year, she volunteered to give an oral presentation to the class on a special social studies project. As you can see, the accent of therapy is one of achieving the desired behavior identified in the goal analysis. In this case, the behavior was easily identified, the client wanted to achieve it (speaking in front of the class), and achievement of the behavior was readily observable.

Another example of a much different form of behavioral counseling is provided by Stilwell (1969), who presents the use of modeling techniques. The client, who in this case did not request the counseling, was a hospitalized autistic child observed to have a narrow range of behaviors, particularly in social skills. He was observed to engage in self-destructive behaviors, seldom spoke, slapped peers, or ran away from them. After observing this child's behavior in many situations, the following goals were established for the client: (1) reduce or eliminate antisocial behaviors, and (2) strengthen desired behaviors, especially pro-social ones. The next step was to identify possible reinforcers and define the situations in which they would be administered. M & M candies, verbal statements, and smiling were selected as positive, consequent events.

Next, the child was taught to follow directions from the counselor. He was rewarded each time he obeyed such commands as, "Put your hands down," or "Sit down." Once his behavior was under stimulus control, i.e., following directions accurately, other target behaviors were identified. This child's approach to other peers was characterized by ambient walking around other children. He cried frequently. When an adult or peer approached him, intensity of crying increased. He refused to interact with others.

The goal was to develop a pro-social repertoire, which included approaching peers. Playing on the slide with others was one of the first goals selected. First, the counselor stood at the base of the ladder of a sliding board and asked the child to come to the ladder. He received an M & M for doing so. He was rewarded similarly for climbing the ladder and sliding to the bottom. This occurred three times during 15 minutes. A peer who had been watching came over and asked for some M & M's. The counselor told him that every trip he made down the slide he would receive an M & M, provided the autistic child followed him with a trip, too. Thus, the peer became a model for the autistic child. Other children wanted to join the activity, and soon six boys, including the autistic boy, were sliding down the slide.

A second goal was to help the child remain near to and interact with other peers. He was given M & M's while in the presence of other boys who previously he shunned whenever possible. He was able to sit with the other boys for up to 5 minutes, during which time he was prompted to give and to receive candy from them. This exchange laid the foundation for learning to share. We frequently think of counseling as talking to someone about their problems, but in this case, counseling took on a much different form.

Examples of counseling used with a wide variety of behavioral problems are numerous. One criticism leveled at behavioral counseling is its difficulties in dealing with feelings, attitudes, and beliefs. The emphasis on specificity, precision, and objectivity tend to cause one to overlook the complexity of human behaviors in its totality.

Empirical-Rational Approach

This approach is related to the behavioral approach in that a change of behavior is the ultimate goal. It is very directive and consists of appeal to the rationality of the client. Through discussion, the client's views are exposed and analyzed. The counselor then helps the client achieve a better understanding of his attitudes and ideas in the hope that these changes will lead to changes in behavior. The counselor points out to the client faulty beliefs in a very direct manner as a teacher would point out grammatical mistakes in a child's composition.

Often, a plan is suggested for the client to follow for improving study habits or taking a positive attitude with people, whatever the case might require. The results of various psychological tests are usually relied on to furnish the counselor with information that might predict success in study or work. The faculty advisor who counsels the student throughout his years in college would use this approach since it relies on rational analysis of needs and requirements.

One current example of this approach is a form of guidance called *Activist Guidance,* a counseling technique recommended by Menacker (1976). Whereas many counseling techniques place the counselor in a reflective role in which the client's activity is key to the beneficial change and the counselor supports the development through conversational activities, "Activist Guidance" has the opposite emphasis. The counselor is very active in eliminating obstacles interfering with the client's adjustment. He encourages the client to be active as well and works together with the client to achieve favorable, environmental conditions. In traditional counseling, the client and her unique psychological state are the focal points of the relationship; but in Activist Guidance, both the client and her unique environment are considered the most important features. The maximum development of the client can be realized only through recognizing and combating environmental elements which stand in the way of the client's goal. Consequently, the active role taken by the counselor, plus an equal emphasis on changing environmental conditions, make this type of counseling much different from other approaches.

Gordon (1967) proclaimed some years ago there should be a much stronger emphasis on rational activism as a means of dealing with problems. He said, "I see no alternative but to discourage the practice of guidance as primarily a symbolic vicarious experience in the exploration of self in relation to a hypothetical or synthetic world . . . Take the emphasis off the counseling relationship and place the emphasis on guidance as a process . . . in which the guidance specialist and the student are continually included in behavioral and environmental manipulation" (p. 84). He felt the student and counselor should actively work together to remove real obstacles in the environment which prohibited the student's progress. The student should be helped to find more acceptable real-life situations using objectives and strategies arrived at through mutual consent. Guidance, in his opinion, should shift from a behavioral science, based on psychology, to a social science framework in which skills of social anthropology and political science are utilized.

Three basic principles are identified as being important in Activist Guidance: First, the counselor becomes actively engaged in projects designed to modify the client's environment. He may organize legal aid counseling for the client or go directly to a school administration in behalf of the client. He may help a student change a professor's conventional, bell-shaped distribution grading system by bringing the matter before the administration. He establishes trust and rapport with the client, not so much through verbal interaction as by his actions. Banks and Martens (1973) put it this way, "Helpers must see that the counselor can and will go beyond passive empathy and actually do something to affect change" (p. 461). This concrete helping relies much more on social science skills than the behavioral sciences.

Second, there must be a mutual counselor-client identification of environmental conditions that may facilitate or retard client goals and self-development. Those conditions which facilitate the client are to be developed, those which retard should be removed. Gordon (1967) states, "I see the guidance worker as a partner with the student in the struggle to make appropriate use of those factors in the environment that best facilitate development and change those factors that retard or obstruct wholesome growth" (p. 84). Here again, when the client's environment is considered as important as his psychological state, the counselor needs a broad range of social science skills to cope with the social and political forces at work in the client's environment.

Finally, Activist Guidance must recognize the distinction between client goals and values and those of the social and educational institutions in which she lives. In some cases, the client's goals might be more appropriate than those of the institution. Solving the client's problem may entail changing the policies of the institution. Recently, I took the role of an Activist Guidance counselor in helping change criteria of a speech department whose graduate program admission policy was based solely on the student's grade-point average. A pupil of mine was denied admission because of an insufficient grade-point average. He complained that because of socioeconomic educational factors in his Mexican-American cultural background, he was denied the kind of education necessary to compete in some math-related courses with other students in the speech department. As a result, his overall grade-point average was slightly below criterion level, but he felt this sole criterion was unfair in his case. We could have reflected about this situation in client-centered counseling sessions but that would have done little to resolve the student's chief problem: admission to graduate school. As a means of assisting the student, I wrote letters protesting the use of a sole grade-point criterion and recommended a committee be formed to develop a different set of criteria which would allow consideration of this student in view of his different cultural background. Other alternatives were suggested including an interview with the vice president which the student negotiated, possible legal options, and contact with lobby groups. I was not only supportive but took an active role in trying to change environmental conditions which were preventing him from being admitted to the graduate program.

In a sense, counselors act similarly to attorneys working for their clients. They spend much time away from their desk interacting with those in the community who are significant to the client. They work outside the school, during evenings, oftentimes on the weekends with no set Monday through Friday schedule. They act as ombudspersons, responsible for the advancement of the client's welfare, even if it conflicts with school policy. The speech clinician might wonder how to apply this type of counseling in the public school setting. Frequently, the clinician must fight for the rights of her students because many schools are teacher, schedule, or program-oriented rather than child-oriented. Attempts to make adjustments in school programs to allow stutterers, for example, to leave class on speaking assignments, may run counter to the administration's policy of compelling students to remain in the classroom. I recall some years ago when a clinician withdrew a child from one class to another because the teacher was unsupportive of the child's language development program. Frequently, speech clinicians must use this counseling approach with young children because they have no ability to change environmental conditions themselves. It is also an effective approach to use with minority students in urban areas as well as with those who are economically deprived.

The empirical-rational approach used in speech therapy: The use of the example of the Activist Guidance approach should not imply that all empirical-rational approaches are of this type. Focus on the intellectual rational approach to problems rather than reflective, insightful approaches are more typical. Johnson (1946) expressed concern about the semantic environment in which speech handicapped people lived. He felt this environment could be improved upon. He resembled an Activist Guidance counselor when he suggested that we should make available to the case the best that environment has to offer. Specifically, he mentioned the following activities: using referral agencies, enrolling the individual in specific courses, acquainting him with organizations for socially useful activities, introducing him to books and magazines, introducing him to influential people, helping find satisfying employment, recreational facilities, and social and leisure time activities. Johnson also suggested educating people who are associated in important ways with the case. Wherever possible, the client should work closely with the counselor in contacting other people who can assist the client in some way. The client should also take some responsibility for his social adjustment by interacting with others. Providing technical information to teachers, parents, and others concerning the nature of the communication disorder is also considered an important role of the clinician. The client may sit in on many of these conferences and would also profit from the discussion. Johnson concludes by stating, "there is a large group who can benefit significantly from environmental alteration providing they are given suitable retraining" (p. 427).

One of Johnson's students, Dean Williams, expanded on some of Johnson's concepts of semantics and described an approach to counseling stutterers which falls into the empirical-rational category. Stressing a rational approach to the way words are used to describe stuttering, Williams (1957) outlined a procedure for helping the stutterer overcome semantic problems in the way he talks about himself and his stuttering. Stutterers who refer to stuttering as "it," or some special entity unique to them, must be convinced that stuttering consists of nothing more than the things they do. Holding their breath, tensing the lips, blinking their eyes, and jerking their heads are behaviors they perform, not things that "just happen" to them. The stutterer is confronted with these behaviors, describes them, and also is made aware of what normal speech is like. He is taught to study the ways in which "normal people" talk in terms of continuous breath stream, pausing, lack of tension, rate, rhythm, and the like. He must learn to stop doing those things that interfere with normal speech flow and begin doing things that facilitate it. The process is one that is very rational throughout and quite directive.

The empirical-rational approach assumes from the onset that the individual will benefit from an instructional, highly directive attack on the problem. It can readily be seen that this approach would be unsuitable for the neurotic or psychotic individual who was unable to perceive his problem clearly, let alone cope with it objectively. Very young children would also not benefit from the appeals to the intellect featured in this approach. But for most students and well-adjusted clients, this approach offers much toward helping them solve problems with the aid of the clinician.

Physiological Approaches

Approaches which concentrate on some form of bodily awareness are placed in the physiological category. The use of drugs and medication would also be considered here, but they are dispensed only by the medical profession. One basic assumption of therapies in this area is that the client has lost touch with his bodily senses, his awareness, and brain wave functions. Gaining control over these functions can lead toward a better understanding of oneself, an enrichment of life through increased sensitivity. A person can learn to relax in tension-producing siutations, control the development of migraine headaches, regulate body functions, eliminate insomnia, and reduce high blood pressure.

Biofeedback has, as one physiological approach, gained popularity in both clinical psychology and medical circles of late. Biofeedback is simply an awareness of different bodily parts or functions (Karlins & Andrews, 1972). Special training, usually with the aid of instrumentation, can allow one to gain a certain degree of control over these bodily functions. For example, Hardych and Petrinovich (1969) used biofeedback to reduce subvocalizations of students whose silent reading rate was too low. Electrodes are attached to the larynx of the reader, and subvocalizations are recorded on an electromyograph. An audible tone is played when the student subvocalizes while reading. The tone terminates when subvocalization stops. Instructed to keep the tone off as much as possible, the student learns to read silently without vocalizing through this biofeedback training in as little as 1 to 3 hours. Budzynski et al. (1970) used biofeedback to induce muscle relaxation as a way to reduce anxiety provoked headaches. Training required 4 to 8 weeks of patient participation, both at home and in the laboratory. Patients no longer required drugs and were able to anticipate and to control the onset of headaches.

Monitoring brain waves as a body function has become a widely used practice among many who practice biofeedback. A variety of machines are available for monitoring alpha and theta brain waves, ranging in price from $100 to $700, and anyone can learn to operate and to use them. Danskin and Waters (1973) suggest biofeedback training could help produce important feedback that could be an aid in counseling individuals. Green et al. (1970) had success in helping people get in touch with their unconscious by teaching them to increase their theta brain rhythm through biofeedback. The individual receives immediate feedback on an internal physiological process through an external source (usually an instrument). This information enables the person to learn how to voluntarily control what would normally be an involuntary function. People who undergo theta brain wave training go into deep states of relaxation which resemble trance-like states. They experience many of the same states brought about by drugs.

Henschen (1976) used theta wave relaxation training as a counseling technique with a woman in her twenties who complained of being lonely and unable to maintain intimate relationships with others. Electrodes were placed on her forehead, and an electromyograph provided audio and visual feedback of theta waves. Throughout seven 45-minute sessions twice a week, she entered a dreamy state, experiencing delirium and hypnagogic imagery. She was encouraged to continue these experiences and was able to produce deep states of relaxation. When she was experiencing these feelings, the counselor probed her attitudes and encouraged her to express her hostilities, fears, and anxious feelings openly. She was able to gain better control over her feelings of insecurity and adapted a much more favorable attitude toward her friends.

Two advantages of biofeedback training are suggested by Henschen. First, the person gains confidence over his ability to control his mental output; and second, the procedure is harmless since no drugs are required and there are no harmful side effects. States of reverie offer more realistic opportunities for counseling than other methods such as dream analysis, although biofeedback is not recommended for everyone since some individuals seem to be unable to reach the deep state of relaxation necessary for reverie.

Biofeedback for stutterers: Biofeedback has also been used in the treatment of stuttering. It is a well-documented fact that almost any event, unpleasant or pleasant, which immediately follows a moment of stuttering tends to decrease the frequency of stuttering. It seems the mere identification of stuttering moments has the effect of decreasing those moments. We also know most stutterers are able to predict instances of stuttering with a high degree of accuracy shortly before stuttering occurs. It is reasoned that identification procedures might be most effective in reducing stuttering if the stutterer's attention is drawn to the earliest possible cues present in the chain of responses which lead to the actual stuttering behavior. The earliest cues consist of increased muscle tension in the jaw and throat area. Some feel stuttering might be generated from this increased muscle tension.

By teaching the stutterer a new adaptive response as soon as the initial muscle tension cue is recognized, it is hypothesized that stutterers can better learn to control their stuttering. Such was the reasoning of Lanyon et al. (1976) when they experimented with biofeedback of muscle tension. By placing electrodes in the masseter muscle and under the chin, stutterers could easily monitor early indications of muscle tension and learn to consciously reduce this tension. A study of eight stutterers revealed that all eight virtually eliminated stuttering on 25 one-syllable words simply by observing a feedback meter registering amount of tension. They learned to consciously reduce the tension to a prescribed level before speaking. Thus, stuttering can be eliminated if speech muscles in the oral region are consciously relaxed while observing biofeedback. Lanyon and his associates have since developed a treatment method for stuttering based upon this principle of biofeedback.

Biofeedback in other areas of communication disorders: Research data reporting the use of biofeedback in other areas of communication disorders is sparse, but we can look forward to its application in a variety of settings. Boone (1977) has reported that biofeedback may prove to be a very useful procedure in helping individuals become aware of laryngeal tension. He is presently experimenting with biofeedback procedures with individuals who have hyperfunctional voice problems. The application of biofeedback with individuals who have hyperfunctional voice problems, especially those diagnosed as spastic dysphonic, will undoubtedly become an area for fruitful research in the future.

Transactional-Communicative Reality Approach

Theories which fall into this category focus on the communication of two or more interested parties, such as between the parent and the child, the teacher and the child, two adults, or even one individual with a group of others. Techniques people use to influence or manipulate others are analyzed, particularly the ways in which some people might distort the communication process. A number of books dealing with "communication games" played by people who try to disguise their true feelings have become popular sellers.

Counseling is directed toward helping individuals develop communication skills to the point where they can relate in a more direct, meaningful way with others. The client is held responsible for his own behaviors as well as the nature of his thoughts. Emphasis is placed upon the verbal honesty of the participants.

Many types of nonprofessional counseling centers have sprung up throughout the United States within recent years. One example would be a group who call their method *Re-evaluative counseling*. The basic assumption is that each of us have had communicative experiences which were thwarted at one time. Many of these experiences occurred early in our childhood, like instances when a mother punished her child unjustly and prevented the child from communicating his ideas. These unsuccessful communication attempts and the frustrating experiences surrounding them have been suppressed in adult life as we learn to put up verbal and nonverbal defenses to protect ourselves from being hurt further and begin to shut people out of our lives. This, of course, leads to poor communication, "game playing," insincerity, and loneliness.

In order to overcome the suppression of the faulty communication experiences, counseling sessions are scheduled to allow the individual to re-evaluate his early communication experiences and through this re-evaluation, cope more effectively with daily problems. Counselors are those individuals who have had training for this type of counseling technique, but college degrees or previous college training are not required. Interested individuals enroll in a program where they meet once weekly for 2 hours. The first hour usually consists of group discussion, whereas the second hour, pairs of individuals team up to counsel each other for an hour. One member of the team is designated listener, the other talker. The listener is accepting and completely nonevaluative. When he perceives the talker has hit upon a sensitive area, one she may wish to avoid, the listener tells her to explore that area more fully, the idea being to analyze and re-evaluate bad communicative experiences. This re-evaluation leads to a better understanding of one's feelings and attitudes toward self and others. The technique is used with children and adults alike.

Speech clinicians have not made use of these techniques, at least the literature does not contain reports of their use. It would not be at all surprising though to find stutterers who have received counseling from some nonprofessionals using techniques of this type. It is difficult to find a technique which has not been used with stutterers (Van Riper, 1973). It is doubtful, I feel, that speech clinicians will utilize approaches which rely upon transactional analysis and similar approaches which utilize nonprofessional counselors and techniques.

Eclectic Approaches

Undoubtedly, most counselors who work with people who have problems adopt an eclectic view with regard to selecting an approach to use. The eclectic approach does not consist of a casual picking and choosing from many different theories, but entails a careful integration and selection process. Eclectic views must be consistent as well as comprehensive and are best suited to meet the various individual needs. It is probably safe to say that in spite of the desire to establish one's own style or individuality in helping others, most people remain rather firmly entrenched with one theoretical position.

Some argue that different people require different types of therapy. Marks and Gelder (1966) believe behavior therapy, insight-oriented psychotherapy, or a combination of these approaches may be suitable for one individual but not for another. On the other hand, they feel there is much "common ground" between many aspects of psychotherapy and behavior therapy.

An attempt to integrate behaviorally oriented and insight-oriented procedures was reported by Katahn, Strenger, and Cherry (1966). They combined group counseling and behavior therapy with college students who had test anxiety. Participants in the study attributed most of their change to counseling interaction, rather than to the behavioral methods used to teach relaxation. Cooper (1963) maintained that behavior therapists can draw beneficially on the traditional forms of insight-oriented psychotherapy.

The term *psychobehavioral* has been used by Woody (1969) to describe the union of insight-oriented counseling-psychotherapy with aspects of behavior therapy. It is not meant to be a "new" position but merely represents a frame of reference from which one can operate to provide more effective services. He cites three reasons to justify this unified approach: (1) Not enough is known about individual differences to assert that one specific theory has universal applicability; (2) While one technique can be applied successfully by one professional, another professional may not experience equal success with the same technique; and (3) Certain techniques may not be as suitable for children as they are with adults. Woody concludes that, "an eclectic approach is undeniably necessary" (p. 146).

Eclectic approach in speech therapy: Speech therapy seldom reports a therapeutic merger of two approaches as widely diverse as psychoanalysis and behavior therapy.

An example of the integration of these two approaches is reported by Fried (1972) as a treatment for stuttering. He states, "there are times when psychoanalysis and behavior theories and therapies not only can but must be integrated" (p. 348). This appeared to be the case in designing a treatment program for a college stutterer. Desensitization was the procedure selected to gain fluency, thereby eliminating the symptom, and psychoanalysis was chosen as the means to accurately diagnose the person. With an adequate diagnosis, the therapist could better structure the anxiety situation hierarchy in the desensitization process, thereby allowing behavior therapy to become more effective. Had Fried been able to continue therapy with the case after he became fluent, he would have then changed to an analytic type therapy to help solve basic inner conflicts that may have contributed to speech anxiety.

Prins (1970) investigated the prevalence of regression in the speech of stutterers who received intensive fluency training and found a high degree of regression when exclusive emphasis is given to attainment of fluency. He felt that maintenance of fluency depended on the management of complex, interpersonal relationships experienced after termination of therapy. If the stutterer is unprepared to cope with these factors in his environment, then stuttering may reappear. He, therefore, recommended more activities directed toward problem- and self-acceptance, the identification and recognition of symptoms, and self-confrontation; in short, insight-oriented counseling.

How the Speech Clinician
Can Use Counseling Techniques

After reviewing the many approaches available to those who help people with problems, you might be totally confused as to what course you should take with regard to counseling others. Certainly, there is not enough information contained in this chapter to prepare you to select an appropriate counseling method. Perhaps now you will be more motivated to seek out counselors or psychotherapists in your school or community. Their professional services can be an invaluable aid when needed. At least now you should have a better understanding of some of the goals and approaches counselors and psychotherapists use. I am sure you have used elements of many of these approaches in the past and will continue to do so in the future.

The purpose of this final section is to present a general counseling strategy individuals in the helping profession should have at their fingertips, whether he or she is a minister, teacher, nurse, social worker, or speech clinician. The suggestions do not fall into any one "camp," but represent elements from a cross section of approaches with the exception of psychoanalysis, which has been excluded. You will find these suggestions helpful not only during the course of your therapy work, but also during those many occasions when you are talking with the wife of an aphasic patient, helping a stutterer cope with his feelings of inadequacy, explaining reasons to a high school student why she should improve her speech, or conferring with a troubled student. All of us will be counseling people. It may consist of a few minutes or may add up to hours. We need to develop these important communicative skills because they constitute effective means of helping people modify and improve both covert and overt behaviors.

What options does a speech clinician have when communicating with another individual? You can simply listen and nod your head, give your opinion, provide information, interpret what you think the person is saying, or reassure the individual. As you might expect, it depends on the situation. Whether you are simply interviewing a parent of a preschool child or consoling the wife of a laryngectomized patient, you will say different kinds of things and use different communication techniques. Brammer (1973) provides general guidelines for learning basic helping skills. He lists three categories: (1) skills for helping people understand themselves and their environment; (2) skills used in comforting individuals in crisis situations; and (3) skills to help individuals take positive action. Using these divisions, he appropriates procedures used in insight counseling and behavioral therapy in a way that makes their use palatable to almost any professional, regardless of her training. Most of the skills listed by Brammer are known and used by everyone, from the local barber to your next door neighbor. But chances are that your barber or your neighbor does not always use these skills to the best advantage of the other party. Careful study of specific communication techniques, plus practice in using them, should provide the speech clinician with more effective ways of interacting and helping to bring about changes in their client's behavior.

Information and Advice-Giving Techniques

One important function performed by the speech clinician is providing *information* and advice to various concerned individuals including parents, teachers, physicians, clients, principals, wives or husbands, students, and psychologists. The following are some typical questions asked of speech clinicians:

What causes stuttering?
How can a person produce speech if his larynx is removed?
How long is therapy required?
Where can I get speech therapy services?
How much will speech therapy cost?
What exercises can I do at home?
How can I help my child?
What did the test show?
Is it wrong to correct him when he stutters?
What is your schedule at Central Elementary School?
How many school children have speech defects?
What is a vocal nodule?
What is a multidisciplinary approach to diagnosis?

Answers to these and similar questions are quite straightforward. They point out the need to be well informed not only about speech and hearing pathology, but also about community resources and referral agencies. Providing necessary information should be done cheerfully and respectfully, not with the attitude of, "What a dumb question," or "Don't bother me with questions like that." If the person did not think the question was important to him, he would not have asked it.

Providing *advice* is somewhat more tricky than giving information since it usually involves giving your opinion as well. Advice may be given in the form of offering alternatives and helping the seeker weigh advantages and disadvantages of the consequences of action. Do not be surprised or discouraged if individuals fail to heed your advice even though you are the expert and supposedly "know" what is best. Many people simply want confirmation of a decision they have already made. If your advice supports their decision, all the better for them. If it runs counter to their decision, they may seek advice from someone else who will support their belief.

Try not to be persuasive in stating your advice. The individual did not ask to be convinced, he simply wants your opinion. Remember, your objective is *not* to change behavior. Also, be alert with regard to leading questions or topics about which you should not offer advice. The following are examples of questions which might tempt you to provide advice:

Should I get a divorce?
What career should I pursue?
Should I take this job?
What should I do to make friends?
If you were me, what would you do?

When questions like those above are asked, you should first explore the person's feelings about the matter of concern. Techniques to deal with feelings will be considered later. The chief task is to determine which questions are honest and direct requests for advice or suggestions, and which ones are expressions of other problems not directly related to the question. Also, beware of giving advice in areas in which you are not qualified. Be prepared to refer the person to someone else who is qualified to provide the advice. If you are unsure of the motives of the person seeking advice, reflect upon what the person says to see if other more significant problems surface.

Finally, be prepared to cope with the individual if he follows your advice and it turns out to be wrong. This might make you more cautious about the freedom you exercise in telling other people what to do. Be especially leery about advising others with respect to values, morals, religious, or political beliefs.

Listening Skills

My experience with speech clinicians has been that they are frequently poor listeners. They tend to be very verbal people, their chief function being to direct others from the diagnostic examination phase through the course of therapy. Once the clinician understands that the listening process is not just a passive act but involves much activity from the listener, perhaps clinicians will perform this task better. Listening skills are basic to all counseling activities, from giving information to psychoanalysis.

The most important skill of listening is learning how to attend to another person. Ivey et al. (1968) identified several components of attending behavior:

1. Contact—attend to the speaker by looking at the eyes of the speaker. That does not mean you should stare at the person. Frequently you may take notes or look away.

2. Posture—leaning slightly toward a person is the natural response when someone is interested in another person.

3. Gesture—folding the arms or leaning backwards is considered to be an indication of rejection. Erratic or flailing gestures may alarm the other person.

4. Verbal behavior—the kinds of things you say to let the other person know whether you are attending or not. Confirming statements such as, "I see what you mean," "That's right," or "I understand," are noncommitting ways of letting someone know you are listening actively. When you attempt to change the subject or interpret the person, the indication is that you are not "listening" well.

Paraphrasing can be used to restate the speaker's basic message in similar but fewer words. This can help the client better understand what he is saying and lets him know you are trying to understand him. It helps if you ask yourself, "What is he trying to say?" Be careful not to overuse this technique. One step beyond paraphrasing consists of attempts to get the speaker to clarify his remarks. You may say, "I'm not sure I understand what you're saying," or "Could you review that point for me again." This technique not only helps you understand what is being said but helps the client pinpoint main ideas.

A further technique used to clarify points is perception checking where you ask for verification of your perceptions about what he said. A comment like, "You seem to be upset with Mr. X, is that correct?" or "Are you saying you are definitely opposed to plan A?" Listening followed by perception checking is an effective way of eliminating confusion in a conversation.

The effect of using listening skills is one of encouraging the speaker to continue verbalizing his ideas. It is one way to help the speaker verbally explore and analyze his own ideas. It has been mentioned that in some cases, a client can solve his own problems if he can only talk out his ideas sufficiently. On the other hand, selective inattention can serve to discourage the speaker from pursuing a topic. Shames (1970) discusses ways to modify thematic content of stutterers' utterances simply by attending to positive comments which the stutterer made like, "I didn't stutter as much today," and not attending to negative comments such as, "Boy, my speech is terrible today." Thus, the clinician can exert considerable influence upon the client's behavior simply by the way listening skills are used. The sole use of listening skills forms the basis of client-centered counseling.

Encouraging Skills

These skills are designed to encourage clients to verbalize their ideas. They are especially valuable in beginning conversations. During the session, they can be used to encourage persons to explore their feelings and elaborate on ideas presented and to encourage clients to remain active and take a major responsibility for expressing themselves verbally.

This can be done directly by focusing specifically on one topic with a comment like, "Tell me more about your job." The purpose is to elaborate or illustrate a specific point that has been mentioned. A second way is more indirect and is used more frequently in beginning a discussion. "What's bothering you today?" or "Maybe we can begin by you telling me how you feel about your speech." Keep these remarks general in nature so as not to start the discussion off in a direction not intended by the client.

Specific questions that begin with the words *how* or *what* tend to evoke more elaborate responses than questions beginning with *are, is,* or *do.* Questions beginning with these latter words tend to evoke yes and no type responses and elaboration is suppressed.

Reflecting on what the client says is another way to encourage verbalization. Reflecting also helps you understand the main thrust of the client's remarks. Reflecting is similar to clarification skills in that the client's remarks are paraphrased. Sometimes the client lacks the vocabulary to express her ideas and your words may help clarify her feelings and stimulate further discussion. Be careful not to reflect every statement or use stereotyped phrases to begin your reflections. Also, be careful not to read more into what the client said than was intended. Reflecting feelings has a way of stopping the conversation if you are not sure what to say next. Often the client will answer a reflection with "Yes" or "No" or "That's right," and then what do you do? You can not reflect that statement again. Be sure you know what to say next.

Summarizing Skills

Sometimes an interview will wander aimlessly. It may be the client's way of dodging an unpleasant subject, or she may have simply gone off the track. When you perceive this happening, provide a summarizing statement of the discussion so far. Pick out the highlights of the discussion, and summarize them in a few sentences. You might say, "Well, Jane, so far we've covered three points—how you feel about stuttering, how you think it affects you, and why you're disturbed about it. I can tell you're not happy about it, are you?" Another summarizing technique is to try to get the client to summarize his feelings or progress up to this point. You may say, "How does it look to you at this point, Bob? Can you summarize for me?"

Summarizing helps both you and the client keep the discussion moving forward and helps the client feel progress is being made. It is also the ideal means of terminating a discussion, especially when time is running out.

Confronting Skills

There is considerable risk involved in confronting the client with a reflection of what you think or infer is occurring. In some instances, the client will feel challenged, threatened, and anxious. He may deny your interpretations, become angered, and terminate the discussion. He may become alarmed or feel trapped into confronting feelings or issues that are extremely unpleasant. He may have to admit he is wrong, confused, in conflict with himself, or perhaps, he has to admit he is an unpleasant person to be around. On the other hand, he may appreciate being confronted with helpful information, no matter how unpleasant. Confrontation may be the quickest and most direct way of helping the client understand the nature of his problem. Sometimes confrontation is used to help speed up the discussion by forcing the client to come to a decision. For example, Bill has discussed advantages and disadvantages of enrolling in a high school speech class to work on his falsetto voice. He is making no special progress toward a decision so you might say, "Well, Bill, it's up to you, do you want to enroll or not?" or "You've been beating around the bush, Bill; why can't you make up your mind? Is it that you feel like a grade-school kid coming to speech class?"

Sometimes during therapy with an unmotivated case, you may confront the individual with whether or not he should continue coming to speech therapy. Brammer (1973) offers several very blunt confrontation statements:

"Your continuing on and on like that is boring me and I find myself getting sleepy." "I feel angry when you talk so much about wanting to hurt other people and not giving a damn about them" (p. 96).

There are some danger signs that you should be aware of when using confronting techniques. If you are working with someone who you perceive is becoming very disturbed or is in an obvious crisis situation, it is wise to terminate your session and either refer them to a professional counselor or seek professional advice. Your role as a counselor is limited, and you should not overstep professional boundaries. In a like sense, you would find it unethical for a counselor to attempt speech rehabilitation with an aphasic patient.

For those well adjusted enough to handle stress situations, confronting clients with your honest reactions about how he affects you can be helpful. Often, it enables the client to change his behavior. Reactions from others help us determine, "Who am I?" But you should provide confronting feedback only at appropriate times. Your personal sensitivity is the only way you have of knowing what an appropriate time is. You might have to ask if he wants your opinions. Don't overlook the fact that confronting feedback can be of a very positive nature. You might say, "You are a much more talented person than you admit. Let's look at the things you have accomplished." People who tend to belittle themselves often require this type of confrontation. In these cases, the risks of confrontation are negligible.

Sometimes it is helpful to ask the client to look at her own behavior in someone else's shoes. "Would you like a person like yourself for a friend?" or "How would you feel if you weren't allowed to help yourself in any way?" or "Do you realize what it would be like not being able to talk?" There are many times when confronting skills can be very valuable.

As I have mentioned before, we have all used these skills in our daily conversation with friends at one time or another. But in a counseling or an interview session, correct timing and selection of the most appropriate phrase is vital to obtaining the desired outcome. Through supervised practice and experience, you can get the "hang" of using effective counseling procedures. Begin by paying more attention to what you say to people during your daily conversations.

Counseling Clients During
the Grief Process

Tanner (1980) in his provocative article, describes the grief process and the speech/language pathologist's role during the time when a client is involved in grief. Those who work with the elderly are in constant contact with individuals experiencing grief through loss of some aspect of the communication process. Loss of hearing, loss of speech, a change in voice quality, or loss of voice frequently accompany other problems experienced by the elderly.

Our role as professionals is to provide appropriate counseling to individuals who are experiencing grief. There are professional counselors who specialize in counseling the elderly and I do not suggest we take over their role. It is important, however, that we understand the grief process. We can, through this understanding, provide support that will help the client to progress through the stages of grief without undue pain. Our help comes through supportive comments, the grief process so one knows what to expect, counseling family members, and knowing when to refer problems to a professional counselor. First, let's consider the stages of the grief process.

The Grief Process

There are two kinds of loss: (1) real, when a person or function, such as speech, is lost, and (2) symbolic, like loss of self-esteem or one's role in the family. Real losses occur when a loved one dies or changes through loss of intellectual facilities. Real loss also occurs when an aphasic woman patient can no longer sew or garden; business men can no longer go to work following a stroke; laryangectomes can no longer converse with their friends; hearing impaired cannot enjoy music. These things are all lost. There is also developmental loss. This may occur as a child grows older and is no longer dependent upon the mother. Older women lose the ability to conceive children. There is also the loss of previous reinforcers. An aphasic may be moved to a nursing home. Children may be moved to foster homes. Loss of self-esteem is experienced by anyone whose speech handicap greatly interferes or limits the way they functioned before.

Grief

A person passes through at least three successive stages during the grieving process, as outlined by Schneider (1974). The first stage consists of attempts to overcome loss. Denial, rage, and bargaining are part of this stage. The second stage is awareness of the loss. Finally, in the third stage the loss is accepted. People pass through all three stages but sometimes they magnify one stage or fixate on it.

Attempts to overcome loss: One's first reaction to loss is to deny it happens. When one is not told the extent of the loss, this may prolong the denial stage. The second part of this stage is anger; the "Why-me" stage. It results from having finally realized the loss. Anger is the natural and predictable reaction to loss. Sometimes the anger is directed at the clinician. Family members must be aware of this anger. Those who have lost their speech may resort to physical violence when displaying anger. Bargaining occurs when the client attempts to reduce the effects of loss. Bargaining involves a commitment by the patient in exchange for the return of what was lost. "If I work really hard, you'll make sure I'll get my speech back, won't you?" the client might say. Clients are enthusiastic and willing to work at this stage, but they may be unrealistic in their expectations. Passing through this stage allows the client time for resolution and is, therefore, desirable.

Awareness of the loss: Once anger and rage have run their course and the person is fully aware of the loss, depression often sets in. The person realizes that the loss will not be regained and may shift from a motivated state, during bargaining, to depression. Depression is a normal reaction to loss. Let the person know this. During this time the client may not respond well to therapy. Sometimes, those who try to cheer up the depressed person only interrupt the grieving process, thereby prolonging grief.

Acceptance of the loss: Acceptance, the last stage of the grieving process, is devoid of feeling. The person is neither depressed nor angry but simply accepts fate as the inevitable result of circumstances. Frequently, counseling is necessary for the family of the patient, since it would appear that the patient is devoid of emotion. At this stage, the patient is usually a good candidate for rehabilitation. Be sure to keep the level of success high at this stage of the grieving process.

Cautions During the Grieving Process

How long does the grieving process last? The typical length is from 6–12 months. The most acute period comes within 2 months after a loss and acute symptoms disappear within 6 months. If it extends over 6 months, the condition may be pathological. It is important to learn to accept irreversible disorders quickly. Our role can be to aid in this process. First, here are ways to avoid interfering with the grieving process.

1. Avoid reinforcing denial statements. Avoidance is an extreme defense and should be replaced as soon as possible. Don't tell a child following the death of her father that daddy just went to sleep. That's denying death. Be honest, open, and tactful. But if there is some hope, let the person know. Fortunately, most communication defects can be improved.

2. Don't punish anger unless it's actually destructive. Inform others that anger is a natural reaction. They are not to blame for the client's loss and his anger is not directed towards them, although it may seem to be at times. But anger is harmful when it's inner directed.

3. Don't bargain with the client by holding out hope for goals that can't be reached. Don't promise miracle cures, such as anything can happen if you have enough faith. You can, however, help set short-term goals. Don't overtax the client in his effort to bargain in regaining what has been lost.

4. Don't provide too much reinforcement for the person who has experienced loss; that is, don't keep pouring out your sympathy. Don't make the person feel so

special that she may not progress through the other grieving stages. Encourage the person to be her own clinician and work out her own grief.

5. Don't rely on drugs and tranquilizers. It delays the normal process. Certain mood-producing drugs may be helpful, but overuse is not recommended. Often the physician relies upon the clinician's observations of the client's behavior to prescribe drugs.

6. Often people recommend distractions and the client immerses herself in a hobby or work. This may delay the grieving process if done too early. Avoid rapid distractions, like taking a trip immediately after a death. On the other hand, don't let the person just sit in a room either.

7. Don't be overly concerned about the person's display of depression. This is a natural part of the grieving process which results from awareness of the loss. Efforts to cheer up the patient may only result in prolonging depression. Often, all that is needed is just being with the person who is grieving.

Ways to Facilitate the Grieving Process

There are several things you can do to facilitate the grieving process. We should be aware that the grief is an experience in growth and transformation. Our job is to help the person go through this process as effectively as possible.

1. Arrange it so the client can have as much control over her life as possible. Avoid making all the decisions for the person, especially if she is institutionalized. Make sure the person participates in planning the therapy and shares the decision-making, such as time or length of therapy.

2. During the acute stages of grief, try to assure the client that things will get better and that these stages must be passed through. Help her understand that things will get better. Arrange for someone else who went through the same experience to visit with the person. Tell the aphasic patient what she is experiencing with language is not bizarre but quite common, and that after time, she will get better.

3. Don't be afraid to fully discuss the loss with the person. Avoiding the subject only prolongs the grieving process.

4. Allow the person to express feelings by being a good listener. Silence is golden in many of these situations. Don't feel you must be a chatterbox. You can't have all the answers to life's problems.

Counseling and the Scientific Method

The use of the scientific method has received major emphasis in this book. In many ways, the counseling procedures in the section just presented and in some of the preceding sections do not appear to follow the rigors of the scientific method. Counseling techniques have come under sharp attack from behavioral scientists because of that fact. I, too, must agree with many of these criticisms of counseling techniques that rely on insight, intuition, and feelings instead of observable behaviors. And yet, I cannot deny that behavior can be modified through simple cartharsis. Certainly, your behavior has a lot to do with the change that occurs. You, as a listener, can provide a host of reinforcers and punishers. These can be delivered under a wide variety of schedules. You can even write behavioral objectives, but for the most part, much of what we do and say in counseling is by educated guess. We can maximize the probability of obtaining desired outcomes of interview sessions by a thorough knowledge of counseling techniques supplemented by practical experience. But before counseling can be considered a science, we need to know a lot more about how humans function.

Behavioral counseling is another matter. Its objectives, methods, and testing procedures come directly from basic, science methodology. *Behavior therapy* is a more comprehensive term which would include behavioral counseling. It will be included in another chapter under the broader scope of behavior therapy.

BIBLIOGRAPHY

Anderson, V. A., & Newby, H. A. *Improving the child's speech,* 2nd ed. New York: Oxford University Press, 1973.

Arnold, D. Counselor education as responsible self-development. *Counselor Education and Supervision,* 1962, *1,* 185–192.

Backus, O., & Beasley, J. *Speech therapy with children.* Boston: Houghton Mifflin, 1951.

Banks W., & Martens, K. Counseling: The reactionary profession. *Personnel and Guidance Journal,* 1973, *51,* 457–462.

Boone, D. R. *The voice and voice therapy,* 2nd ed. Englewood Cliffs, N.J.: Prentice-Hall, 1977.

Brammer, L. M. *The helping relationship: Process and skills.* Englewood Cliffs, N.J.: Prentice-Hall, 1973.

Brammer, L. M., & Shostrom, E. L. *Therapeutic psychology: Fundamentals of counseling and psychotherapy,* 2nd ed. Englewood Cliffs, N.J.: Prentice-Hall, 1968.

Bryngelson, B. *Clinical group therapy for problem people.* Minneapolis: Dennison, 1966.

Budzynski, T., Stoyva, J., & Adler, C. Feedback induced muscle relaxation: Application to tension headaches. *Journal of Behavior Therapy and Experimental Psychiatry,* 1970, *1,* 205–211.

Cooper, J. E. A study of behavior therapy in thirty psychiatric patients. *British Medical Journal,* 1963, *1,* 1222–1225.

Danskin, D. G., & Waters, E. D. Biofeedback and voluntary self-regulation: Counseling and education. *Personnel and Guidance Journal,* 1973, *51,* 633–638.

Fitzgerald, P. W. The professional role of school counselors. In J. W. Loughary, R. O. Stripling & P. W. Fitzgerald (Eds.), *Counseling, a growing profession.* Washington, D.C.: American Personnel and Guidance Association, 1965.

Fried, C. Behavior therapy and psychoanalysis in the treatment of a severe chronic stutterer. *Journal of Speech and Hearing Disorders,* 1972, *37,* 347–372.

Froeschels, E. Stuttering and psychotherapy. *Folia Phoniatricia,* 1951, *3,* 1–19.

Glauber, I. P. The nature and treatment of stuttering. *Social Casework,* 1953, *24,* 162–167.

Glauber, I. P. The psychoanalysis of stuttering. In J. Eisenson (Ed.), *Stuttering: A symposium.* New York: Harper, 1958.

Gordon, E. W. (Ed.) The socially disadvantaged student: Implications for the training of guidance specialists, in College Entrance Examination Board. *Preparing School Counselors in Educational Guidance.* New York: CEEB, 1967.

Green, E., Green, A., & Walters, E. Voluntary control of internal states: Psychological and physiological. *Journal of Transpersonal Psychology,* 1970, *2,* 1–26.

Gustad, J. W. The definition of counseling. In R. F. Berdie (Ed.), *Roles and relationships in counseling.* Minneapolis: University of Minnesota Press, 1953.

Hahn, E. Indications for direct, nondirect and indirect methods of speech correction. *Journal of Speech and Hearing Disorders,* 1961, *26,* 230–236.

Hardych, C., & Petrinovich, L. Treatment of subvocal speech during reading. *Journal of Reading,* 1969, *12,* 361–368.

Hejna, R. *Speech disorders and nondirective therapy.* New York: Ronald Press, 1960.

Henchen, T. Biofeedback-induced reverie: A counseling tool. *Personnel and Guidance Journal,* 1976, *54,* 327–328.

Honig, P. The stutterer acts it out. *Journal of Speech and Hearing Disorders,* 1947, *12,* 105–109.

Hosford, R. E. Overcoming fear of speaking in a group. In J. D. Krumboltz & C. E. Thoresen (Eds.), *Behavioral counseling.* New York: Holt, Rinehart & Winston, 1969.

Ivey, A., et al. Micro-counseling and attending behavior. *Journal of Counseling Psychology,* 15, Monograph Supplement, 1968, 1–12.

Johnson, W. *People in quandries.* New York: Harper & Row, 1946.

Karlins, M., Andrews, L. M. *Biofeedback.* New York: Warner Books, 1972.

Katahn, M., Strenger, S., & Cherry, N. Group counseling and behavior therapy with test-anxious college students. *Journal of Counseling Psychology,* 1966, *30,* 544–549.

Katz, M. *Counseling—secondary school.* Educational Testing Service Research Memorandum 67–7. Princeton: The Service, 1967.

Krumboltz, J. D. Behavioral goals for counseling. *Journal of Counseling Psychology,* 1966, *13,* 153–159.

Krumboltz, J. D., & Thoresen, C. E. (Eds.), *Behavioral counseling.* New York: Holt, Rinehart & Winston, 1969.

Lanyon, R. I., Barrington, C. C., & Newman, A. C. Modification of stuttering through EMG biofeedback: A preliminary study. *Behavior Therapy,* 1976, *7,* 96–103.

Lemert, E. M., & Van Riper, C. The use of psychodrama in the treatment of speech defects. *Sociometry,* 1944, *7,* 190–195.

Low, G., Crerar, M., & Lassers, L. Communication centered speech therapy. *Journal of Speech and Hearing Disorders,* 1959, *24,* 361–368.

Luper, H. L., & Mulder, R. L. *Stuttering: Therapy for children.* Englewood Cliffs, N.J.: Prentice-Hall, 1964.

Marks, I. M., & Gelder, M. G. Common ground between behavior therapy and psychodynamic methods. *British Journal of Medical Psychology,* 1966, *39,* 11–23.

McGowan, J. F., & Schmidt, L. D. (Eds.), *Counseling: Readings in theory and practice.* New York: Holt, Rinehart & Winston, 1962.

Menacker, J. Toward a theory of activist guidance. *Personnel and Guidance Training,* 1976, *54,* 318–321.

Moncur, J. P., & Brackett, I. C. *Modifying vocal behavior.* New York: Harper & Row, 1974.

Moses, P. J. *The voice of neurosis.* New York: Grune & Stratton, 1954.

Patterson, C. H. Comment. *Personnel and Guidance Journal,* 1964, *43,* 124–126.

Prins, D. Improvement and regression in stutterers following short-term intensive therapy. *Journal of Speech and Hearing Disorders,* 1970, *35,* 123–134.

Rogers, C. Significant aspects of client-centered therapy. *American Psychologist,* 1946, *1,* 415–422.

Rogers, C. *Client-centered therapy: It's current practice, implications and theory.* Boston: Houghton Mifflin, 1951.

Rogers, C. *On becoming a person.* Boston: Houghton Mifflin, 1961.

Schneider, J. *The stresses of living: Loss.* Paper presented at Michigan State University, 1974.

Shames, G. H. Operant conditioning and therapy for stuttering. In M. Fraser (Ed.), *Conditioning in stuttering therapy.* Memphis: Speech Foundation of America, 1970.

Smith, D. C. Counseling and psychotherapy in the school setting. In J. F. Magary (Ed.), *School psychological services in theory and practice: A handbook.* Englewood Cliffs, N.J.: Prentice-Hall, 1967, 142–170.

Snyder, W. U. An investigation of the nature of non-directive psychotherapy. *Journal of General Psychology,* 1945, *33,* 193–223.

Steffire, B. Research in guidance: Horizons for the future. *Theory into Practice,* 1963, *2,* 44–50.

Stilwell, W. E. Using behavioral techniques with autistic children. In J. D. Krumboltz, & C. E. Thoresen (Eds.), *Behavioral counseling.* New York: Holt, Rinehart & Winston, 1969.

Tanner, D. C. Loss and grief: Implications for the speech language pathologist and audiologist. *Asha,* 1980, *22,* 916–928.

Thoresen, C. E. Revelance and research in counseling. *Review of Educational Research,* 1969, *39,* 263–281.

Thorn, K. 'Client-centered' therapy for voice and personality cases. *Journal of Speech and Hearing Disorders,* 1947, *12,* 314–318.

Trogan, F. A. A new method in the treatment of stuttering: The kinetic discharge therapy. *Folia Phoniatrica,* 1965, *17,* 195–201.

Van Riper, C. *Speech correction: Principles and methods,* 2nd ed. New York: Prentice-Hall, 1947.

Van Riper, C. *Speech correction: Principles and methods,* 4th ed. Englewood Cliffs, N.J.: Prentice-Hall, 1963.

Van Riper, C. *The treatment of stuttering.* Englewood Cliffs, N.J.: Prentice-Hall, 1973.

West., R., Ansberry, M., & Carr, A. *The rehabilitation of speech,* 3rd ed. New York: Harper & Row, 1957.

Williams, D. A point of view about stuttering. *Journal of Speech and Hearing Disorders,* 1957, *22,* 390–397.

Winder, C. L. Psychotherapy. *Annual Review of Psychology,* 1957, *8,* 309–330.

Wolpe, J. The systematic desensitization and treatment of neurosis. *Journal of Nervous and Mental Diseases,* 1961, *132,* 189–203.

Woody, R. H. *Behavioral problem children in the schools.* New York: Appleton-Century-Crofts, 1969.

UNIT 6 STUDY QUESTIONS

1. To what extent has counseling been used in speech therapy?
2. Differentiate between guidance, counseling, and psychotherapy.
3. Why is it so difficult to define constructs used in counseling?
4. How would a psychotherapist use counseling techniques?
5. How do psychoanalysists treat the problem of stuttering?
6. What basic assumption about the individual does Rogers make in his theory of client-centered therapy?
7. What is the counselor's major contribution to the therapy process according to Rogers?
8. How has the client-centered approach been used as a treatment for speech problems?
9. What role do counseling techniques play in the area of speech therapy?
10. List and define four essential features of behavioral counseling.
11. How do behavioral counseling procedures differ from client-centered counseling approaches?
12. List seven common problems the behavioral counselor is likely to face when attempting to set goals.
13. What is the chief objective of the behavioral counselor?
14. What main feature typifies activist guidance?
15. What type of individual is best suited for empirical-rational counseling?
16. Explain how bio-feedback has been used to decrease stuttering behavior.
17. What reasons are given for using eclectic approaches to counseling?
18. Explain three reasons to justify the speech pathologist's use of counseling skills.
19. In what areas should one be very cautious about giving advice?
20. Why are reflecting skills an important aspect of counseling?
21. When is it important to summarize a discussion?
22. What risk is there in confronting an individual with her problem?
23. What type of counseling best meets the rigors of the scientific method?
24. Describe the steps people go through during the grief process.
25. What should be the speech clinician's role in helping a person who is experiencing grief?

Unit 7

The Instructional Process: Theoretical and Practical Applications

Objectives

The objectives of this unit are (1) to introduce you to the area of instructional planning and (2) show by practical application of case studies how behavior therapy is conducted. You should be able to identify four components of a system designed to optimize the instructional process. Also, you will be able to identify how key elements of the behavior therapy process are administered in speech therapy situations.

Suggested Assignment

The assignment of this unit is to read the material included in chapters 11 and 12. No study questions are provided.

11

A Psychology
of Instruction

So far, the major thrust of this text has been to review and to explain major contributions from current theories of learning as they apply to therapeutic procedures used in speech pathology. Theories of learning are essentially descriptive in nature and have developed from psychometrics, one of the two major areas of psychology. Emphasis among the various branches of psychometrics has been placed on the application of practical techniques with little attention given to theoretical concerns. This work is best represented in the fields of educational psychology, industrial psychology, and human engineering. The paramount task among psychologists and educators engaged in these fields has been that of relating the knowledge gathered from research in the behavioral sciences to the problems of education.

The second major area of scientific psychology is experimental psychology. From this branch has developed a psychology of learning based upon theoretical constructs, giving little attention to the design or application of practical techniques as they apply to the modification of human behavior. Complex learning models such as those reviewed by Johnstone (1974) represent the theoretical approach to problems in education. The theoretical model systems he reviewed ranged from simple arithmetic computational models to those requiring very sophisticated mathematical computations. They include four basic model types: deterministic, Markov chain, regression, and mathematical programming models.

Two books may serve as illustrations representing each of these two major areas of scientific psychology. One presents a practical application approach to education.

Competency Based Learning: Technology, Management, and Design (Davies, 1973) offers a *learn-by-doing* approach to learning and teaching. It introduces students to task analysis, writing behavior objectives, and implementing teaching strategies in the classroom. The second book, *Learning Theory: Instructional Theory and Psychoeducational Design* (Snelbecker, 1974) reflects the theoretical point of view. It provides an objective description of contemporary as well as historically important ventures in psychology of learning with little concern for the practical application of theory to instructional settings.

The dichotomy between these two extremes, one being the practical application of knowledge, the other involving theoretical constructs in psychology, has been recognized since the turn of the century. John Dewey (1900), in his presidential address before the American Psychological Association in 1899, expressed a desire to bridge the differences between psychological theory and practical work with what he called a *linking science*. Dewey warned that many teachers, without such a linking science, would be inclined to fall back on routine traditions of school teaching or to adopt the latest fad of some pedagogical theorist who publishes an article about an educational panacea.

Further concern about the apparent dichotomy between the theorist and the practical worker was voiced by Thorndike (1922). His answer to this problem centered around the development of a single set of theories from which practical application to educational settings could be made. You may recall the discussion in the beginning chapters of this text which dealt with the various laws of learning Thorndike formulated. His three primary laws—the laws of effect, exercise, and readiness—formed the theoretical construct of stimulus-response bonds from which practical techniques of transfer of training and reward were incorporated into teaching strategies. He applied his theory and findings directly to the teaching process.

Glaser (1976) points out that Dewey's plea for the link to connect theory and application is somewhat different from Thorndike's translation of science into the practice. Whereas Dewey sought a special structure, a new branch of psychology intervening between scientific theory and practical application, Thorndike was concerned with the direct and immediate application of what he knew about learning theory to the actual business of teaching. He did not bother formulating the link between the two.

Thorndike's approach to instruction is highly individualistic in that it represents a unique combination of a theoretical scientist and the applied scientist. His influence on educational methodology has been more extensive than any single person in this century. Of course, close behind Thorndike is Skinner, who like Thorndike, put his theory into practice, resulting in the current surge of interest in behavior therapy.

But to rely on the work of certain key individuals as the sole cornerstone of educational methodology could interfere with the development of that link between theory and practice Dewey so aptly sought some 80 years ago. Reliance solely on the schemes of individual psychologists can lead to a noncumulative collection of practices which could actually inhibit the development of a unified body of knowledge (linking science). Rather than the development of a sound, systematic structure, what usually results from such highly individualistic approaches are procedures which lack wide parameters of application. Frequently, educators follow instructional fads whose application may be very superficial and dependent on the sporadic interests of individuals.

It was not until the late 1950s and the 1960s that interest was rekindled for developing a theory of instruction as the missing link between theory and practice. Bruner (1964) summarized the feelings of many contributors to the 1964 *Yearbook of the National Society for the Study of Education* in a challenging article calling for the development of a theory of instruction. He clearly distinguished such a theory from the more common theory of learning which describes, after the fact, the conditions under which learning has taken place. A theory of instruction, on the other hand, sets forth rules and criteria which specify ways of achieving performance or knowledge. Such a theory entails a *prescriptive* science, as opposed to a theory of learning that is primarily *descriptive*.

Anyone familiar with Skinner's work and his interest in the technology of teaching will realize that he also was interested in developing procedures for prescribing conditions for learning. His work with programmed learning models, along with efforts of many other professionals, has been aimed at developing instructional settings which almost guarantee that learning will occur. And yet, most approaches that are based on theoretical and empirical description have not been concerned with the development of a prescriptive science.

Simon (1969) pointed out the traditional role of scientists within university settings was to describe how things are and how they *work*. The areas of physics, mathematics, and biological sciences are concerned with describing the various aspects of our environment. The professional schools, such as medicine, architecture, engineering, law, and education, are concerned with a different role, that of *designing* and making things. One of the chief functions of a medical doctor is to prescribe medicine for the ailing. An architect prescribes a certain type of living space for inhabitation. A lawyer outlines his case in an attempt to persuade the jury toward his views. And an educator designs a program of instruction for a school system. Design is the central core of all professional schools. But according to Simon, prescriptive design is less prominent in professional school activities than it should be.

It would appear that the professional school curricula have drifted more toward the activities of the descriptive sciences. Certainly, descriptive theory and analysis is considered to be much more intellectually tough than activities which involve design and application. The latter is often thought of as more intellectually soft, more instinctive, or somehow below descriptive science. The first thing that comes to one's mind when contemplating design strategies is some kind of an educational "cookbook" process to be followed in step-by-step fashion.

But such a "cookbook" procedure is not at all what a psychology of instruction entails. The central purpose of a psychology of instruction is to devise courses of action aimed at changing existing situations into desired ones. Given (1) a set of alternative goals, (2) the constraints of the situation, and (3) a function that describes the relationship between these two factors, the quest is to discover a set of values that provides the best solution to the attainment of a selected goal.

Simon provides an illustration of this paradigm by showing how one might solve a problem with diet. Suppose you wish to lose x number of pounds. That clearly defines the goal. There are several constraints, such as availability of certain foods, food prices, nutritional content of the food, nutrient and energy requirements of your particular body, and the like. There is also a relationship between the cost of a diet, calories per day, and minimum needs for nutritional requirements. The problem is to find the kinds and quantities of food necessary to reduce weight from the present weight minus x number of pounds within a given time frame. Once this solution to the weight problem can be found for a given individual, and the solution would be quite different from one individual to the next, the diet program is administered. The result would be the anticipated loss of x number of pounds, providing all conditions would be met.

This same paradigm could be applied to the prescriptive treatment of communication disorders. Suppose you selected 98% fluency as a goal, among other goals, for an individual who stutters. The constraint would consist of the amount of time the individual can spend in therapy, how well motivated he is, his past history of success in therapy, his age, the severity of the communication problem, type of speech clinician available, and so on. Also, given the relationship between the motivation of the individual, the cost of therapy services, and the amount of time the clinician has available to provide therapy, the task is to select the therapy technique and clinician that will be most appropriate for achieving the stated goal of 98% fluency. On the basis of this prescribed solution, the treatment plan can be executed.

The prescriptive treatment plan described above is often not followed as a standard procedure for dealing with problems involving modification of stuttering in many university training centers. What one commonly finds students learning is a highly individualistic and stylized approach, taught by one professor who has developed his own pet theory about the nature and treatment of stuttering. In the long run, such an approach can only result in the development of separate "camps," or schools of thought. The treatment procedures may be highly successful for some, but for others, they may be of little value. If the clinician has few alternatives as possible remedial techniques or goal statements, this places severe limitations on his ability to meet the needs of a wide variety of individuals. Furthermore, this highly individualistic approach to the treatment of stuttering will not result in the identification of a unified set of principles from which a theory of instruction could be developed.

The matter of chief concern here is that we cannot be satisfied with simply coming up with a solution to a problem; we must search for the most appropriate assembling of all components involved. These components consist of a number of alternative procedures and an a priori selection of those that seem most promising. Those deemed least appropriate are rejected. These alternatives then need to be tested against practical requirements, constraints, and values peculiar to the unique individual and his environment. This approach to the instructional process is quite different from the intuitive, one-shot designs so often found in education.

Again, turning to the treatment of stuttering, one can find a wide variety of procedures which can be used to modify stuttering. Rather than focus on finding "the" method most popular at the time or that claims to result in success with most stutterers, the focus should be one of selecting from a variety of alternatives the procedure and set of conditions which seem best suited to the needs of the particular individual. For one individual, a goal could be set to eliminate stuttering behaviors from her speech; for another, reduction of certain feared speaking situations might be most appropriate. For still another, it may be necessary to teach more acceptable coping procedures, knowing that the client may always continue to "stutter."

A case in point is that of a male stutterer I treated recently at the Arizona State University. This young man had received speech therapy while enrolled in several programs but was disappointed with his progress because he continued to stutter. He had little confidence in student speech clinicians and felt he knew a great deal more about the subject of stuttering than they did. He had learned a type of "slowed speech" pattern and coped with airflow blockages with an easy onset type of vowel and consonant prolongation. Yet, stuttering still caused him much concern, and he sought remedial help. The type of program I outlined for him was totally different from one for another individual I worked with who had received little remedial help and demonstrated severe blockages of airflow. This individual was quite naive about the nature of stuttering. He was willing to attend an intensive treatment program for 3 months. Also, we could expect a great deal of support from his family. The conditions relating to both individuals were quite dissimilar and called for radically different remedial procedures. The thorough analyses of the parameters and constraints of each situation, followed by the selection of one among a number of remedial procedures as the most likely set of therapeutic alternatives, constitutes the core of the psychology of instruction.

To many well-trained speech clinicians, this approach to the treatment of communication disorders is not a new one. The sole purpose of a thorough, diagnostic procedure is to aid the clinician in selecting the most appropriate therapy procedure. This same process is called prescriptive teaching in some educational circles.

One of the first attempts toward the development of a psychology of instruction was reported by two psychologists, Atkinson and Paulson (1972). They presented examples for perfecting simple paired-associate list-learning skills commonly required for initial reading tasks or in learning vocabulary words of a foreign language. The examples they provided were illustrative of how one might proceed from a theoretical learning process to the specification of an optimal strategy for carrying out instruction. They outlined a set of clearly defined steps necessary for deriving and testing instructional strategies. They stressed that educators and psychologists should focus their efforts on the detailed study of simple learning situations. Using this information, we should be able to generalize and to develop prototypical procedures for analyzing more complex learning problems and generating workable instructional strategies.

Components
of a Psychology
of Instruction

In an effort to identify the components of an emerging psychology of instruction, Glaser (1976) lists four essential parts required for optimizing instruction or for deciding between several possible instructional alternatives. These components include the parameters, the constraints, and the functional relationships which must be considered in developing a psychology of instruction.

Analysis of Competent Performance

The first component of the design of a psychology of instruction, as set forth by Glaser, is the problem of task analysis. We must decide the exact nature of what is to be learned or what skill is to be mastered. It is first important to identify the distinguishing features of skills those who can perform the task in question have in contrast to individuals who cannot perform the task. This component is closely tied to what many educators call behavioral objectives.

Learning language skills could serve as an illustration here. If we analyze the skill of the 8-year-old child who has good control over language skills, we find that she is acquainted with thousands of words as well as a set of rules for putting them together in an orderly fashion appropriate to the situation at hand. Given certain information or a particular situation, she has a set of many possible alternatives she could use in response to the situation. Her search for the correct sentence is based on her perceptual ability to recognize the informational pattern set before her. For example, if a classmate asks her for a pencil, and she does not wish to give it to him, a number of appropriate answers are available such as, I need it, I'm using it, no, ask someone else, where's yours, bug off, be quiet, you should take care of your pencils, and so on. Literally hundreds of possible responses could be appropriate, but millions more would not be appropriate such as, where's your dish, behind what barn, chew your gum, black is the color of coal, to sleep perchance to dream, ad infinitum. But for one who has mastered the use of language, only a few patterns would be appropriate. The selection of one phrase is done quickly and almost automatically.

This simple act, answering the question, "Can I use your pencil?" requires a vast repertoire of words, syntactic patterns, and the knowledge of which set of words are appropriate to the situation. This knowledge, as simple as it might seem, requires years of practice to build the familiar language patterns required to speak appropriately at the automatic level. The acquisition of language skills requires a vast accumulation of words and their use in a variety of situations. A psychology of instruction must address itself to a careful analysis of both the informational content, and the skills of the competent performer as well as the novice speaker.

One way of analyzing tasks is to study the behavior of a competent or skilled individual in order to determine how he functions. By specifying the structures and processes by which competent individuals perform tasks, this knowledge may help us better understand how to teach these processes to other individuals. Another way to view task analysis is through what Gagné (1970) described as "learning hierarchies." His system for a rational task analysis is based on a cumulative learning model where simple tasks must be mastered before more complex ones can be learned. For example, concept learning is a prerequisite for rule learning, and rule learning is a prerequisite for problem solving. It is through this step-by-step learning procedure that complex skills are acquired.

A number of speech pathologists have approached the teaching of articulation by establishing task hierarchies. First, the child is taught the sound in isolation, then in nonsense syllables, in combination with words, phrases, sentences, and finally, as a part in the conversational speech of the child. Others take a more Gestalt-oriented approach and recommend correcting articulation first at the sentence level and working backward, if necessary, to the sound at the isolation level. What we do not know is whether or not the articulation learning process is best learned by first teaching the individual, component parts of simple articulation patterns, which when combined, result in the ability to use the sound consistently in conversational speech, or by beginning at a low task level and building on the behavioral movement patterns as they are hierarchically related to one another in sequenced progression. This type of question is most appropriate for research efforts within the field of instructional psychology.

Description of Initial State of the Individual

Whereas the first component of a psychology of instruction dealt with a careful analysis of the task to be learned, the second component suggested by Glaser is concerned with an accurate description of the individual as a unique person. In order for instruction to be effective, much must be known about the learner, specifically his abilities, weaknesses, previous history of learning, repertoire of experiences, motivational state, and the like.

Speech pathologists have access to a wide battery of tests and assessment devices which can be used for this purpose. Unfortunately, many clinicians use this information primarily for evaluating and classifying individuals, rather than as information which can be used to guide instruction. For example, some clinicians administer the Illinois Test of Psycholinguistic Ability without the faintest notion about how the information derived from this test could assist them in terms of providing instruction. Worse yet are those clinicians and teachers who drill a child on memorizing lists of numbers after that child has been observed to score low on the auditory digit-span memory section. During the past few years, there have been some fairly successful attempts to generate prescriptive instructional strategies based on score patterns obtained on this particular test. These attempts to carefully assess cognitive strengths and weaknesses of an individual represent current trends toward developing a psychology of instruction.

All too often in the past, educators have used tests, usually intelligence tests or aptitude tests, as psychometric predictors of future academic success; but they have been of little value to teachers whose chief concern is to provide remedial instruction to individuals who attain low scores on these tests. What teachers are concerned with is what can be done to increase the likelihood that these low-scoring children will succeed.

One case in point is illustrated by Estes (1974) who investigated the digit-span test in the Stanford-Binet Intelligence Test. It is well known that high scores on this test correlate very well with academic achievement. It is also suspected that there may be certain abilities tapped by this test which account for the fact that the individual will or will not succeed academically. Estes points out that a careful analysis or assessment of those skills necessary to perform well on the digit-span test may reveal what instruction the individual requires to enable him to succeed in academic ventures. First, he analyzed the task involved. It was found that in order to remember a number of sequence of 691472, the individual must be able to sequence the ordinal numbers 1, 2, and 3. When asked to repeat the series, two chunks of information must be recalled (691 and 472), each in turn producing the individual set of sequentially ordered numbers. Upon assessment of an individual's performance, it may be found that an appropriate strategy for grouping numbers has not been developed. This would prohibit one from separating out "chunks" of numbers. Estes contends that the digit-span test might be used to identify certain deficiencies among learning strategies used by some children. An analysis of performance on this test may also suggest ways of improving these skills. A test which previously held predictive value may now be employed as an indicator of how deficient performance in that task and similar ones could be remediated.

One of the central targets speech pathologists should pursue is a diagnostic approach which will result in the development of prescriptive teaching strategies. Many current speech and language tests assist us in classifying children into groups so we know which ones have what problems, but they provide us with little information concerning what instructional strategy to follow. One of the most deficient areas is assessment of the individual who stutters. Several clinicians have developed tests that describe the act of stuttering or the frequency of occurrence of moments of stuttering; but obviously, this provides us with little useful information about planning therapy. As I mentioned earlier, several predictive tests of articulation abilities have been developed to determine who may require therapy; but here again, they tell us little about how instruction should proceed. Of more help are inventories used to analyze the feelings and attitudes stutterers have about their speech and various speaking situations. With this information, the clinician can at least generate a list of fear hierarchies, which can serve as a guideline for desensitization therapy. But we have no way of knowing whether we should select an instructional program designed to establish normal fluency, take a counseling approach regarding the individual's fears, or teach the person alternate techniques to cope with the problem.

Hunt et al. (1973) adequately summarized the need for making more careful assessments of individuals when they stated, "Hopefully [this] new viewpoint . . . will lead to measuring instruments which are diagnostic, in the sense that they tell us how the institution should adjust to the person, instead of telling us which people already are adjusted to the institution" (p. 120).

Conditions That Help Foster the Acquisition of Competence

So far, an analysis of special features of the task as well as the unique characteristics of the learner have been considered in the design of instruction. The third concern is the teaching method, or what is done to the environment to bring about prescribed change. What little we know about teaching methodology is strictly in terms of descriptive science. Chiefly, the work done in behavior modification has led to attempts at using what we know about learning in designing the conditions of instruction. For the most part, these attempts have dealt with rather simple, cognitive performances. The need is for designs aimed at discovering how to maximize outcomes of learning for different individuals. What we need to know is, given a particular task plus a unique individual, what is the best teaching methodology possible for that situation? Glaser contends we need to test existing learning models so we can determine which ones best fit the nature of the task and the individual who is supposed to learn the task. He maintains that we need a theory which will encompass how an individual acquires increasingly complex behaviors by assembling the present components of his repertoire, by deliberately altering the environmental conditions, and by using his knowledge of how he learns.

One concept educators have toyed with for some time has been the "learning to learn" phenomenon, or learning in the absence of direct or complete instruction. Some suggest instruction in these processes might be a way of increasing the individual's generalized learning-to-learn abilities. One practical application here would be in the area of stuttering. By making the individual more aware of the role environmental cues play in evoking the disfluent response, stutterers might be taught ways of anticipating and analyzing cues that cause disfluency. Recognition of these cues may prompt effective action, which will lead to reduction or elimination of the cues which provoke stuttering. This type of self-regulatory behavior, the learning-to-learn concept, could be a major contribution toward the remediation of stuttering for some individuals. The application of self-reinforcement may even enhance self-regulatory behavior. Thus, very careful consideration must be given the type of teaching methodology used as it is matched to the task and to the individual.

Assessment of the Effects of Instructional Implementation

The final component of Glaser's psychology of instruction is assessment. Assessment includes those evaluative devices used before instruction begins, often while instruction is in process, and later as follow-up evaluations.

These assessment procedures have already been discussed in previous chapters, but their importance in a developing science cannot be overstressed. Many speech pathologists are still caught in the traditional framework of administering only norm-referenced tests. The test items in such tests are usually external to the instructional process and provide very little input into instructional design. Far more important is the use of intrinsic assessment devices, which allow one to pinpoint deficiencies and strengths of the instructional process. These criterion test results allow us to accurately diagnose and troubleshoot weaknesses in an instructional methodology and help identify aids for maximizing learning.

The role of assessment in instruction is illustrated by results of our early work in developing the S-PACK (Mowrer, Baker, & Schutz, 1968). At first when children missed an item, we gave them a chance to repeat it. If they produced /s/ correctly on the second try, the examiner said "Good" and gave them a token. The result was there were a lot of first-try misses and second-try hits. This increased instruction run-time and seemed to generate numerous error responses. We were assessing the effects of instruction in terms of error response rate, correct response rate, and program run-time. Bob Baker conceived of the notion that while allowing for a second chance, instead of giving a token contingent on the correct /s/ production, we should only say "Good" and proceed to the next item. Tokens were reserved for first-try hits only. Upon changing the instructional design slightly to incorporate Bob's suggestion, assessment of the data from the next 10 children revealed he was right. The number of error responses decreased sharply as did runtime. Thus, it is clear how careful assessment of student response plus some insightful thinking and planning can result in instructional design changes which maximize the effects of the instruction.

The use of follow-up assessment procedures is important too. My initial experience in running the S-1 stuttering program was very positive. At least all the assessment indicators employed during program administration lead me to believe high levels of fluency were achieved. The instructional program was obviously doing the job for which it had been designed. Those who administered the program, as well as the individuals to whom it was administered, were convinced this program was the answer to fluency. But several months after these individuals were dismissed from the program, I began to receive reports that stuttering had reappeared. Long-term assessment following dismissal from therapy revealed the instructional program alone was not sufficient to fully eliminate the problem. Currently I am supplementing the fluency approach with an individually tailored counseling approach, and preliminary results are favorable. The point to remember is that short-term assessment procedures may not provide us with accurate data for instructional design input. We are compelled to make long-term assessments as well.

The emphasis of assessment procedures must be discovering those factors about learning which will allow us to improve instruction. We must search for those characteristics of the learner's performance attainments and capabilities that can be linked to the various, available educational options. Many currently used assessment procedures fail to come close to this objective. It is simply not sufficient only to describe a child's articulation skills apart from the instructional process. Factual description of disfluencies, normative data concerning a child's language competencies, or an evaluation of voice quality may be quite beneficial when comparing one individual's communication skills to another's, but if these data are not related to the instructional process, they are of limited value. Assessment data must be aimed at helping the clinician decide on appropriate courses of instruction.

A close approximation to Glaser's concept of the link between theory and practice can be found in the 10 steps White and Haring (1976) outline as the process of teaching. These 10 steps plus a brief description of each are found in Figure 11–1. The authors maintain that teaching is a process of manipulating environmental factors in order to achieve pre-set instructional goals designed for a particular child. In order for this to occur, the teacher must be in the position to make accurate assessments of the child's progress. New programs or instructional strategies develop from these assessments. While it is not exactly the linking science between theory and practice that Dewey had in mind, it does represent an attempt to approach the art of teaching as a science.

There are still those, especially among humanists, who will maintain good teaching is an art, that it should never be a science. Perhaps this may be true in some areas of creative instruction. But when we consider the types of problems and goals we in speech pathology have, it becomes imperative that we apply a scientific approach

1. *Goal setting:* specifying what *should* be taught. It is important to involve all interested people in the specification of goals.

2. *Objective setting and sequencing:* breaking the overall, general goals down into specific statements of what each child should be able to do and in what sequence the child should learn to perform those skills. Usually specialists in each area perform or assist the teacher in this step in the process.

3. *Preparation of assessment devices:* finding or making assessment devices that will determine what objectives each child has already met. Although some prepublished assessment materials may be useful, we must take care to select and use only those materials which are directly related to the objectives and goals we have specified. Many times this will necessitate making new materials which are unavailable through commercial sources.

4. *Conducting initial assessments:* after meeting the child and making the child feel at ease, assessing the child on all of the objectives which relate to his or her general educational level. Assessments are conducted individually, allowing plenty of time to get a good assessment of the child's skill in each part of the curriculum.

5. *Analyzing the results of assessment:* comparing each child's performance against the standards specified in the objectives. This will pinpoint the place where instruction should begin with each child.

6. *Developing a plan:* with knowledge of the child gained through the assessment, through interaction with the child, and from other people who know and work with the child, developing a plan for his instruction. The plan should include descriptions of the setting which will be used for the program, the materials required, the cues and instruction that the teacher will provide, the behavior in which the child is supposed to engage, and the consequences (if any) which should be arranged to encourage the best possible performance.

7. *Implementing the plan:* implementing and following the plan as closely as possible.

8. *Collecting progress information:* collecting daily information about the progress of the child. The performance of the child during the program is certainly as important as his performance during the initial assessment, if not more so. Information on both the accuracy and the fluency of the child's performance are collected.

9. *Charting progress:* immediately charting the information collected on each child to form a picture of the child's progress. This chart enables quick, simple, and timely decisions to be made concerning the effectiveness of the instructional plan.

10. *Changing the plan:* using the chart to predict when a child will reach his aim so that another program can be ready at the right time or using the chart to determine if a child will *not* reach his aim in time so that the plan can be changed *before* the child fails and the problem grows to insurmountable proportions.

FIGURE 11–1. Ten Steps In The Process Of Teaching (Reprinted By Permission
Of Charles E. Merrill, From O. R. White & N. G. Haring,
Exceptional Teaching, 1976)

to the study and treatment of communication problems. Perkins (1977) stresses that to him, at least, speech pathology is an applied, interdisciplinary behavior science. He, too, strongly supports the notion that one of our most important goals is to develop solid theory rather than just a workable methodology. We should aim at developing principles that can unify the seemingly unrelated series of events we observe.

Although it may be some time before we will have a well-developed psychology of instruction available to us in speech pathology, recent advances in the field of psychology suggest it is forthcoming. The development of psychological instruction as described by Dewey and Glaser will require considerable research effort by speech pathologists. Through continued research effort, we may be able to devise instructional prototypes which fulfill all of those components suggested by Glaser. But until this occurs, speech clinicians will be required to use their best judgment in selecting appropriate instructional procedures. Hopefully, this judgment will be based on a sound, empirical foundation, not blind acceptance of some new educational fad.

BIBLIOGRAPHY

Atkinson, R. C., & Paulson, J. A. An approach to the psychology of instruction. *Psychological Bulletin*, 1972, *78*, 49–61.

Bruner, J. S. Some theorems on instruction illustrated with reference to mathematics. *Theories of learning and instruction. The Sixty-third Yearbook of the National Society for the Study of Education*, Part I, 1964, *63*, 306–335.

Davies, I. K. *Competency based learning: Technology, management, and design.* New York: McGraw-Hill, 1973.

Dewey, J. Psychology and social practice. *The Psychological Review*, 1900, *7*, 105–124.

Estes, W. K. Learning theory and intelligence. *American Psychologist*, 1974, *29*, 740–749.

Gagné, R. *The conditions of learning*, 2nd ed. New York: Holt, Rinehart & Winston, 1970.

Glaser, R. Components of a psychology of instruction: Toward a science of design. *Review of Educational Research*, 1976, *46*, 1–24.

Hunt, E., Frost, N., & Lunnebory, C. Individual differences in cognition: A new approach to intelligence. In G. H. Bower (Ed.), *The psychology of learning and motivation* (Vol. 7). New York: Academic Press, 1973.

Johnstone, J. N. Mathematical models developed for use in educational planning: A review. *Review of Educational Research*, 1974, *44*, 177–201.

Mowrer, D., Baker, R., & Schutz, R. Operant procedures in the control of speech articulation. In H. Sloane & B. MacAulay (Eds.), *Operant procedures in remedial speech and language training.* Boston: Houghton Mifflin, 1968.

Perkins, W. *Speech pathology: An applied behavioral science*, 2nd ed. St Louis: C. V. Mosby, 1977.

Simon, H. *The sciences of the artificial.* Cambridge, Mass.: MIT Press, 1969.

Snelbecker, G. E. *Learning theory: Instructional theory and psychoeducational design.* New York: McGraw-Hill, 1974.

Thorndike, E. L. *The psychology of arithmetic.* New York: Macmillan, 1922.

White, O. R., & Haring, N. G. *Exceptional teaching.* Columbus: Charles E. Merrill, 1976.

12

Application of Behavior Therapy Techniques: Selected Case Studies

The purpose of this chapter is to illustrate how behavior therapy techniques are used in changing specific behaviors associated with various communication problems. By studying the examples provided, you will learn how the principles of behavioral management you have read about in the previous chapters have been applied. These cases are not hypothetical cases. They are actual cases the authors have worked with recently, one for each of the following areas: articulation, stuttering, voice, and language.

Modifying Articulation Skills

We spend a great deal of our time teaching children how to articulate sounds they have not yet learned to produce or produce incorrectly. The behavioral model I'll use to demonstrate how to achieve changes in articulation skills is not complex. Teaching a child how to articulate sounds in words is a relatively easy task providing there are no muscular or neurological anomalies.

The first point I would like to make before presenting the case study is the importance of differentiating between the type of therapy used and the method of presenting that therapy. The central focus of this book has been the method of presentation i.e., behavior therapy. You may select one or a combination of several different therapy methods to change articulation (phonetic placement, motokinesthetic, sensori-motor, stimulation, or key word approaches). But several essential procedures must be followed when we present the method of our choice if we choose to use the behavior therapy model. These procedures would include stating behavioral objectives, charting behaviors, changing reinforcement schedules, reinforcing selected behaviors, extinguishing undesired behaviors, planning for generalization, and maximizing transfer of training. For the following presentation, I'll place emphasis upon these important aspects of behavioral management.

Diagnosis

When I first met Clifford, who was five years old, his speech was unintelligible. He was enrolled in kindergarten located in a small rural community. Results of an articulation test revealed that he used only the consonants /b, d, f, l/. The remaining consonants were omitted or one of the consonants present was substituted. Analysis of his phonological system resulted in the following areas of need:

1. frication /h, s, z, θ,   ð, v, w, ʃ, dʒ /;
2. combination frication-plosive /tʃ, dʒ /;
3. velar plosives /k, g/;
4. liquids /ɝ, j/ and consonantal /r/;
5. cluster addition.

The oral and hearing examination revealed no problems that might contribute to his poor articulation skills.

Baseline

Clifford's articulation was sampled two more times during a 2-week period before therapy was initiated. A graph of the baseline behavior for one phoneme, /s/, is shown in Figure 12–1. Baseline data for other missing consonants were also graphed.

Delivery of Instructions

Since Clifford lived in a rural community and could not attend speech therapy sessions, a phone amplifier was installed in his home. Thus, the clinician could deliver instructions using the phone and could be heard by both Clifford and his mother.

Behavioral Objectives

The behavioral objectives were derived from five need areas identified in the diagnostic evaluation. The first need area was frication. One of the most effective ways to establish frication is to teach production of the sounds containing this

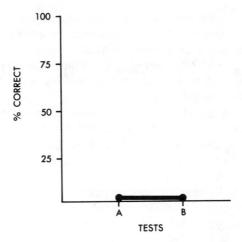

100

75

% CORRECT

50

25

A   B

TESTS

FIGURE 12-1. Baseline Record Of /s/

feature: /s, z, θ, ð, ʃ, ʒ, v/; /f/ was already present. According to Crocker's (1969) model of sound development, /s/ and /θ/ production would be a logical place to begin. Two instructional programs, the S-PACK (Mowrer, Backer, & Schutz, 1974) and a similar /θ/ correction program were sent to Clifford's mother so she could follow the instructions and assist in judging adequacy of the response. The clinician read the instructions to Clifford using the telephone.

The first behavioral objective was: Clifford will use /s/ and /z/ in words containing these sounds with 100% accuracy in all speaking situations. Bear in mind that the chief objective was to establish the feature of frication in his phonological system. I was not concerned with only the /s/ and /z/, but also the /v, θ,ð, ʃ,ʒ/ and the fricative elements of /tʃ, dʒ, t, d, k/. The term aspiration better describes the element of frication present in /t, d, k/.

The objective stated for /s/ and /z/ is too complex to accomplish during the first session, so sub-objectives need to be identified. I have listed several objectives that are to be accomplished early in the program.

(1) Clifford will say /i/ once on the first attempt given the following instruction: "Close your teeth and say /i/." (2) Clifford will say /is/ once when instructed to "Look in the mirror and try it again." (3) Clifford will say /s/ once when instructed to "Say it quickly." (4) Clifford will say five /s/-vowel syllables following the clinician's model of the five /s/-vowel syllables.

As you can see, writing each of these objectives is laborious and time-consuming. You must identify the objectives you wish to accomplish and the order in which they are to be presented, but it is not necessary to write each sub-objective in detail. It would be better to write one objective we wish to accomplish by the end of one session. Such an objective would be as follows: Clifford will say /s/ in one and two syllable words containing /s/ in the initial position when shown pictures of objects by the clinician and asked to name them. He will say /s/ in at least 8 out of 10 of the words presented.

If Clifford achieves this objective, an objective for the second session is stated. The instructional program is designed to reach the second objective. If the first objective is not reached, the program is repeated, altered, or even terminated.

Following three sessions using the S-PACK program, Clifford's mother was instructed to continue an /s/ follow-up program. The follow-up program required her to provide Clifford with 15 additional training sessions over a 3-week period. Each lesson contained a behavioral objective.

The next sound to be introduced was /θ/, presented in a similar program format. Behavioral objectives were written for this sound in much the same way as they had been for /s/. Following four instructional sessions, Clifford's mother was asked to continue a second follow-up program for /θ/ and /ð/ while she also administered the follow-up program for /s/ and /z/.

After two weeks of therapy, it was apparent the fricative sounds were being produced with greater ease. The clinician decided to begin work on the second major objective which was addition of the velars /k/ and /g/, a place problem. A program for introducing /k/ and /g/, patterned after S-PACK, was initiated. The behavioral objectives were similar to those stated previously.

Space does not permit a detailed presentation of the behavioral objectives written for the remaining three main objectives. Once you have planned objectives for many individuals, there is no need to spend time in actually writing a long series of objectives.

Management of Consequent Events

When Clifford is asked to repeat a sound, we know that he will respond either correctly or incorrectly. We need to identify the consequence for each response. If he is correct, he will be reinforced immediately with a positive verbal statement such as "good," "fine," or "right." Also, his mother will give him a token when she hears the clinician's positive statement. When Clifford has 50 tokens, he gets one prize point which he can exchange for a toy. A package of toys, mostly G.I. Joe equipment which Clifford prized, was sent to his mother who in turn showed them to Clifford. He was told he could earn the toys by exchanging prize points earned during his speech class. Each toy was worth a certain number of prize points. Working for prize points provided the motivation needed to maintain Clifford's interest in the speech activities.

The schedule of reinforcement was altered as follows: At first, when a new articulation skill was being learned, continuous reinforcement was given. As the sound was used more frequently, the schedule was changed to a variable ratio. Clifford had to say two or three sounds correctly before the clinician said "good." This can be accomplished easily when phrase and sentence drills are used. When working on /s/, the clinician said "good" following each correct word he repeated correctly (an FR-1 ratio). Later when he repeated a sentence like "Sally took her sister to the zoo," only one positive statement was given providing all three /s/ sounds and the one /z/ were correct. At other times, two or perhaps three /s/ or /z/ sounds would be included in a phrase. This would best be described as a VR-3 schedule. Later, when he was conversing, a VR-10 schedule was used. At this point in therapy no attempt was made to count every response. Probe samples were taken periodically. The number of correct and incorrect responses were counted and graphed.

What about incorrect responses? Extinction is one technique used to decrease the frequency of a response. One simply ignores the incorrect response. The problem with this consequence is that it requires considerable time before you can see the effects of its use. It is more effective to follow an incorrect response with a simple statement, such as "no" or "that's wrong." It is even more effective to tell the child what was done wrong or how to do it correctly. For example, when Clifford omitted /s/, he was told, "No, Clifford, you didn't hiss that time. Now try it again and hiss like this, *pass.*" Often he was simply told, "Nope, try it again." He would usually say the sound correctly on the second try. He needed more consistent feedback in the form of cues when he was first learning a sound, but after a week of practice, "try it again" was sufficient to evoke the correct response.

In summary, make sure you provide appropriate consequences following correct and incorrect responses. These consequences must be immediate and consistent.

Recording and Graphing Data

The practical aspects of recording and graphing data can be an extremely burdensome task, like writing behavior objectives. You can go to the extreme by giving more attention to keeping data than to teaching. In Clifford's case, I had to find an effective way of keeping track of the 16 sounds that were taught plus numerous consonant clusters in a variety of speaking situations.

A practical solution is to take frequent probes of the target sounds. For example, when /s/ was taught, each correct and incorrect /s/ attempt was not recorded. After the first 100 instructional items were given, a 10-item probe test was administered to determine if criteria for the first objective had been met. The data form showing baseline performance (pretest), the three probes (parts I, II, and III), and a posttest are shown in Figure 12–2.

Clifford's mother recorded data using the form shown in Figure 12–3 when she administered the 3-week parent program for correction of /s/.

These data were transferred to a graph showing percent of accuracy. The graph for /s/ performance is shown in Figure 12–4.

A similar record keeping procedure was used for /θ/ and /k/ as they were taught. No distinction was made between voiced and voiceless cognates. /z/ was counted as /s/, /ð/ as /θ/, and /g/ as /k/ since the voicing feature was not a problem.

A large portion of the therapy involved repetition of phrases to assist Clifford in acquiring coarticulation skills. Several sounds he had been working on at the word stage were imbedded into phrasal units such as: "Make a suit," "It's a book," "There's a sock," "He's the one," "Cook the soup," and "Think about it."

The first phrase contains /k/ and /s/ target sounds, the second /s/ and /k/, the third contains /ð/, /s/ and /k/. You could easily place a check beside each correct phrase, or a circle around each incorrect target sound, compute the totals, and graph these data. I don't feel that keeping such minute data is really helpful. It is much more convenient to sample the behavior at periodic intervals and record the percent correct for each target sound. You can get so involved with record-keeping

CRITERION TEST SCORE SHEET

Child's Name: Clifford

Administered by: DM

X = right
O = wrong

Date	11-15-78	11-20-78	11-21-78	11-23-78	11-23-78
Test	Pretest	Part I	Part II	Part III	Posttest
Items	1 O 16 O	1 X	1 X	1 X	1 X 16 X
	2 O 17 O	2 X	2 X	2 X	2 X 17 X
	3 O 18 O	3 O	3 X	3 X	3 X 18 X
	4 O 19 O	4 X	4 X	4 X	4 X 19 X
	5 O 20 O	5 X	5 X	5 X	5 X 20 X
	6 O 21 O	6 X	6 X	6 X	6 X 21 X
	7 O 22 O	7 O	7 X	7 X	7 X 22 X
	8 O 23 O	8 X	8 X	8 X	8 X 23 X
	9 O 24 O	9 X	9 X	9 X	9 X 24 X
	10 O 25 O	10 X	10 X	10 X	10 X 25 X
	11 O 26 O				11 X 26 X
	12 O 27 O				12 X 27 X
	13 O 28 O				13 X 28 X
	14 O 29 O				14 X 29 X
	15 O 30 O				15 X 30 X
Total right	0	8	10	10	30

Recommendation: Parent Program

FIGURE 12-2. Data Sheet For Probe Testing Of /s/

428

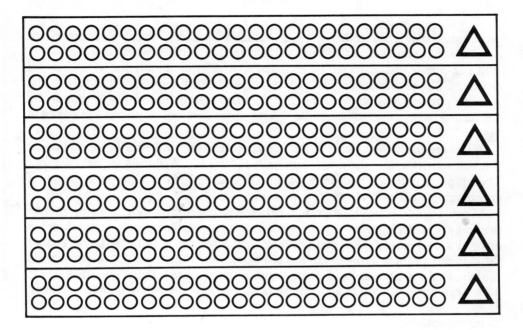

FIGURE 12-3. Data Sheet For Recording Performance Of Parent Administered Program

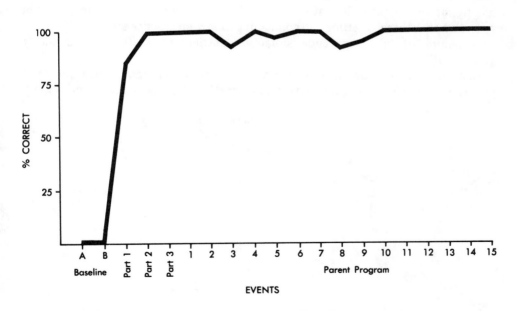

FIGURE 12-4. Graph Showing Percent Of Accuracy Of /s/ Attempts During Baseline, The Three-Part
S-PACK, And The Parent Program Of S-PACK

procedures that they interfere with valuable teaching time. The procedure developed to keep track of Clifford's phrase practice activities was to end the session with a 12-phrase test. Each phrase included several target sounds that were circled if incorrect. The phrase probe included 15 /s/ sounds, 8 /θ/ sounds, and 11 /k/ sounds. Another phrase probe may include 12 /s/ sounds, 11 /θ/ sounds, and 14 /k/ sounds. By converting these scores to percentile figures, these data can be graphed as shown in Figure 12-5.

How were these data used? If the correct responses fell below 80%, additional practice activities were provided, especially for this sound, during the next session. The graphed data were also shown to Clifford and his mother as a means of encouraging their efforts.

As new sounds were added (/r, h, ʃ, tʃ/) I wasn't concerned about keeping data on the original target sounds (/s, θ, k/) since the original target sounds were seldom in error. I kept records of correct and incorrect attempts at the new target sounds through test probes, in much the same way as I had done with the original target sounds. Had I kept records of every target sound Clifford spoke, my office would have been covered with charts! There is no need to keep such detailed records.

Generalization

Speech clinicians frequently complain that although they do not find it difficult to evoke the correct response in the therapy room setting, many children do not use the sound correctly in other environments (classroom, playground, and home). I had the unique advantage of providing therapy in Clifford's home, where he does most of his talking, because I called him at his home. I was able to solicit his mother's aid in attending each therapy setting and conducting follow-up practice sessions. Thus, the very nature of the therapeutic situation contributed greatly to maximizing generalization.

Also the use of common phrases aided generalization. Rather than contrived phrase patterns like "May I spin the spinner please?" or "I would like to pick a card,"

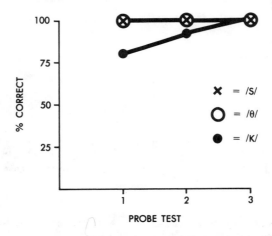

FIGURE 12-5. *Graph Showing Results Of Phase Probe Test Of Three Target Sounds: /s/, /θ/, And /k/*

phrases such as "It's a," "he's as," "make a," "there's a," "who's going," "where's the," and "I see a," were used. If you listen to children talk, you'll discover they use certain phrases over and over. These are the types of phrases I used in therapy.

Along these lines, I often reserved about 3 to 5 minutes at the end of the session to chat with Clifford about his rabbit, his trip to the dentist, what happened at school, how he helped his father, and so on. I recorded these conversations and transcribed those phrases in which errors occurred. For example, when asked what he had for lunch, he said, "I ad a amburger," omitting /h/. The next day we practiced a series of phrases using variations of these words: "I had a hamburger," "I had a ham," "I had a burger," "I had some milk," "I had a bun," "I had some ice cream," and "I had a hamburger." We practiced these phrases until he could say five consecutive phrases correctly. Then I asked him what he had for lunch today, what he had for breakfast, and what he had for supper last night. The strategy was to help him practice the target sounds in the context in which he uses these sounds.

As I mentioned before, I had the luxury of providing therapy in the home (via telephone) as well as his mother's aid. This is seldom the case in school. In these settings I try to provide therapy in a variety of situations outside the therapy room. I may ask the child to repeat words or phrases outside the therapy room, on the playground, in the lunchroom, in the classroom, or even in the principal's office. I try to solicit the aid of class members who will help monitor speech, send assignments home for the mother to complete, or request the child to speak with several people on the school grounds who will provide consequences for correct or incorrect articulation (school bus driver, custodian, secretary, cafeteria worker, etc.). In order to achieve carry-over, you must plan a number of different speaking activities designed to assist the generalization of the new response in a variety of speaking situations.

One simple reminder was to provide Clifford with a speech pencil for each sound he was practicing. (Speech pencils are available from IDEAS, Box 741, Tempe, Arizona 85281.) Written on the pencil was a brief speech practice lesson that he could review from time to time during daily activities when he used a pencil. This was another procedure used to remind him to use the target sound.

Retention

Once a new articulation response is learned and used consistently in conversational speech, there is little need for retention activities. Rapid articulation becomes an automatic process that requires little thought or attention. But during the time when the response is unstable, it is wise to engage in activities that aid in retention. You may recall three factors that increase retention: overlearn the material, provide frequent instruction, and use meaningful material.

A conscious effort was made to insure all three factors were employed during therapy. First, we kept reviewing the target sounds he had learned as we practiced the phrase routines. I was always conscious of his /s/, /θ/ and /k/ productions long after I had stopped teaching them. Often, I called Clifford's attention to the fact that he was saying these sounds correctly.

Secondly, I provided therapy three to four times weekly. His mother provided daily follow-up lessons which maintained practice sessions on a frequent schedule.

Of course, Clifford didn't object because more practice meant more points and the cost of the toys was going up. Inflation? No, just a change in the reinforcement schedule!

Finally, every attempt was made to use meaningful material during the practice sessions. I never used tongue twisters or contrived unnatural phrase or sentence patterns. The best source of practice material was Clifford's own speech samples taken during conversations with him.

Thus, the three factors known to contribute to retention were deliberately used throughout the sessions to curb forgetting. I believe all clinicians can make use of these three factors in almost every therapeutic setting.

Summary

Therapy for Clifford was begun in late November and terminated in March. His progress was steady and rapid. He was always interested in the sessions and was eager to participate. His mother was a willing participant who contributed significantly to Clifford's progress. The fact that the phone was used to deliver much of the therapy is not, in my opinion, an important variable. I feel I could have accomplished the prescribed goals just as well had I seen him in person during therapy. The use of the phone did result in substantial time and financial saving for the parents, though.

Clifford was dismissed when he had mastered the five target need areas with 80% or better accuracy in conversational speech. I felt that once he was using target sounds with that degree of accuracy, no further therapy would be necessary. His phonological system had been altered sufficiently that consequences of natural speaking conditions at home and at school would be sufficient to modify any remaining errors in his speech.

An itinerant speech-language pathologist examined Clifford during the fall and felt the few articulation errors noted did not require her services. I saw Clifford one year later and his articulation was satisfactory. No trace of his original errors remained.

Modification of Stuttering Behavior

Working with clients who stutter often involves a considerable amount of behavioral counseling. Mike, whom I have chosen to discuss, received behavioral counseling as well as a programmed approach designed to establish fluent speech. You will see how both therapy techniques can be used simultaneously to achieve a common objective: fluent speech.

Diagnosis

Mike, age 25, began stuttering when he was six years old, following his mother's illness. He was told not to talk with his mother and subsequently remained mute for two months. Following this event, he said he began to stutter and has stuttered ever since. When he was nine, he received help for his stuttering in the form of reading therapy, but it was not effective. He was expelled from high school for fighting, which was related to his speech problem. He was working as a mechanic when he enrolled for speech therapy.

Analysis of conversational speech revealed a speaking rate of 42 words per minute, 25 of which were disfluent. Reading rate was 19 words per minute, 11 of which were disfluent. Disfluencies consisted chiefly of repeated interjections (2.5 interjections per intended word) consisting of the following: ya know, ah, tadee, and, OK, that would be, on, in, then, that, and throat-clearing. A rising intonation was present on about one eighth of the interjections.

The Ryan Stuttering Interview (Ryan, 1974) was administered. The summary of this test revealed Mike stuttered on 13 words per minute and exhibited 3.3 stuttering behaviors per minute. Results of Erickson's attitude scale (Erickson, 1969) revealed that 92% of Mike's responses matched those of other confirmed stutterers.

Baseline

I felt there was enough information contained in the Ryan Stuttering Interview form to suffice for baseline data, so no further probes were taken. Ryan's test samples speech in 14 different speaking situations. Mike stuttered in every situation with the exception of singing.

Behavioral Objectives

The obvious behavioral objective with anyone who stutters is to help them learn to talk fluently, or if this seems unlikely, help them to learn to stutter less often and with less tension. Gregory (1980) summarized the content of two different therapy goals. One technique seeks to establish fluent speech patterns, whereas the other focuses upon modifying the moment of stuttering.

I chose to establish a fluent speech pattern and selected the S-1 program (Mowrer, 1975b) to accomplish this goal. This program is described in detail in Mowrer (1975a, 1975b). The strategy is to increase the mean length of utterance while maintaining a high fluency level.

The behavioral objective of the first program is *Objective A:* To read 120 groups of three-word combinations (360 words) with 95% fluency within 10 minutes without the assistance of cue signals.

In order to reach this objective, nine tasks must be mastered to a specified criterion performance. There are nine sub-objectives to be met in order to reach the first program objective. The first objective was *Objective A–1B:* Mike will read aloud one word from a list of monosyllabic words in any order he wishes following a beep that occurs every 5 seconds. Criterion is met when he reads 360 words within 30 minutes with no more than 18 disfluencies. The program is terminated if this objective is not met by the time 960 words have been read.

The objective was not met, so I wrote another objective describing an easier task. It is difficult to talk about objectives without discussing response data. The accuracy of the client's responses dictate what the objectives will be and vice versa. You will better understand this interplay as you read the section concerning recording and graphing responses. The second objective substituted whispered speech for reading the words aloud. Surprisingly, Mike did not meet the criterion set for this objective.

Since the S-1 program did not list objectives below the whispered speech level, I constructed the following: *Objective A-WS1:* Mike will whisper one word from a list of monosyllabic words simultaneously with the speech clinician following a beep that occurs every 5 seconds. Criterion will be met when 240 words are read within 20 minutes with no more than 12 disfluencies.

Mike reached this objective during his first attempt maintaining fluency at the 97% level. The objective was then written as: *Objective A-WS2:* Mike will read aloud simultaneously with the clinician one word from a list of monosyllabic words in the order selected by the clinician following a beep that occurs every 5 seconds. Criterion will be met when 240 words are read within 20 minutes with no more than 12 disfluencies. At the end of his second day in therapy, 6 hours, Mike met this objective. During the third day he met criterion for the fourth objective (A-WS2). Achievement of the third objective (A-WS1) was the target, followed by the second objective (A-1B), and finally the first objective (A-1), the original starting point. Objective A-1 was reached after 8 hours of therapy and repeated readings of the same list of words on the fourth day. The first objective (A-1) was reviewed before moving ahead to objective A-2 but criterion was not met. I backed up to the fourth objective again and followed the sequence of third, second and first objectives. Finally, after 15 hours of therapy, criterion was met for objective A-1 again and I moved to *Objective A-2:* Mike will read aloud one word from a list of monosyllabic words in the order they are presented on a word list following a beep that occurs every 5 seconds. Criterion is met when he reads 240 words within 20 minutes with no more than 12 disfluencies.

Mike met this objective on the first attempt; but when the objective was changed to include two words read aloud together, Mike was not able to meet this objective, even after 20 hours of therapy using the same word list!

Perhaps I should have realized sooner that the thrust of this therapeutic approach was inappropriate for Mike. I decided to give up the attempt to establish fluent speech. I tried to teach Mike how to reduce the frequency of stuttering and modify the stuttering act. Van Riper (1973) views this approach as teaching fluent stuttering and describes the procedures to be used in teaching controlled stuttering. Ryan (1974) outlines a series of program steps to be followed for those who wish to use Van Riper's cancellation and pull-out procedures to modify the moment of stuttering.

Space does not permit description of the objectives written for the second part of this program. The interested reader may consult Ryan's (1974) text, pages 69–70. Ryan presents an outline of the objective for this program.

A third major therapy thrust involved behavioral counseling to assist Mike in learning to take responsibility for his speech behavior. I wanted him to monitor and purposely control certain aspects of his speech behavior rather than rely upon a clinician to provide feedback. Behavioral objectives were not so clear cut, neither were the criteria for meeting them. As a result of poorly defined objectives and inadequate data-keeping, one easily slips into more traditional "gut level" therapy techniques. This is characteristic of reports in which master clinicians describe therapy procedures with clients. When objectives are vague and data are not kept, it becomes impossible to replicate procedures or identify the independent variables responsible for behavioral change. We become susceptible to adopting superstitious behaviors or continuing ineffective procedures. We are not always as diligent in therapy as we should be.

An attempt was made to write behavioral objectives for the counseling sessions. These consisted of a list of do's and don't's Mike was to follow during speaking activities.

Do's

1. Plan what you want to say.
2. Focus on the first word and first sound of the word in the sentence.
3. Place your tongue and lips in position to say the first sound.
4. Gently produce the air stream and voicing (if present) to initiate the first sound.
5. Slowly produce the first sound and following vowel, then complete the word.

Don't's

1. Don't use interjections.
2. Don't take a deep breath.
3. Don't wrinkle your forehead and look up.
4. Don't stop breath stream in mid-sentence.

This list does not meet the requirements of a behavioral objective. The list of *Don't's* do not tell him what he should do and the list of *Do's* do not specify the conditions or the accuracy statement. We could keep data regarding how often he showed evidence of terminating one of the *Don't* behaviors and initiating one of the *Do* behaviors, but we had no idea of what criterion should be met or when to advance to another objective. Consequently, we could not show the client progress is being made.

It is not too difficult to write behavioral objectives "after the fact" but often times while experimenting with different procedures, it is easier to use a subjective, hit-or-miss approach to therapy. I'm not implying this subjective approach is better than the objective approach in which all behavioral objectives are clearly stated beforehand. I try to use the objective approach whenever possible, but sometimes it isn't.

The point I wish to make is that you should not get the idea that a behavior therapist is a human computer, never deviating from the exact rigors of scientific methodology. Although we should attempt to follow these principles as much as possible, there are times when we may not.

Management of Consequent Events

Managing consequent events consisted of the following. When Mike was fluent the clinician praised him. Frequently, he was also shown a graph of the number of fluent and disfluent utterances. While the first program was being administered the reinforcement schedule was FR-1, changing to a FR-2 when program A-4 was used. When the S-1 program was terminated, the clinicians who worked with Mike (five graduate students and I served as clinicians) praised him frequently when he was fluent but no specific schedule of reinforcement was used. Often, we praised Mike immediately after he demonstrated control over one of his *Don't* behaviors by using the list of *Do* behaviors, but again, a pre-arranged reinforcement was not used. Verbal praise occurred spontaneously and varied in frequency and intensity with each clinician.

When Mike stuttered during the S-1 program, he was simply told no and a zero was recorded on the score sheet. Later when the goal of therapy was shifted to modifying the moment of stuttering, verbal cues such as "What are you supposed to do?," "Follow your instructions," or "Look out" were provided. These cues were not provided following every disfluent utterance. I would estimate that they were provided following about a third of the disfluencies.

Recording and Graphing Data

When the S-1 program was being used, each of Mike's utterances was scored and recorded as either fluent or disfluent. A disfluent utterance was defined as a verbal hesitancy in speech, a sound or word repetition or prolongation, and an unusual body mannerism or extraneous vocalization. A fluent utterance was defined as containing none of the above deviancies.

The score sheet, shown in Figure 12–6 was used to record data when the S–1 program was being used. Percentage scores of fluent utterances in each group of 120 responses (a cycle) were then plotted on a graph (Mowrer, 1979). The results of the first 7 days of therapy (3 hours daily) are shown in Figures 12–7 through 12–9.

As I have already mentioned, there is a close interplay between what the data show and how you choose behavioral objectives. The decisions you make are based solely upon how you interpret the data. In Mike's case, I set certain criterion standards I felt were necesssary for him to meet before he should progress to a more difficult task. He had to maintain a fluency of 95% on a specified task. It could be argued that this criterion was too high. I based these criterion standards upon past experience with other individuals who stutter and have progressed through the program successfully. Unfortunately, there are no universal criterion standards that meet the needs of all individuals. We may fail with some cases but, generally, I have found the 95% accuracy rate an effective criterion to use.

Keeping accurate data when the objective was changed to modifying the moment of stuttering became a problem. This was partly because we were monitoring several behaviors at once and were unable to specify when he used elements of his *Do* list and when that wasn't necessary. We attempted to keep score of times he engaged in *Don't* list behaviors but, since no criterion standards were established for success, we were unable to determine when he was performing adequately and when he wasn't. Judgment of these factors was subjective. I did not have sufficient experience using this objective with stutterers to know what to expect from Mike in terms of accuracy. I found this to be a distinct handicap in my attempt to conduct a behavior therapy approach. It is an area I hope to remedy.

Behavioral objectives must be well specified and data must be kept to determine if the objectives are met, otherwise we run the risk of conducting therapy that takes up time but seldom results in steady progress. On the other hand, often therapy progresses very well without written objectives and without keeping data. Many

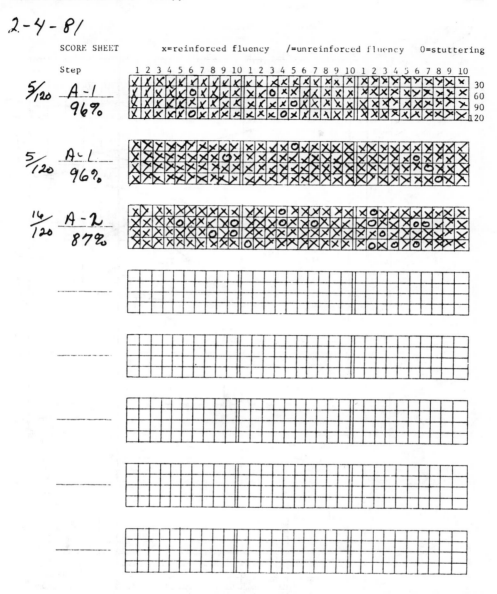

FIGURE 12-6. *Sample Score Sheet Used To Record Fluent And Disfluent Utterances Produced During The S-1 Program*

clinical reports of successful cases were presented long before the common use of behavioral objectives or keeping data. But I do feel that writing objectives and keeping data adds greatly to our clinical effectiveness and we should attempt to follow the behavior therapy model.

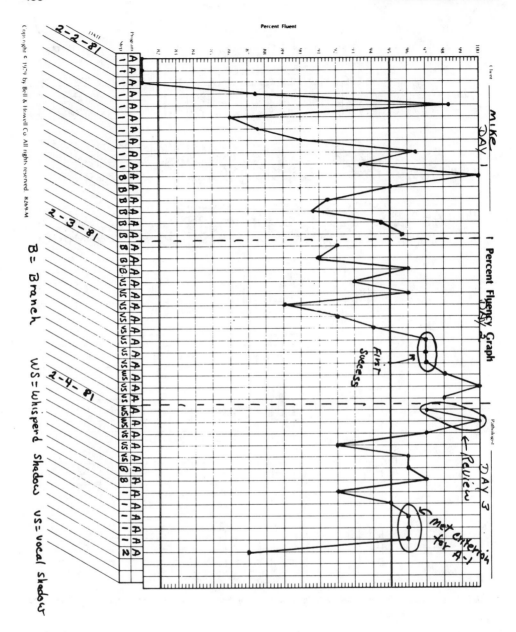

FIGURE 12-7. Graph Showing Percent Of Fluent Utterances During Days 1 To 3

Generalization

The most effective technique used to aid in generalizing newly learned speech skills is
the practice of new skills in many other environments. I believe these generalization
activities should occur as early as possible. Just as soon as a new skill is learned in the

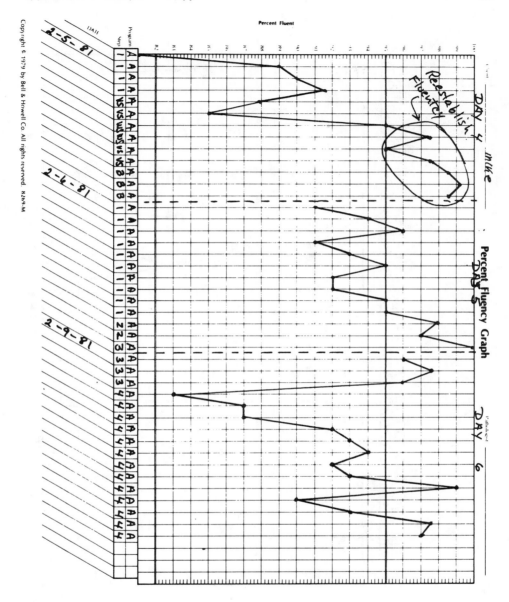

FIGURE 12-8. *Graph Showing Percent Of Fluent Utterances During Days 4 To 6*

clinic, it should be practiced in other environments. One of the major faults of past therapy programs was the belief that fluency should be achieved first in the clinic. The person then would be ready to use this new speech outside the clinic. Often, this did not occur. The client maintained two behaviors: a fluent way of speaking while in the clinic and the old pattern of stuttering outside the clinic.

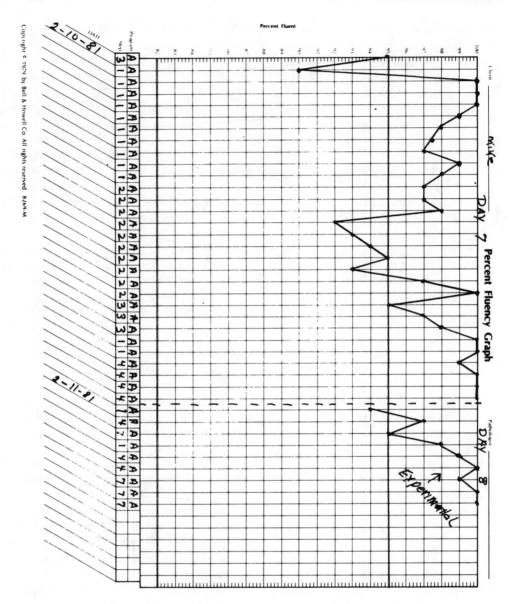

FIGURE 12-9. Graph Showing Percent Of Fluent Utterances During Days 7 And 8

Near the beginning of Mike's therapy, a student clinician and I ate lunch with him at the garage where he worked. Frequently, a customer would enter to ask about a car, Mike received phone calls, or his boss would come in to chat. We were able to observe firsthand how Mike coped with these speaking situations. We could count the number of his disfluencies and the number of times he began a sentence or phrase with a fluent utterance. We taped these sessions and reviewed the tapes during a subsequent therapy session. He was encouraged to identify occasions of stuttering and demonstrate how he could have spoken more fluently. We offered suggestions to his boss regarding the cues he could give Mike following an occasion of stuttering. He was also instructed to praise Mike occasionally following fluent utterances. We also spoke with Mike's parents, offering suggestions about consequences they could provide to aid Mike in maintaining fluent speech.

Using the telephone was especially difficult for Mike, yet his job demanded he use it frequently. We began a generalization program by practicing sentences he regularly used on the phone at work when speaking to customers. Next, we used these sentences when speaking on a toy phone. This was followed by talking to the clinician from another room on the clinic phones. Then we began calling various car-part agencies from the clinic. Finally, we monitored his phone behavior on the job. Through this desensitization program, Mike was able to generalize the fluent pattern of speech he learned using the clinic phone to other phone situations, such as calling his parents, his relatives, and his customers.

We also attempted to achieve generalization of the newly learned behaviors by conversing with students and employees on the college campus. He was asked to practice his list of *Do* behaviors and avoid the list of *Don't* behaviors in these situations.

Thus, generalization was accomplished by using fluency producing behaviors in as many real life situations as possible. Just as soon as he learned a new skill in the clinic, we helped him use it outside.

Retention

Retention at this point in therapy means keeping the gains that have been made and being aware of old behaviors that return (interjections, distorted breathing, facial grimace). Although Mike is not ready for dismissal, we cannot assume the newly learned skills needed to assure his fluent pattern of speaking will automatically be present. There are numerous stimuli that can and do trigger stuttering and if left unchecked, Mike may quickly generalize these old behaviors to many other situations.

As in the case of Clifford, frequent instruction is an effective way to increase retention of the new behaviors. We have been seeing Mike 2 hours daily during the past several months. Obviously he gives high priority to his speech work.

In terms of overlearning, Mike receives considerable supervised practice speaking in a more fluent manner. I am not sure to what degree overlearning is important in stuttering therapy. Developing proper attitudes may be more important than speech practice, but the two undoubtedly are closely related.

Finally, using meaningful material is a third characteristic of programs that stress retention. The word lists used in the S-1 program did not contain meaningful material. Meaningful material was used only when we visited Mike on his job, engaged in speaking on the campus, and used the telephone. One student used a carburetor as a discussion topic in some of her therapy sessions. Mike labeled various carburetor parts for her, explained how to service it, and how to rebuild it. Topics related to cars were discussed frequently. A spinoff benefit was that several students learned how to tune their cars, but the chief value was in conversing with Mike about topics he discussed daily with his boss and with customers. It was felt retention of fluent speech patterns would be more effective if we chose topics related to auto mechanics as opposed to topics of little interest to Mike, such as politics, economics, philosophy, or art.

Summary

I have tried to point out the value of using behavior therapy procedures in Mike's program even though, at times, therapy was much more subjective than objective. When one lacks criterion standards and is not quite sure of what the therapy objectives should be, it is difficult to follow a tight behavior therapy model. Although I attempt to follow this model most of the time, I sometimes deviate from it. I couldn't say these deviations result in better or worse therapy than that had I followed the behavior therapy model. But without data, it is difficult to come to any valid conclusions.

The end of the semester report concerning Mike's progress is very encouraging. Pretest and posttest video tapes reveal a positive change has occurred in Mike's manner of speaking. Words spoken per minute increased to 112 while disfluencies per minute decreased to 6. When one compares these data to the original 19 words read per minute and 11 of those words stuttered, there can be little doubt concerning the progress obtained during the 3-month period.

Vocal Nodules*

Neal J., a 12-year-old boy, was referred by a local otolaryngologist. The physician's statement indicated that Neal had bilateral vocal nodules and generalized swelling of his vocal folds. He was referred for a complete evaluation of vocal habits and possible therapy to eliminate any habits which had caused his voice disorder. The otolaryngologist also stated that he was concerned about the possible need for psychological counseling because of "Neal's aggressive personality." He asked for an opinion on such a recommendation.

Diagnosis

Neal was accompanied to the clinic by his mother, who provided information about Neal's case history. She stated that Neal was the youngest of three boys and, as a result, seemed to always come out on the losing end of family arguments. Neal's mother stated that the whole family had a tendency to be aggressive and competitive in daily interactions and that Neal constantly had to yell and speak intensely just to compete with his dominating brothers. Most arguments occurred with the brother just older than Neal.

According to his mother, athletics played an important part in Neal's life. He was large for his age and well coordinated, making him a leader in team sports. Although

---

*The case is written and presented by James L. Case, Ph.D., associate professor in the Department of Speech and Hearing Science, Arizona State University.

Neal found this was satisfying, it seemed he was constantly yelling "instructions" at other boys on his team, a significant factor in the development of his vocal nodules. Considerable time was spent on Neal's case history to determine specific instances of vocal abuse associated with these athletic events.

As a result of the case history, the following specific items of vocal abuse were identified:

—intense verbal interaction with family members, especially his brothers;
—intense verbal arguments with his older brother;
—yelling and screaming on the playground and as an athletic team leader;
—excessive muscular tension in his neck area when speaking, particularly when angry;
—constant clearing of his throat in an abusive manner;
—hard or abrupt onset of voicing, especially when yelling or screaming (hard glottal attack);
—a tendency to call people to him rather than make an effort to get closer to the person being sought;
—miscellaneous instances of vocal abuse when playing army, motorcycles sounds when riding his bike, and in general play activities.

After identifying the above factors of vocal abuse, each was ranked in a hierarchy of severity from the lowest factor of vocal nodules etiology to the highest. This ranking took into consideration frequency of occurrence, effect on the vocal folds (based on clinical experience), and ease of modification. Therefore, the lowest factor on the hierarchy was the form of vocal abuse considered the easiest to eliminate but which would have the most significant effect on eliminating vocal abuse. The above list represents the hierarchy established by this method of analysis.

The next part of the evaluation involved obtaining a baseline audio recording of Neal's voice to establish pitch, vocal quality, and loudness characteristics. He was asked to state his name, age, the date, count from 1 to 20, prolong the vowels /a/ and /u/, prolong in maximum duration the /s/ and /z/ sounds to obtain the S/Z ratio, and to read a few lines from the "Rainbow Passage."

Analysis of this baseline recording revealed the following factors:

—*Habitual pitch:* F_o = 349 Hz (F in the fourth octave on a musical scale).
—*Optimal pitch:* could not be determined because of excessive hoarseness.
—*Quality:* judged as extremely tense and breathy (hoarse). According to the Frank B. Wilson Voice Profile: $+2-2$ laryngeal opening, with a severity factor of 6 (Wilson & Rice, 1977).
—*Loudness:* -2 on intensity scale of the Voice Profile.
—*Prolongation of* /s/: 11 seconds; /z/: 7 seconds; ratio: $-.64$ This ratio is typical of patients with vocal nodules and other laryngeal disorders in which voiced and voiceless sounds cannot be prolonged in equal duration (Boone, 1977).
—*Spectrograms* were made of Neal's voice on the /a/ and /u/ vowels. The spectrographs showed significant aperiodic vocal fold vibration and excessive breathiness on the voice spectrum.

Baseline

The baseline factors in Neal's voice disorder constituted the audio recording of Neal's voice and spectrograms of /a/ and /u/. No attempt was made to determine the baseline occurrence of the abuses identified since the information was obtained from case history rather than observation.

Management

Therapy for Neal involved identifying instances and types of vocal abuse and systematically eliminating each type. It was decided that Neal, with the help of his parents and brothers, would choose a group of abuses and *count* each occurrence. By counting each abuse Neal was to learn to anticipate when an abuse was likely to occur and therefore avoid or prevent it from happening. He was given a small pencil and a 3 × 5 card to use for data collection. He was instructed to begin counting and, hopefully, eliminate the lowest three abuse forms on his hierarchy: miscellaneous instances of vocal abuse while playing, such as motorcycle sounds when riding his bike; calling people from a distance; and hard or abrupt onset of voicing (which was demonstrated to him). His card was marked for each abuse so a daily tabulation could be recorded.

As reinforcement, his parents paid him 50¢ each day he attempted to record his abuse data; when an abuse form had been essentially eliminated for 2 consecutive weeks, he was allowed a night out with a friend to see a professional baseball game; and he would receive a new first baseman's glove when the doctor confirmed that his vocal nodules were gone. After showing Neal and his family slides of vocal nodules, and telling them exactly how they developed, an appointment was made for Neal to return in 4 days. It was also decided that I would call him at least every other day between visits to see how he was doing with his charting and abuse elimination.

When Neal returned in 4 days, another recording was made of his voice for serial comparison of voice quality. An analysis of his data card indicated that on the first day Neal counted seven instances of random playing noise such as the motorcycle sounds, four instances of yelling from one room to another, and 10 instances of using a hard vocal attack. The next day his data showed instances of four, two, and eight abuses respectively. The day before coming to his appointment, vocal abuse was reduced to two, two, and three respectively. The day of his appointment, Neal indicated that no instances of abuse had occurred in the categories being managed. His mother agreed with Neal, as well as she could tell. The recording of Neal's voice indicated no significant change in voice quality. Neal had earned $2.00 for data collection and was paid by his mother during the therapy session.

Neal was then instructed to continue to count the abuses of the past 4 days with an additional category, constant clearing of his throat. An appointment was made for therapy in 4 days. Phone calls of encouragement were made on two occasions before his next visit. When he returned, his data showed near elimination of the first three forms of vocal abuse, and a progressive reduction of the newly added category, throat clearing: first day, 15; second day, 10; third day, 4; fourth day (day of appointment), 1. Once again, Neal was paid $2.00 for data collection. Analysis of Neal's voice recording revealed slightly less breathiness, although this was not analyzed spectrographically. He was told that if he could continue to eliminate the first three categories of vocal abuse until the next appointment, he would earn a night out with a friend to see a ballgame.

During the next two months, Neal's therapy sessions essentially followed the same format: voice recording and analysis, data evaluation and reinforcement when appropriate, identification of target abuses to be counted during the following days, and general encouragement about the process. There were times when Neal seemed pleased with his efforts, particularly when he was paid for data collection or when he was about to win a night out, but there were also times when he seemed discouraged. For example, the hardest form of abuse to eliminate was yelling while playing in a team sport (baseball). Although he reported on his data card that he was not yelling while playing baseball, his mother seemed to have a different opinion. It seemed to make Neal angry when confronted by this difference of opinion. When this occurred, I made an effort to reinforce the fact that his mother was only trying to help him improve his voice and also to earn his new baseball glove. Neal seemed to accept the advice, but with some resistance.

Generally, Neal's therapy progressed nicely with constant progress being made to eliminate his vocal abuse. On three occasions, his brothers were asked to attend therapy to encourage their support for Neal, particularly when Neal's mother indicated that arguments were frequent in the home. It seemed that for a few days after his brothers came to therapy the tension lessened in the home. However, the intense nature of this family seemed to be a significant factor in Neal's voice disorder. At one time, I discussed the possibility of establishing a schedule so his brothers would be reinforced for *not* fighting with Neal, but this was never formalized.

Approximately 3 months after Neal began therapy, I was sure that a significant change had occurred in Neal's vocal habits. He was still an intense boy and inclined to erupt vocally when angry, but generally he was in control of the vocal habits which had been identified as abusive. He returned to his otolaryngologist who confirmed a "normal appearance of his vocal folds and surrounding tissues. No nodules were noted." Neal received his baseball glove.

During the session following his visit to the otolaryngologist, another recording was made of Neal's voice using the baseline format. The following results were obtained:

—*Habitual pitch:* F_o = 274 Hz (approximately C# in the fourth octave, a pitch which is essentially normal for a 12-year-old boy who had not begun puberty).

—*Optimal pitch:* same as habitual.

—*Pitch judgment:* 1 on the Voice Profile (normal).

—*Quality:* judged slightly hoarse with a slight amount of breathiness still present. Voice Profile: -2 on laryngeal opening, severity of 2.

—*Loudness:* 1 on intensity scale of Voice Profile (normal).

—*Prolongation of /s/:* 12 seconds; /z/: 12 seconds; ratio: 1.00 (normal).

—*Spectrograms of /a/ and /u/* were made and found to reveal slight aperiodicity but diminished breathiness on the spectrum.

It was decided to have Neal return to the clinic for periodic checkups, at which time a voice recording would be made and compared and vocal habits discussed. At the time of this writing, Neal has been seen for three checkups with no significant evidence of a relapse. He has also been seen once by the referring otolaryngologist who found a normal and stable larynx. So far, a successful case management.

Using Behavior Therapy with a Language Case*

Behavioral management is a procedure for controlling the events immediately prior to and following desired behavior. In order to control these events, clinicians engage in activities such as task analysis, pretesting, writing behavioral objectives, and planning lessons. They also use management techniques that have proven successful in influencing both nonspeech (social) and speech-language behaviors: being consistent, being positive, ignoring inappropriate behaviors, keeping the pace moving, and using correction procedures.

In order to determine if the behavior management techniques you use are effective, it is important to have direct and frequent measurement of the behaviors to be changed. Prior to beginning therapy you will need to decide which behaviors to observe and record, how often data will be collected, the method to use collecting data, and what type of data best represents the behavior to be changed. Collected data will be used to decide the effectiveness of your therapy. If your therapy was not effective, the data will indicate this and aid you in selecting appropriate aspects of your lesson to modify.

I used a production approach to change the language of a 5-year-old girl, Ann. Similar behavior management and data collection techniques could be used with clients who exhibit a variety of disorders, even though different therapeutic techniques were used.

Diagnosis

When Ann came to the clinic on January 15 for a speech and language evaluation, she was 5 years old. Based upon the test results, Ann's hearing, intelligence, and articulation were appropriate for her age. Results of the Northwestern Syntax Screening (NNST) indicated a receptive language score at the fiftieth percentile and an expressive language score at the fifteenth percentile. A spontaneous language sample was collected and analyzed using Lee's (1974) Developmental Sentence Scoring (DSS). Ann obtained a score of 6.52, placing her expressive language performance at the tenth percentile. Ann's syntactical errors were characterized by the omission of copulas and auxiliaries and the substitution of objective pronouns for subjective pronouns. These parts of speech are used at the 96% accuracy level by the average 4-year old (Menyuk, 1963). It was recommended that Ann receive therapy to improve the syntactical aspects of her expressive language.

---

*This study was conducted and written by Kathryn Kenney, clinical supervisor in the Department of Speech and Hearing Science, Arizona State University.

Objectives

Ann was scheduled to begin therapy to remediate her syntactical errors on January 29. Based upon the results of her evaluation, the objectives I selected were the correct use of copula, auxiliary, and subjective pronouns. When formally written each objective was composed of four parts: learning, behavior, condition, and criterion. Learning was a statement of the desired outcome. Behavior was the overt response that I used to measure that outcome. Conditions stated exceptions or limitations on the performance of the behavior. Criterion indicated the level of accuracy necessary for an objective to be considered attained. Ann's objectives were to demonstrate her understanding of the copular forms (is, are, am, were, and was) by using them correctly in spontaneous discourse with 95% accuracy. She would demonstrate her knowledge of the auxiliary forms (past and present tense) by using them correctly in spontaneous discourse with 95% accuracy. Finally, Ann would demonstrate her understanding of subjective pronouns (person and number) by using them correctly in spontaneous discourse with 95% accuracy (see Table 12-1).

Table 12–1.
Conjugations of Copula for Person, Number, and Tense

Person	Singular	Present Tense	Past Tense
1	I	am	was
2	you	are	were
3	he/she	is	was

Person	Plural	Present Tense	Past Tense
1	we	are	were
2	you	are	were
3	they	are	were

Task Analysis

Next, I completed a task analysis for each of the objectives. A task analysis is a process in which you identify, isolate and sequence the essential subtasks of an objective. The subtasks are described according to their content and to the response domain. For example, the content of the subtasks for correct use of copula would include description of all the different conjugations of the copula (person, number, and tense). Similar content analyses would be made for the auxiliary and subjective pronouns.

Next the subtasks would be described in terms of their response domain. A response domain identifies the stage of learning, that is, the accuracy, mastery, or generalization, and the behavior response used to produce the learning. Certain types of behavioral responses are associated with each stage of learning. During the accuracy stage when you are trying to establish a correct response, imitation, delayed-imitation, and drill activities are common responses. Mixed-practice drills and answers to questions are common responses during the mastery stage when you are trying to increase the response rate while maintaining accuracy. Finally, story retelling, monologue, and discourse are examples of responses typically used during the generalization stage, where the goal is to broaden the response classes and encourage more spontaneity. You have completed a series of learning specifications when you organize the subtasks by content and response and add the criteria. These specifications are shown in Table 12–2.

Table 12–2. *Specifications for Present and Past Tense Copula*

| | Response Domain | | |
Target Behavior	a. Accuracy (% data) Materials: probe sheets picture cards puppets	b. Mastery (rate data) Materials: probe sheets picture cards	c. Generalization (rate or % data) Materials: long sample
1. Use first person singular copula in sentence (am).	1a. 95%	1b. 1 minute 48 correct 2 errors	1c. 95%
2. Use third person singular copula in sentence (is).	2a. 95%	2b. 1 minute 48 correct 2 errors	2c. 95%
3. Use second person singular and plural in sentence (are).	3a. 95%	3b. 1 minute 48 correct 2 errors	3c. 95%
4. Use first and third person plural in sentence (are).	4a. 95%	4b. 1 minute 48 correct 2 errors	4c. 95%

Once the analysis for the production of the copula is written, probe tests for each of the tasks must be devised. These probes are initially used to determine where the client should begin in the hierarchy, and later, to determine when she should proceed to the next task. The probes for appropriate task analysis could be used again with many other clients.

The probe for subtask 1a consisted of 10 sentences in which "I am" was used. Some examples were I am red; I am small; I am up high; I am under the table. The clinician and the child both had similar puppets. The clinician instructed the child to "make her puppet say what the clinician's puppet said."

The probe for subtask 2b consisted of 20 items. The clinician presented 10 pairs of picture cards. Each pair consisted of a boy and a girl. The clinician asked questions such as, "Who is bigger?", "Who is fatter?", "Who is taller?", etc. The child was to answer the question using a complete sentence. Similar probes were written until there was one for each subtask. At this point I was ready for our first session.

Baseline

In order to plan Ann's therapy more efficiently, I collected baseline information during the first 30-minute session. I administered probes until she scored between 10–30% on three subtasks. I felt I could work effectively on no more than three subtasks in any given session. Also items with a 10–30% accuracy were not likely to be spontaneously correct. Results of the probes are shown in Table 12–3. Based upon the probe results, I decided to begin working on accuracy of "is" (b), mastery of "are" (a), and generalization of "he/she" (c). The points were plotted on graphs as baseline data (see Figure 12–10).

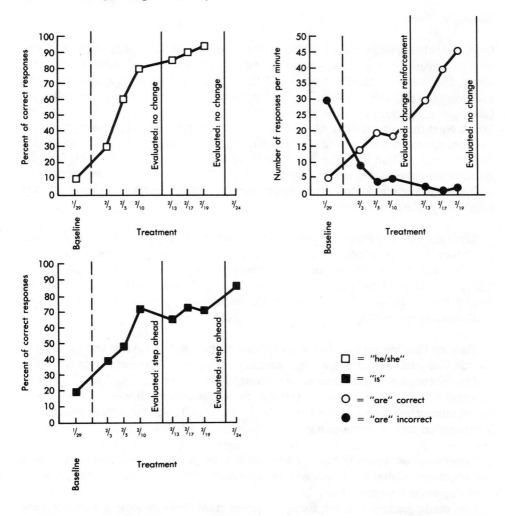

FIGURE 12-10. Data Points Of Ann's Baseline And Therapy Performance For Selected Language Targets

Table 12–3.

Copula		Level	Auxiliary		Level	Pronouns		Level
am	(95%)	c	am	(90%)	c	I	(100%)	c
is	(20%)*	b	is	(5%)	a	he/she	(10%)*	c
are	(70%)	a	are	(20%)*	a	they		
was	(0%)	a	was	(0%)	a	you		
were	(0%)	a	were	(0%)	a	we		

*Targets selected for remediation.

Therapy Plans

Once the subtask was selected as a target for therapy, I could write therapy plans and begin intervention. My therapy plans were divided into three main sections: (1) what was done prior to the child's response, (2) the child's response, and (3) what was done following the child's response. The therapy plan that I used reflects these divisions (see Figure 12–11). First, the general setting, materials, and procedures used are listed. Next there is a statement about the client's target behavior. Finally, there are the consequences and criterion. When writing the therapy plans, first transfer the relevant information from the task analysis to the therapy plan form. This includes information about the subtask and criterion. Then decide on the therapeutic technique to use and fill in the setting, materials, and procedure. The last section to complete is the consequences.

Accuracy Therapy Plans: When writing accuracy therapy plans, be sure to include models or demonstrations of accurate behavior as a procedure. This is to enable the child to identify correct behavior. As the consequence, give precise feedback, such as "You said 'are'. You know how to use the word 'are' correctly." Continuous reinforcement is given. Also, elaborate correction procedures are needed to facilitate correct responses.

Mastery Therapy Plans: The procedures incorporate few models and cues will be faded. The goal is to evoke a large quantity of accurate responses from the child.

The consequence statements are reduced to single words, "yes," "right," "correct." They are delivered at a ratio of one consequence to five correct responses. Correction procedures are less elaborate. The data collected are usually based upon a prescribed rate of responding.

Generalization Therapy Plan: The child will be provided with new occasions to use his target. Usually the task will be less structured, consisting of a spontaneous monologue or discourse.

The consequences will be social reinforcement delivered on a variable ratio schedule. Correction procedures are minimal.

Methods of Data Collection

I used my therapy plans as guidelines for my prescriptions for Ann. Subtask probes were administered after each session. The data were then transferred to a graph (see Figure 12–10). These activities took about 5 minutes. A dotted line was drawn to isolate baseline from treatment data.

These data were used to make decisions about changes in therapy. Every 3 days the trend of the progress was evaluated to determine the effectiveness of the therapy plans.

The guidelines used to evaluate my prescriptions were (1) If the performance progressed during three consecutive sessions, the same plan was continued for three more sessions, then re-evaluated. (2) If the child's performance was 0% correct, I would back up or branch to an easier subtask. (3) If the child's performance stopped progressing or became highly variable, the consequences would be altered or items from the next subtask included (step ahead) to increase the child's motivation.

These changes would be written on the same lesson plan. A line would be drawn on the data chart to indicate when a new method was being initiated. Data would be kept for 3 days then progress re-evaluated. The task analysis, probes and therapy plans used for Ann could easily be reused with another client. Writing these programs, although initially time consuming, can save therapy time in the long run.

Figure 12–11. *Examples of Therapy Plan.*

Client _____ Clinician _____ Date _____ Time _____

Settings & Materials	Procedure	Subtask (3a)	Consequences	Criterion	Data
10 minutes in small therapy room with clinician and child. No materials needed.	Play "Simon Says" with the student. Comment on what they are doing, e.g., you are standing, you are sitting, etc. Then switch roles.	Use of second person singular auxiliary in a sentence, "are".	*Correct:* That's right, you said "are," or, you used "are" correctly, or, you remembered to say "are." *Incorrect:* Cue = raise hand, and model correct answer 2 times; ask child to repeat.	95% correct.	
Clinician seated across a small table from student 50 pictures of professional people, objects, animals.	Present a picture, tell child, "I want you to answer my question using a complete sentence." Questions would include: What color is it? What is this? What is he?	Use of third person singular copula "is" in a complete sentence.	*Correct:* That's right. *Incorrect:* Ignore if less than 5%. If > 5%, cue as in previous stage.	*Pass probe:* 48 correct, 2 errors in 1 minute.	

| Table, chairs, sequence cards

The clinician is seated next to the child. | Provide child with sequencing cards and have him tell a story about the boy or girl. | Use of third person singular personal pronouns in spontaneous discourse. | *Correct:* Social statements on a variable ratio 1:10.

Incorrect: Use cue established in previous stage. | 95 % accuracy |

BIBLIOGRAPHY

Boone, D. *The voice and voice therapy.* 2nd ed. Englewood Cliffs, N.J.: Prentice-Hall, 1977.

Crocker, J. A phonological model of children's articulation competence. *Journal of Speech and Hearing Disorders,* 1969, *34,* 203–213.

Erickson, R. L. Assessing communication attitudes among stutterers. *Journal of Speech and Hearing Research,* 1969, *12,* 711–724.

Gregory, H. Contemporary issues in stuttering therapy. *Journal of Fluency Disorders,* 1980, *5,* 291–302.

Lee, L. L. *Developmental sentence analysis.* Evanston, Ill.: Northwestern University Press, 1974.

Menjuk, P. Syntactic structures in the language of children. *Child Development,* 1963, *34,* 407–422.

Mowrer, D. E. An instructional program to increase fluent speech of stutterers. *Journal of Fluency Disorders,* 1975a, *1,* 25–35.

Mowrer, D. E. *Technical research report S–1: Reduction of stuttering behavior.* Tempe, Ariz.: Ideas, 1975b.

Mowrer, D. E. *A program to establish fluent speech.* Columbus: Charles E. Merrill, 1979.

Mowrer, D. E., Baker, R., & Schutz, R. *S-PACK.* Tempe, Ariz.: Ideas, 1974.

Ryan, B. *Programmed therapy for stuttering children and adults.* Springfield, Ill.: Charles C Thomas, 1974.

Van Riper, C. *The treatment of stuttering.* Englewood Cliffs, N.J.: Prentice-Hall, 1973.

Wilson, F. B., & Rice, M. *A programmed approach to voice therapy.* Austin, Tex.: Learning Concepts, Inc., 1977.

Subject Index

Name Index